Assessment of Autism in Females and Nuanced Presentations

Terisa P. Gabrielsen • K. Kawena Begay
Kathleen Campbell • Katrina Hahn
Lucas T. Harrington

Assessment of Autism in Females and Nuanced Presentations

Integrating Research into Practice

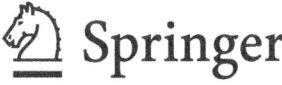 Springer

Terisa P. Gabrielsen (iD)
School of Education
Brigham Young Univeristy
Provo, UT, USA

K. Kawena Begay (iD)
School of Education
University of Washington Tacoma
Tacoma, WA, USA

Kathleen Campbell (iD)
Developmental and Behavioral Pediatrics
Children's Hospital of Philadelphia
Phildelphia, PA, USA

Katrina Hahn
Developmental Assessment Clinics
University of Utah
Salt Lake City, UT, USA

Lucas T. Harrington
Autism Center
University of Washington
Seattle, WA, USA

ISBN 978-3-031-33968-4   ISBN 978-3-031-33969-1   (eBook)
https://doi.org/10.1007/978-3-031-33969-1

This Springer imprint is published by the registered company Springer Nature Switzerland AG
The registered company address is: Gewerbestrasse 11, 6330 Cham, Switzerland

Paper in this product is recyclable.

For Avery, Brielle, Cielo, Jessie, Gina, Haley, Mollie, Natasha, and Natalie, thank you for teaching me. Always and forever, for Gabe. TPG

For Chip, Dakotah, Dallas, and Cheyenne. You are my heart. For Jane, thank you for a lifetime of unfailing support. KKB

For Ben, Will, and Lily—always, no matter what. For Pat, thank you for teaching me to be comfortable in my own skin. KH

For my colleagues who have dedicated themselves to doing right by my community. And for Vanessa Castañeda Gill, who is shining a light for autistic girls everywhere. LTH

Foreword

Girls and women with autism have been missed and neglected for far too long. *Assessment of Autism in Females and Nuanced Presentations* is the first book combining the newest research with autistic women's perspectives and insights. Historically, autistic individuals' input has not been sought when trying to better understand autism. Instead, knowledge based on behavioral observations and clinical judgment of researchers has been the basis for guidelines, often far removed from lived experiences of autistic individuals. This has led to a lack of understanding of the autism spectrum as a whole, but especially "less noticeable," or nuanced autism often found in females.

Dr. Terisa Gabrielsen is an established researcher and clinically trained school psychologist who has come to understand the difficulties of "measuring" autism in this complex and easily (dis)missed population. We both started our graduate education at the University of Utah's Department of Educational Psychology, studying autism, but our paths diverged. Where I personally worked in public schools and an inpatient psychiatric setting before leading a university autism clinic and later a private practice, Dr. Gabrielsen worked in schools, as part of interdisciplinary hospital teams, clinical researcher, and graduate student trainer. Eventually, our paths converged again, leading us to work with similar populations in clinical practice and a university research setting respectively.

Dr. Gabrielsen and her interdisciplinary team have made tremendous efforts to connect with autistic women, truly hearing their stories and understanding their lived experience and linking that information to the most current research in the field. Drs. Begay, Harrington, and Campbell, and Ms. Hahn bring extensive professional and personal experience throughout. In our collaborations in clinical and research settings, we have attempted to better characterize this population and provide much-needed support. Dr. Gabrielsen and colleagues have met a critical need for both clinicians and researchers by creating this desperately needed resource.

Assessment of Autism in Females and Nuanced Presentations is a must-have resource for clinicians, individuals, and families affected by female or nuanced autism, and students in the field of autism. Rather than looking for ways to "treat autism" with a single strategy, such as applied behavior analysis (ABA), this book embraces autism, while offering understanding necessary to truly support and respect the varied needs of autistic individuals. It provides a lens to see and better appreciate the many challenges they experience throughout the lifespan. Its chapters cover topics ranging from interdisciplinary assessment procedures, communication and language differences, difficulties with sleep and sensory profiles, co-occurring psychiatric conditions, learning differences, sexuality, and gender identity. Woven throughout the book are case studies and narratives, giving the reader ongoing glimpses into what female and nuanced autism "looks and feels like" while connecting the case studies to current research findings, leading to an in-depth understanding of the issues at hand. In addition to connecting research with the lived experience of autism, the case studies also make the book a pleasure to read.

As a clinician specializing in the assessment of autism in girls, women, and others with more nuanced or "less noticeable" autism, I am aware that good resources have been scarce. Until now, reading books written by autistic women and listening to countless women and others with nuanced autism talk about their experiences have been my "go to" strategies when trying to better understand how to assess and support this particular autism presentation in my clinical setting. While these resources have been immensely informative, many clinicians may not know where to look for help or may not be aware that they need more information. I work with this population in an assessment capacity as well as in long-term therapeutic relationships, and it has been a frequently disheartening experience. Many clients have struggled as they have been dismissed, misdiagnosed, judged, and labeled, in some cases leading to frustrations, and in others to repeated traumatic treatment experiences. This occurs no matter the age or specific personal situations, ranging from schools to psychiatric inpatient settings. It has been eye opening that even though I am an expert on these issues, I am also often dismissed by school teams and providers in inpatient psychiatric settings that my clients at times need to access.

Unfortunately, psychiatric care in the 2020s is as traumatizing for autistic women as ever. One client who participated in a day treatment program recently was told she was only allowed to communicate verbally, even though she experiences brief periods of time when she is unable to speak at all (combination of autism and trauma). She was told that it was unacceptable for her not to talk in therapy groups and was labeled as "resistant" instead of being accommodated or supported, leading to an increase in trauma and anxiety symptoms before she opted not to return to the program. Another recent experience in an inpatient setting was that a client was not allowed to have a small fidget or sensory tool because then "everyone would want one." This continued even after I called the program, explained the situation, and asked for my client to be accommodated. A third recent example is that of an autistic woman who was admitted to another inpatient facility, where she was not given her medications, leaving her in severe pain from leg cramps. She ended up being physically restrained and told if she "toughed it out," her cramping would subside, and she would be okay.

The following brief quote from the chapter regarding burnout in the autistic population describes a "pervasive lack of autism awareness in people who are in a position to help" (see p. 212). This is a more profound statement than one might initially realize. It lies at the core of the problems thus far when it comes to accurately diagnosing and supporting girls, women, and others with nuanced autism presentations. This is illustrated by my clinical experience supporting female clients through the past decade in which lack of awareness extends even to me as a provider with extensive school, in-patient, and out-patient experience being dismissed in favor of the status quo. I have been left feeling powerless while possessing knowledge and skills that could quickly and easily improve clinical care for individuals in distress, who need to be heard, validated, and supported. This volume has the potential to start lifting the veil on nuanced autism and lead to a paradigm shift in clinical practice so desperately needed by many. We know that autistic individuals are at least 7.5 times more likely to die by suicide than neurotypical peers. Recent studies indicate even higher risk if the person has above-average cognitive abilities and if she is an autistic female (Casten et al., 2023, Hirvikoski et al., 2016, 2020); the time is now to spread awareness and understanding. We have finally reached the point of greater awareness for early identification and support of more "classical" autism over the past two decades. The time is now to see the (so-far) largely invisible population on the autism spectrum and continue to learn how to more accurately identify, better understand, and legitimately support them.

This book will become a trusted companion for clinicians and researchers attempting to truly grasp the vast differences and nuances in autistic presentations. With engaging and illustrative case studies and quotes from stakeholders tied to current research, I believe this approach accurately represents the vast complexity of nuanced autism and the needs of this population and it is long overdue.

Director, The Autism Clinic   Julia Connelly, PhD
Salt Lake City, UT, USA

References

Casten, L. G., Thomas, T. R., Doobay, A. F., Foley-Nicpon, M., Kramer, S. Nickl-Jockschat, T. Abel, T. Assouline, S. , Michaelson, J. J. (2023). The combination of autism and exceptional cognitive ability is associated with suicidal ideation. *Neurobiology of Learning and Memory, 197*, 107698. https://doi.org/10.1016/j.nlm.2022.107698.

Hirvikoski, T, Boman, M, Chen, Q, D'Onofrio, B. M., Mittendorfer-Rutz, E., Lichtenstein, P., Bölte, S., & Larsson, H. (2020, July), Individual risk and familial liability for suicide attempt and suicide in autism: a population-based study. *Psychological Medicine, 50*(9), 1463–1474. https://doi.org/10.1017/S0033291719001405. Epub 2019 Jun 26. PMID: 31238998.

Preface

This book is released at a unique moment in time. Had it been released any earlier, the wealth of research conducted since 2020 would not have been included. The flood of information about nuanced autism and autistic female experiences will undoubtedly continue to grow, so this manuscript is the first step toward changing how we think about autism identification. The change we hope to accomplish is to bridge the gap between autistic people seeking support and understanding and the professional communities who have previously been positioned as gatekeepers for diagnostic decisions.

Autism has always been characterized as a spectrum, but that conceptualization has not been an exact fit with existing diagnostic practices. In the medical model (including mental health diagnostic models), the idea of "autistic enough" based on "counts" of "deficits" and "dysfunction" that have a certain "look," exemplars, or presentation ignores the reality and complexity of individual autistic traits. Daily experiences in a society that does not expect or accommodate autistic traits very well can be difficult to capture in a set of data—particularly for measures based primarily on one subset of the population. This is a problem not unique to autism but has life-altering consequences just as significant as missed diagnoses of a heart attack in a woman whose symptoms do not match up or appear to be the same as a man's (because females had not been well represented in research).

The solution to this problem is probably easier than some may think. Joining the autistic and professional communities together to solve the problem can be as simple as taking more time to listen. Reaching beyond cutoffs and checklist approaches to complicated diagnostic decisions can lead to more informed diagnoses, more individualized approaches for supports, and better advocacy for acceptance and inclusion of neurodiversity as something that is known and expected in the world rather than an aberration from a norm.

Data from first-person narratives are included here along with data from scientific research, integrated into a comprehensive approach to assessment. As a group, we represent professionals and stakeholders. We are autistic and parents and grandparents of autistic children across all genders. We are clinicians who diagnose and provide support for autistic people. We teach and train the next generation of professionals in a very different way than we were trained originally, informed by experiences across communities over the years. We first planned this resource based on our own clinical experiences, but in the intervening years, evidence to substantiate our clinical observations is now well established. We are incredibly hopeful about this moment in time.

Checklists are supposed to be succinct descriptions of what is. But in the case of autism, most sounded more like one-dimensional prescriptions for how autistic people were supposed to behave. If it swims like a duck, walks like a duck, follows Mama Duck, it's probably a duck. Unless its the Ugly Duckling—a.k.a. the swan who's failing at being who/how others say he ought, instead of being a natural at being himself. And let's face it, he's probably going to have a much better explanation for what he was doing all along than would a duck who had watched him struggle with his lack of duckiness. (Jennifer O'Toole, 2018, p. 9)

Provo, UT, USA   Terisa P. Gabrielsen
Tacoma, WA, USA   K. Kawena Begay
Philadelphia, PA, USA   Kathleen Campbell
Salt Lake City, UT, USA   Katrina Hahn
Seattle, WA, USA   Lucas T. Harrington

Reference

O'Toole, J. C. (2018). *Autism in heels: The untold story of a female life on the spectrum.* Skyhorse Publishing.

Acknowledgments

We gratefully acknowledge the contributions of chapter reviewers:

Kirsten Aalberg, DPT
Board-Certified Clinical Specialist in Pediatric Physical Therapy

Natalie Buerger, PhD, NCSP
Clinical Director, University of Utah Huntsman Mental Health Institute's Autism Spectrum Disorder Clinic

Julia Connelly, PhD
Director, The Autism Clinic

Rebecca Cramer, EdS
School Psychologist, Autism Team, Jordan School District and Stakeholder Parent

Elizabeth Cutrer-Párraga, PhD
Associate Professor, Special Education, Brigham Young University

Victoria Hatton, PhD, NCSP
School Psychologist, Granite School District

Heid Vogeler, PhD
Licensed Psychologist, Counseling and Psychological Services, Brigham Young University

We are also grateful for the contributions of our research team and facilitators:

Kathy Donahey Bingham, EdS
Robyn Orr, EdS
Greer Finster, EdS
Laurel Bishop
Kylie Burdge
Linda Cheng
Paul Crenshaw
Rachel Koster
Taylor Stirland
Austin Stirland

Book Description

This book examines the characteristics of autism that may be different than expected, or nuanced. These characteristics are increasingly found in females, but also in others, and are likely to be missed or misdiagnosed when identification and support are needed. Chapters follow a lifespan framework to guide clinicians through comprehensive assessment processes at any age. Interpretation of standardized measures, new information from scientific literature, and information from first-person accounts are integrated to provide a more nuanced and sensitive approach to assessment. Implications for improved treatment and supports based on comprehensive assessment processes are also discussed. Case studies within each age range are included to consolidate and illustrate the assessment.

Key Areas of Coverage Include the Following:
- Interdisciplinary assessment processes including psychology, speech-language pathology, education, and health-care disciplines
- Lifespan approach to a comprehensive assessment of autism in females/ nuanced autism
- Guide to an interpretation of standardized measures in females/nuanced autism
- Additional assessment tools and processes to provide diagnostic clarity
- Descriptions of barriers in diagnostic processes from first-person accounts
- Intervention and support strategies tied to assessment data
- In-depth explanations of evidence and at-a-glance summaries

Assessment of Autism in Females and Nuanced Presentations is a must-have equity resource for clinicians, professionals, and policymakers in psychology, speech-language pathology, medicine, education, social work, mental health, and all interrelated disciplines as well as researchers, professors, and graduate students.

Contents

List of Figures

List of Tables

About the Authors

Terisa P. Gabrielsen, Ph.D., NCSP is an associate professor of School Psychology in the School of Education at Brigham Young University and a licensed psychologist. She has 15 years of interdisciplinary clinical and research experience in toddler, pre-K-12, hospital, clinical, and research settings. Her specialties are early identification of autism, social skills interventions, and building community capacity in autism services.

K. Kawena Begay, Ph.D., NCSP is an assistant professor in the School of Education at the University of Washington Tacoma. She is a licensed psychologist and nationally certified school psychologist with 20 years of experience working in culturally and linguistically diverse PreK-12, university, and clinic settings. Dr. Begay has served in a variety of roles, including classroom teacher, counselor, school psychologist, licensed psychologist, trainer, and consultant. She specializes in culturally responsive evaluation practices, with a special emphasis on autism evaluations.

Kathleen Campbell, M.D., M.H.Sc., is a pediatric fellow, training in developmental and behavioral pediatrics at the Children's Hospital of Philadelphia. She has clinical experience in autism intervention, pre-school, and medical settings and has published research relating to screening, diagnosis, and medical care of autistic children.

Katrina Hahn, M.Ed., CCC-SLP, is a speech and language pathologist with the University of Utah Developmental Assessment Clinics. She has 23 years of experience in various capacities in early intervention, Pre-K-12, and clinical settings. Ms. Hahn specializes in the identification, evaluation, and therapy planning for social-emotional development and pragmatic language for individuals with autism.

Lucas T. Harrington, PsyD is a licensed clinical psychologist at the University of Washington Autism Center. He is autistic and personally experienced the challenges of seeking evaluation as an adult who was assigned female at birth. Dr. Harrington provides neurodiversity-affirming services for autistic people and their supporters in a variety of areas, including diagnostic evaluation, individual therapy, parent coaching, and consultation/training.

Chapter 1
Sex, Gender, Autism, Assessment, and Equity for Females

Introduction

For those with years of experience, much of this text will resonate with past assessment of nuanced autism, particularly in women and girls. Some clinicians may be new to the idea of the differences that mark nuanced autism. Others have asked if there will ever be a separate set of diagnostic criteria for "female" autism (which is not likely). All can agree, however, that

> *"While all psychiatric and neurodevelopmental conditions can present in various ways, ASD is rather extreme in its variability,"* (Duvall et al., 2021, p. 1174).

Terminology

There are diverse preferences for language to describe the experiences of individuals. In this text, "autistic" and ". . . with autism" are both used to address preferences for either identity-first or person-first language. We have focused a lot on females here to allow us to report research findings, but have also included research about transgender men, non-binary individuals, and other aspects of gender diversity. It is probable that you may also encounter some cisgender males who may present in the nuanced manner consistent with many females. Our intent is to be respectful in our use of language, but in the case of quoted material, original language is preserved, including first-person narratives, mention of Asperger syndrome, and some medical model language (e.g. "disorder," "risk," "symptom").

> *"We call upon researchers, clinicians, and advocates to work together to identify other terms for this profile – terms inclusive and respectful of gender-diverse youth who may not identify with female gender* (Strang et al., 2019)" (Strang et al., 2021, p. 224).

T. P. Gabrielsen et al., *Assessment of Autism in Females and Nuanced Presentations*, https://doi.org/10.1007/978-3-031-33969-1_1

We are striving to be inclusive and respectful of the gender variability that describes many in the autism community and understand that language can be hurtful. We hope to avoid this as much as possible. Finally, non-autistic individuals are referred to as neurotypical, typically developing, or allistic according to the original source authors' terminology.

Evolution of Autism Diagnostic Criteria

The early history of autism and prevalence monitoring throughout the world are important considerations for clinicians regarding not only *how* to identify autism but *how well we are doing* in our efforts to identify autism. The diagnosis was first described by Leo Kanner and Hans Asperger in primarily male samples (Asperger, 1944; Kanner, 1943). See Rosen et al. (2021) for a history of autism as a diagnosis from its first appearance in the *Diagnostic and Statistical Manual of Mental Disorders*, Third Ed. (DSM-III; APA, 1980), through each subsequent edition of the DSM. Differences in presenting characteristics for females were briefly mentioned in the DSM-5 (2013), but further described in the DSM-5-TR (APA, 2022). The terms have changed from Asperger's syndrome, autistic disorder, and pervasive developmental disorder-not otherwise specified to the all-encompassing "autism spectrum disorder" in the United States. The term used in the United Kingdom is currently autism spectrum condition, all of which are referred to here as simply "autism."

Prevalence Studies

ADDM Prevalence Studies

In the United States, the Centers for Disease Control and Prevention (CDC) and the Autism and Developmental Disabilities Monitoring (ADDM) Network sponsor studies to sample populations with similar methodology over time, beginning in 2002. Estimated prevalence rates have increased dramatically from 1:150 to 1:36 over the last two decades (Maenner et al., 2023). These studies sample selected populations by extracting samples of medical and/or educational records to evaluate descriptions of characteristics, traits, and concerns mentioned in these records. Records flagged with multiple signals for autism are evaluated by autism specialists to determine "caseness," so as to not restrict the study to children with formal autism diagnoses in the hopes of not introducing diagnostic bias to the prevalence data. Using this methodology, the ratio of males to females has not changed significantly from the current estimated 4:1 ratio among 8-year-olds. This suggests that parents and providers are not really documenting autism traits in females in medical or educational records as much as their male peers, at least prior to age 8. Trends suggest a shift in the identification of more girls, however. Girls with autism (8-year-olds) are now at least 1% of the sampled population in the CDC/ADDM studies. In the most recent study of 4-year-olds, the ratio is 3.1:1 (Shaw et al., 2023). This may be due to improved early identification, but may also reflect the fact that more apparent presentations of autism in females are more likely to be recognized at younger ages, whereas more nuanced autism is not recognized in either males or females until later ages, perhaps after age 8. The good news from the pre-COVID prevalence study is that children just 4 years younger than the 8-year-olds surveyed in the same year were 50% more likely to have been identified before age 48 months, so earlier identification seems to be an overall trend (Shaw et al., 2021).

Worldwide Prevalence Studies

In a recent systematic review of all studies of autism prevalence worldwide, a median rate of 100/10,000 was found (Zeidan et al., 2022). This converts to a ratio of 1:100 compared to the most current US rate of 1:36 (Maenner et al., 2023). The ratio of males to females, however, is strikingly similar, with the global median reported to be 4.2:1 (range 0.8–6.1), similar to the US overall ratio of 3.8:1 (Maenner et al., 2023). Studies reporting IQ consistently reported higher proportions of girls with autism and intellectual developmental disorder (IDD) than autistic boys in the past, with Maenner et al. (2023) as the first to report *no* significant differences in IDD and autism across genders. This suggests that girls with autism and IDD have been more easily identified in the past. In most studies, as with the United States, overall estimated autism prevalence has increased over time, while the ratio of males to females has remained relatively stable (Maenner et al., 2023). In the 2022 Lancet Commission on the Future of Care and Clinical Research in Autism, the lopsided gender ratio suggests that at least some proportion of autistic females are under-recognized and underdiagnosed (Lord et al., 2022).

Parent Report Prevalence Studies

Although parents are reporting more cases of autism than the sampling studies, they are recognizing autism in females at the same rates shown in the CDC/ADDM studies. The 2019–2020 National Survey of Children with Special Health Care Needs in the United States asked parents about autism diagnosis in their children and identified a higher prevalence rate of 1:34. The approach of this parent report study gives us a much broader sample (nationwide, ages 3–17), but relies on parent report of diagnoses which is a different methodology than expert review of records or direct assessment. Both approaches are informative. The overall prevalence rate in these studies has not increased as much over time as the ADDM rates described above, suggesting that more clinicians are documenting autism traits in medical and educational records over time in the CDC/ADDM studies to match what parents have been reporting all along. Prevalence for males in the parent report study is 1:22, while prevalence for females is 1:83, representing a ratio of 1566 boys to 400 girls (3.9:1) in a total sample of over 60,000 children, equally divided male and female (Child and Adolescent Health Measurement Initiative, 2022).

Prevalence by Gender Internationally

Although more autistic children are being identified, with some improvement in earlier ages of identification in recent years, the overall ratio of males to females identified with autism may not be changing much. It is possible for autism to be reliably diagnosed as young as age 14 months (Pierce et al., 2019), but what is possible in a specialty clinic does not necessarily reflect what is happening in communities. Gender differences in age of diagnosis have not been found in some studies (Mussey et al., 2017), and in other studies, older average ages of diagnosis are documented for females (Giarelli et al., 2010; Shattuck et al., 2009), perhaps more related to differences in the samples than to progress over the years. Rutherford et al. (2016) identified delays (later referrals) in the diagnosis of females in a small Scottish sample, with less disparity as the age of diagnosis increased (i.e., as children got older, the ratio of males and females became more balanced). As one of many themes that will be repeated throughout this text, Russell et al. (2011) found that even when females had the same level of autistic traits, males were more likely to receive a diagnosis than females. Jensen et al. (2014) looked at trends over time and found a reduction in the male/female dominance from a ratio of 5:1–3:1 over 15 years in Danish populations. A Finnish study found ratios of 1.8:1 (Mattila et al., 2011), and in South Korea, a ratio of 2.5:1 was observed (Kim et al., 2011), in cohorts of 8-year-olds and 7–12-year-olds, respectively. The wide variability in the male/female ratio in the context of fairly consistent prevalence rates suggests that identification of females is a worldwide issue.

Prevalence of Autism and Gender Identity Issues

Most individuals identify with their gender assigned at birth, although among individuals with autism, there is higher occurrence of gender diversity. Bejerot et al. (2012) commented that the co-occurrence of autism and gender diversity was "striking." They described autism as more of a "gender-defiant" condition and concluded that gender variance in adults with autism is somewhat expected (Berjerot et al., 2012, p. 122). The intersectionality of autism and gender issues may confuse clinical conceptualization or obscure one or the other set of traits and support needs, as specialized professional and support communities don't necessarily overlap. Strang et al. (2021) found that transgender autistic adolescents reported significantly higher levels of internalizing symptoms than either transgender-allistic or cisgender autistic peers. "Gender development is a complex process involving biological, psychological, and cognitive elements that are influenced by social norms. As such, individuals with ASDs may present with variance in their gender identity and expression that may defy easy categorization" (Janssen et al., 2016).

Strang et al. (2021) found 20% of their transgender youth sample had clinically significant autism-related difficulties. Mental health concerns in this group (transgender and at the margin of autism diagnosis) are similar to those of transgender youth meeting autism criteria. The subthreshold group in this study included primarily transgender men (assigned female at birth). This is just one of the issues with limiting the nuanced type or subthreshold type of autism as a "female" profile when it is seen across the gender spectrum. Within this transgender group, elevated mental health problems were the same in youth with subthreshold and in those with higher measures of autistic traits, indicating a similar level of supports needed regardless of the extent of autism traits (Strang et al., 2021).

In a 2021 "road map" for the differential diagnosis of autism, Duvall et al. (2021) cited prevalence of gender diversity in autistic youth as between 4% and 5.4%, compared to a rate of 0.7% in neurotypical youth (Janssen et al., 2016; Strang et al., 2014). These rates were further substantiated by de Vries et al. (2010) at 7.8% and between 2.3% and 9.3% by Spack et al. (2012). Walsh et al. (2018) found 15% transgender and non-binary individuals in their Netherlands autism sample, the majority of whom were assigned female at birth (AFAB). Warrier et al. (2020) examined item-level data in their study of both autistic and neurotypical youth and found autism trait scores to be higher in transgender and gender-diverse youth regardless of autism diagnostic status. Specific scores noted as high were systemizing (analysis and organization of rule governing systems) and sensory sensitivity. Janssen et al. (2016) also found autistic youth to be 7.76 times more likely to report wishing to be the opposite sex than non-autistic youth.

Theories on Prevalence Differences

Kreiser and White (2014) presented several theories about gender differences in autism. One is that the way we measure differences can vary quite a bit across the spectrum. Autistic children with measured cognitive abilities in the low ranges do not differ much across genders. When autism diagnosis is examined across genders with typical cognitive and language performance, however, the disparities are striking, suggesting that autism is more difficult to identify in females without co-occurring conditions such as intellectual developmental disorder or language disorders. They noted the three most prevalent theories, or models, have been the brain differences model (systemizing as something male brains do better and empathizing as something female brains do better; Baron-Cohen, 2004), the greater variability model (there is more variability in the classic male presentation than the severely affected females; Wing, 1981), and the liability/threshold model (higher genetic loads are required for autism to manifest in females; Tsai et al., 1981). Among these theories, the genetic differences in female genotypes have subsequently shown the most evidence of effect in many ways. Kreiser and White explored the social contexts and cultural factors that may better explain the differences between ease of diagnosis for males and more difficulties in identifying females. Even when females are showing similar traits as male peers, the male is more likely to receive a diagnosis than the female.

Importance of Equity Issues in Identification: First-Person Narratives

My head had been spinning all my life with trying to make sense of why these things happened to me, why I was so odd, why I couldn't live like other people. The diagnosis stopped my head from spinning. I was able to breathe a sigh of relief and relax. Woman with autism. (Hendrickx, 2015, p. 118)

Kurchak felt that diagnosis was important because she wanted to feel differently about her childhood, that is, she wanted to feel proud instead of beating herself up for her failures, as she puts it. (Nerenberg, 2021, pp. 179–180)

I think women tend to be diagnosed later in life when they actually push for it themselves ... when you're a child, you don't realize that you're anxious and depressed . . [that] your education is going to suffer because of that and I think that if I had known, and if people had helped me from earlier on, then life would've been a whole lot easier. P07 (Bargiela et al., 2016)

Having never been identified as anything other than gifted, I had nothing to raise my suspicions,... I tried instead to manage on my own, even when my troubles continued to mount... My real difficulty came when I began to tell myself my differences were not just superficial incidentals, but cracks in my dignity. (Willey, 2014, p. 53)

I know in my heart and in my head, that if I had owned more AS knowledge, if I had been able to objectively understand that terms like rigid thinking, semantic pragmatic disorder, social impairment, echolalia, bilateral coordination problems, sensory integration dysfunction and auditory discrimination, were very real words that defined who I was, I would have made small changes in my course. . . I would have realized I had a different set of needs and wants that set me apart from many of my classmates, but that never meant I was undeserving or incapable. And most important, I would have asked for the support I really needed. (Willey, 2014, p. 63)

Because we don't sense danger and can't. That's one reason. I think you not reading people to be able to tell if they're being creepy, you're that desperate for friends and relationships that if someone is showing an interest in you, you kind of go with it and tend not to learn from other's safety skills. P07 (Bargiela et al., 2016)

One woman explained that, from her perspective, there is subtle interaction between two sets of issues. 'Problems related to the [autism] spectrum are combined with problems of society's expectations of women. How one looks, what one wears, how one is supposed to relate socially, that a woman is supposed to have a natural empathy towards others, expectations about dating and marriage...' Women are affected by autism in the same ways as their male counterparts; however, they are doubly challenged by the added assumptions that society places on the female gender. Catherine Faherty (Attwood et al., 2006, p. 12)

Is it important to have a diagnosis if the individual is doing well enough without one? I don't really have the answer to that question, but I do believe you don't have to have a diagnosis to take advantage of any learning tools you can find and apply. It is very important to remember that many adults learn how to hide their challenges exceptionally well. But I like to think they shouldn't--at the end of the day the exhaustion levels and stress from doing so can be debilitating. In my opinion, everyone should know how to use her Asperger syndrome as a gift that enriches without exhausting. (Willey, 2012, pp. 151–152)

Barriers to Timely Identification

Barriers to identification have been identified in the first-person literature to inform clinicians. Researchers have also investigated the lived experiences of autism in detail to better inform diagnostic practices. Although the themes are nominally different, there are common threads in the narratives and research findings.

Even when exhibiting similar symptoms, boys are more likely to receive ASD diagnosis than girls
So, who gets to have a diagnosis in the first place? Well, we can discuss privilege, to begin with. If you have good insurance and access to genuinely nonjudgmental psych specialists, you might be in luck. That already is leaving a lot out of the population. People with low income or limited access to healthcare have a lower likelihood of getting in through that front door. Victoria M. Rodríguez-Roldán (Ballou et al., 2021, p. 86)

There are several professional criteria designed to measure whether or not a person has an ASD. Yet females remain largely underrepresented in these measurement tools. Until our researchers and institutes of higher education decide females really are on the spectrum in numbers far larger than they recognize, it will be up to us, the laypeople, to identify and support our girls and women. (Ballou et al., 2021, p. 147)

The female profile of autism describes an experience and presentation of autism that is unique and different from male individuals. Assumptions about autism, and diagnostic tools often do not reflect these sex-based differences, leading to underdiagnosis and late diagnosis of autistic female individuals. (Brown & Stokes, 2020, p. 735)

Regarding diagnosis, general expectancy biases and gender-stereotypes may impede timely recognition of autism in females. Appreciating the multilevel sex and gender impacts on presentation, development, and diagnosis is key to sex-equitable and gender-equitable care for autistic individuals. A holistic approach to understanding the person in the contexts of sex and gender is essential for timely and accurate diagnosis and support. (Lai & Szatmari, 2020, p. 117)

None of the barriers described above or listed below are insurmountable. Awareness, training, and continued research already exist, but need to be more prominently featured and updated in professional communities to improve equity of access to appropriate care and supports. See Chap. 13 for more discussion of advocacy.

Male Bias in Research and the Search for a Female Phenotype

Many researchers in the past decade have been working on the analyses of existing datasets to find the answers to the question of why females are not identified as autistic as often or as early as males. As each historical dataset is mined for data, all acknowledge that the selection bias in these studies has created a distinctly cisgender male version of autism as the definitive profile (Rosen et al., 2021). Bourson and Prevost (2022) cite the contributions of Kopp and Gillberg (1992) and Kirkovski et al. (2013) to the acceptance of the idea that there is a particular female profile or a behavioral phenotype of autism that is different between males and females. Given the heterogeneity of autism, it is not surprising that a single description might not be found in any one study. Kreiser and White (2014) also identified more internalizing than externalizing behaviors in females than males with autism as they looked at social and cultural factors. They acknowledged that these differences may not represent a different subtype of autism, but that females are more likely to be missed for diagnosis due to lack of awareness of these subtle differences. Less noticeable repetitive behaviors (Charman et al. 2017; Frazier et al., 2014; Lai & Szatmari, 2020) as well as possibly more sensory traits have frequently been noted (Øien et al. 2018; Tang et al., 2021). Several other studies are referenced throughout this work as they identify particular areas of difference. In general, however, the details of the female phenotypic profile are still somewhat unclear (Bourson & Prevost, 2022). Ratto et al. (2018) analyzed female traits in typical assessment measures used in research and concluded that some autistic females are likely to be missed by current assessment batteries and diagnostic procedures.

Genetic Load and "Protective" Effect

Because the autism prevalence ratios have always been lopsided (more males than females), many have speculated on the possibility of a female genetic effect usually referred to as a "protective" effect, but this may not be the best term. Most have concluded that the genetic load (cumulative differences) must be significantly higher for females to show traits of (or be recognized as having) autism. A large consortium study found autism spectrum-associated genes interacted with sex differential processes, supporting the theory of autism "looking" different according to sex. Specifically, that "cumulative, genome-wide risk for ASD differentially impacts the male and female brain," (Lawrence et al., 2022, p. 384). Jack et al. (2021) examined genetic and neuroimaging data together (the neuro-endophenotype) regarding the interpretation of social motion perception and concluded that higher copy number variant (CNV) counts were found in autistic females, consistent with the female effect theory and other studies (Lawrence et al., 2022; Wigdor et al., 2021). Effects on brain structures due to these genetic differences happen early in brain development. Typically developing (TD) females were perceiving the social motion data differently from all other groups, but female differences (between TD and autistic) were not in the same areas as differences between TD males and autistic males. Although brain function was similar in both autism groups, the genetic load in terms of CNV in autistic females was higher (Jack et al., 2021):

> Our finding that girls are relatively shielded from the impact of polygenic risk on salience network functional connectivity with sensorimotor regions thus raises the intriguing possibility that girls may exhibit fewer repetitive behaviours and ultimately be less likely to receive an ASD diagnosis, precisely because this neural circuitry is protected. (Lawrence et al., 2022, p. 384)

Another recent study found females need a greater "load" or accumulation of genetic differences (variations from neurotypical) than males in order to be identified as autistic. Multiple genetic factors produced different sets of behavioral traits and effects that differed by sex within the very large sample. Higher genetic loads were also found in parents of autistic children, particularly mothers (Wigdor et al., 2021).

Different Profiles and Patterns

Given the gender bias that exists, what do clinicians do to identify females? In one study, 70% of expert clinicians reported that they perceive differences in core traits in autistic females that are most apparent in school age and adolescence, with fewer differences in early childhood autism traits (Jamison et al., 2017). Sedgewick et al. (2019) looked for differences in friendships and socialization and found that autistic girls had more friend conflict and found it more difficult to manage conflicts than their neurotypical female peers, but that their friendships and social experiences were self-reported to be consistent with typical female reports of friendship and more different from both autistic and neurotypical male friendships (see Chap. 6). There are many studies indicating lower scores on ratings of special interests and stimming behaviors in females (see Chap. 5 for more details) and conflicting findings on social communication skills—seemingly better at younger ages, more apparent difficulties appeared with increased age. See Chap. 3 for more details on these studies. Some studies examining differences between genders also acknowledge differences between genders in neurotypical samples (Lawrence et al., 2022).

Milder, Less Apparent Differences Become More Apparent Over Time

Jamison et al. (2017) concluded that the perceptions of differences in presentation for females reflected less severe social difficulties, but gaps between neurotypical and autistic females grew more apparent over time. As young children, differences across genders are less pronounced (arguing for earlier evaluations), but a child may be advanced in some areas (e.g., an early reader), which may reduce concerns about development in other areas. In their "road map" analysis, Duvall et al. (2021) coined the term "pink flags" to indicate the more nuanced signs within the diagnostic criteria that clinicians can learn to look for and recognize as indicators of autism. This lowered or alternative threshold approach is consistent with the issue raised by Constantino and Charman (2016) regarding subtle or nuanced autism and the idea of clinical threshold. They described the tension between expert clinician judgment and the clinical thresholds that may not have incorporated the evolution of what we know about autism as a spectrum condition. Meng-Chuan Lai stated in a 2020 editorial that autism may not be a binary yes/no condition in ways that are easily quantified, but a condition comprising multiple spectra in which manifestations may vary yet still remain within the core definition of autism.

Comparisons to the Wrong Reference Group(s)

DaWalt et al. (2020) proposed that choosing appropriate comparisons when judging differences is critical. Rather than focusing on the differences between males and females with autism in identification, we may limit the historical bias effects if we instead compare autistic females to neurotypical females (gender-specific norms).

> "For women with ASD, the way that their autism symptoms interact with typical patterns of female social behavior may be significantly more impairing than their autism symptoms alone [e.g., Bargiela et al., 2016; Kanfizer & Collins, 2017]" (DaWalt et al., 2020, p. 2160).

One example of this is often noted in restricted and repetitive interests and stereotyped behaviors (hereafter may also be referred to as special or intense interests and stimming behaviors), which may be closer to those of neurotypical females than they are to those of autistic males, yet still be different in how they are expressed in autistic females (Bourson & Prevost, 2022). It is also possible that gender expectations for females may be different than for males in conversation, and clinician gender bias is always possible. The consistent evidence of genetic load differences in autistic females tells us that if we are looking for an appropriate comparison group, other females are a closer genetic comparison, so they may be a more appropriate phenotypic comparison (Jack et al., 2021). It may be that we need to consider which groups we compare autistic females to, as they are likely different enough from TD females that identification may be easier with gender-specific comparisons.

Parent Perceptions and Positive Traits Invalidating Consideration of Autism

Many women identified with autism in adulthood report that they were somewhat unaware of their own differences until they began to seek help for their children (Ballou et al., 2021; O'Toole, 2018; Willey, 2014). Duvall et al. (2021) described an example of parents characterizing their children as empathetic when examples given clearly indicated generosity, caring, and somewhat rigid ideas about fairness.

> Consequently, when working with individuals with more subtle presentations, it is also not unusual for an affected parent to remain undiagnosed and have a limited awareness of his or her own social challenges. Even when they are aware of their child's difficulties, they may normalize them, because they had (or have) them as well. (Duvall et al., 2021, p. 1188)

Due to stereotypes about autistic people lacking empathy, these strengths may be incorrectly seen as contraindicating autism. Especially in the absence of siblings, cousins, or friends of similar ages, reporters may not realize that the person still struggles with specific social skills that are expected for their age. Another likelihood is that some autistic traits observed in nuanced autism are seen as positive or advanced development, overshadowing difficulties that may be present but overlooked. Some examples include being honest or truthful, following the rules, making sure things are always fair, being detail-focused, and having analytic insights (Eckerd, 2020). Precocious and voracious reading is recognized as gifted and possibly quirky when it might be a special interest (see Chap. 7). Some may have high standards of performance that might reflect black-and-white or binary thinking. Children who struggle with back-and-forth imaginative collaboration may still have strong pretend play (see Chap. 5), which can include trying to re-play social situations or enjoying a solitary world free from criticism (Grandin et al., 2019). In other words, if they are successful in any domain, that is often all the evidence a parent or provider needs to not consider autism as a possible reason for any other difficulties or differences.

Camouflaging Behaviors

Although camouflaging is not a trait of autism and is not exclusively found in females (Fombonne, 2020), the phenomenon of imitating others in an effort to fit in and be accepted (or not bullied) is cited as a barrier to identification (Rosen et al., 2021). Based on better imitation skills than expected (given the male autistic profile), females (and others with nuanced autism) work very hard to do what peers are doing, but may not understand the underlying social context, so may not get it quite "right" at times (Hull et al., 2020). Identifying camouflaging (or seeing the person without camouflaging) may be easier when assessment extends across settings. Teachers and parents may have very different perceptions of a child who shows different behaviors involving attention, compliance, and/or emotion regulation, play, etc. according to setting and context. Duvall et al. (2021) suggested that one reason the child may appear to be very different at home than school or vice versa is that parents may have adapted by reducing demands and/or increasing supports at home, resulting in fewer difficulties at home. On the other hand, some children thrive best in the structure of school, with schedules, routines, clear rules, etc., and don't do as well at home (Grandin et al., 2019):

> *"I was unbearable with my mother, but at school, I was perfect"*. *P09* (Bargiela et al., 2016, p. 3286)

Camouflaging (or compensatory coping) plays into this scenario as children work really hard to "hold it together" at school, but the stress and effort have used up all resiliency by the time they get home, so their ability levels look very different across settings (Hull et al., 2020). One term we have heard to describe this is "after-school restraint collapse." This may seem to violate the clinician's expectation of difficulties that "should be" consistent across settings, confusing the presentation with seemingly discrepant reports of behavior. As females grow up, the emotional and psychic toll of needing to pretend to be someone else to be accepted can overwhelm their abilities to maintain and cope. Bourson and Prevost (2022) described camouflaging as typically being more effective and efficient in females with higher cognitive abilities, but even with that advantage, it is not necessarily easier for them. Many if not most are eventually overtaken by expectations from society and by relational issues during adolescence. Within the rather unique context of neuropsychological assessment, it is possible that eye contact and social skills may seem to be typical because of the restricted, highly structured environment and the adult social partner (Duvall et al., 2021). Casual conversation or non-goal-directed activities may provide a clearer sample of social behavior.

"They may also engage more successfully with tests that are clearly structured and struggle with more open ended, imprecise questions and directions, particularly if they include nonliteral, abstract or metaphorical language" (Duvall et al., 2021, p. 1187).

Clinician Expertise

Straightforward or unambiguous presentations of autism may be easily diagnosed by clinicians with generalized training in community practice, with or perhaps without the comprehensive evaluations discussed. "Clinicians need to be aware of the potential for under-recognition of signs of autism in women and girls and different expressions in particular sign and symptom clusters" (Lord et al., 2022).

Sociocultural factors also play a role in how clinicians apply diagnostic criteria in females according to their own perceptions and biases (Rosen et al., 2021). See Chap. 8 for more about the diagnostic odyssey autistic women typically have to travel before they find a clinician with sufficient awareness, experience, and training to pick up on nuanced autism traits through comprehensive evaluation. This expertise crosses many disciplinary lines and includes speech and language pathologists, school psychologists, clinical psychologists, neuropsychologists, pediatricians, and other specialists in diagnostic roles. "Even when an adult woman suspects she might have ASD, professionals often dismiss the idea when the woman presents it. One woman commented, 'When I mentioned the possibility to my psychiatric nurse, she laughed at me'" (Eckerd, 2020, p. 37).

Regardless of discipline or experience, each clinician is likely to bring their own lived experience to their clinical decision-making and may not have enough perspective or experience to recognize autistic differences as such, particularly if they share some of the autistic traits:

> The point is how do clinicians interpret the criteria rather than changing the criteria? […] The key is asking the right questions and sadly that only comes from experience and knowledge about the female presentation of the condition. Educating professionals as we do in our diagnostic training is one of the ways forward (Gould, 2014, personal communication). (Hendrickx, 2015, p. 34)

Rosen et al. (2021) described subtle qualitative differences in presentations of core autism traits in females among their reasons for missed diagnoses. Clinicians accustomed to looking for "red flags" for autism need to become more aware of the "pink flags" such as those outlined by Duvall et al. (2021) that are milder and less apparent in casual observation. In each of the chapters that follows, "pink flags" will be discussed as they have been identified in the research and first-person literature.

Interviewing is a critical element of evaluations when nuanced autism is the question, but as with most of the assessment process for females or other nuanced autism, adjustments are likely needed. Eckerd (2020) summarized some important considerations in diagnostic interviewing for clinicians as follows:

- Verbal response rate might be slower than expected to allow for processing.
- Open-ended questions can be confusing.
- Specific, clear, and direct questions are easier to answer.
- Reports of social relationships may reflect acceptance, inclusion, and rejection rather than the quality or reciprocity in the relationship.
- Ask directly about sensory and executive function and disruption in routines.
- Difficulties described may not seem to be significant, but they likely are significant to the individual.
- Assess daily and occupational functioning from the client's perspective.
- Consider possible camouflaging or masking; bolster with other informants or data.

See Chap. 13 for the complete listing of nuanced characteristics from Duvall et al. (2021).

Gender Diversity and Autism

The concept of "spectrum" applies as much to gender diversity as it does to autism. No discussion of assessment or supports for autism is complete without consideration of gender diversity beyond gender assigned at birth. The DSM-5-TR describes higher rates of gender variance in autistic females (assigned female at birth) compared to autistic males (assigned male at birth) and also compared to the general population (APA, 2022).

Gendered Social Expectations

Cooper et al. (2018) described a pattern of gender identity in autism females that was opposite the pattern across gender neurotypical groups—autistic females (AFAB) showed less social identification with their gender and had more negative feelings about a gender group than autistic males assigned male at birth (AMAB) or cisgender females. Overall cognitive levels are generally average or higher than average in the nuanced type of autism in females and others, which is one reason why autistic females may not rise to the attention of teachers or parents as being different or needing support. It is important to look beyond the overall results, however, and look at the *variability* within the cognitive profiles as a more accurate assessment of cognitive strengths and differences. Many of the first-person narratives describe systematic thinking processes that may be expected more of males in general than females. George and Stokes (2018) commented on this traditionally male-associated thinking and behavior as a possible pathway for some autistic females to perceive themselves as masculine relative to non-ASD females.

Strang et al. (2018) set forth some clinical guidelines for the assessment of autism with gender variance. The first is that specialists in both autism and gender be involved or that each of the specialities collaborate. Consistent with our recommendations throughout this text, assessments need more time to allow for clinicians to discover more about the individual across settings. A general recommendation for gender clinics is to screen for autism in all of their patients. If screens indicate further autism assessment, an autism specialist should conduct the type of comprehensive evaluation described in the following chapters, starting with Chap. 2. Strang and colleagues recommend that gender assessment include structured interview by a gender specialist to assess dysphoria over time, including intensity and pervasiveness. Interviews with parents are also key, especially if the individual has difficulty with communication, self-awareness, and self-advocacy. Strang et al. (2018) also found that gender dysphoria in autistic youth was typically enduring and in need of support, contrary to the possible assumption that gender issues are not "real" but a manifestation of special interest, concrete thinking, etc.

First-Person Narratives About Gender

One adult Asperger Syndrome service in Brighton reports that…at the time of first contact with the service almost all of the trans people who approached them for support were undiagnosed with autism. Many stated that their gender identity issues had masked their autism. (Hendrickx, 2015, p. 157)

Sometimes I feel like a third gender, not in a nonbinary way. I feel so rejected and judged by other women, and so alien and undesirable to men, that I feel like a subwoman-- not a man, in a female body, but with none of the mystique and allure that is supposed to accompany womanhood. [User] whaletuuune (22 years old), 2021

My gender came in question at that time—the boys would say, "You aren't like other girls. You don't cry when you get hurt, so you are better than other girls, but you aren't a boy, so you are a Mary Margaret." Of course it was lonely being given a category to myself and it taught me to hate my gender. It would take feminist readings many years later to move me out of my male-identified position. MM (Miller, 2015, p. 50–51)

For some of us here, our lives, outlook, and behavior don't have much of a sense of gender at all. I myself live a somewhat femme life but it feels in some sense detachable, like a costume. I was an androgynous kid and most clearly perceive the world in a non-gendered way. Jean (Miller, 2015, p. 51)

In many ways, as the social theorists point out, gender is a performance that is enacted. Learning one's gender role (how to enact it) has been the key channel through which girls have become value added social participants. That's what make-up is about, for example. Jane (Miller, 2015, p. 55)

It was as if everyone else had studied a script and learned their parts beforehand. In fact, of course, they were improvising brilliantly, thanks to the social code capacity programmed into their brains and to the natural ease with which they acquired their gender identity from the culture around them. Jean Meyerding (Miller, 2015, p. 183)

I can tell you that it's probably because if you have a spectrum disorder, where you're not concerned with social norms, you probably won't care about the gender norms pushed on everyone, so it's easier to explore your gender. I personally forgot I had a gender back in the mid-2010s, and I haven't been bothered to care about it since. Mallory Cruz (Ballou et al., 2021, pp. 163–164)

In one of the psychology books I read it pointed out differences in male and female thinking and strengths. I realized I had a lot of male areas of talent strengths. I began to wonder if I had a male mind. (April Griffin, 2016)

Transgender and Non-binary 101

For readers who are not familiar with transgender/non-binary/gender-diverse terminology and concepts, this section will provide a brief introduction. Gender identity is a very complex topic, and this discussion may not capture all of the nuances found in gender-diverse individuals.

When an infant is born (barring some intersex cases), they are given an *assigned gender at birth*. An infant born with a penis is assigned male gender, and an infant born with a vagina is assigned female gender. "Assigned gender" is now considered more appropriate than "biological sex" for a variety of reasons, including the fact that the brain is also a biological characteristic and some sex characteristics (e.g., genital shape and facial hair) may be changed through medical intervention.

If the person continues to identify with this assigned gender throughout their life, they are said to be *cisgender*. If the person determines that a different gender is more appropriate, they are generally said to be *transgender*. This may be a straightforward transition from male to female or vice versa. However, some people determine that they have no gender, multiple genders, or something else entirely. People who fall outside of the "only male" or "only female" binary are generally described as *non-binary*.

It is important to note that many people enjoy activities that cross traditional gender lines (e.g., men wearing dresses) while still identifying with their assigned gender. In addition, transgender or non-binary may not present as expected, such as a transgender woman who prefers to grow a beard or keep her penis intact. It is important to respect individuals' self-reported gender identities rather than attempting to assign categories based on assumptions. Gender identity is also separate from sexual/romantic orientation; a transgender or non-binary person may be gay, straight, asexual, or any other orientation.

Considerations in Instrument Use and Norms

While we have generally assumed that diagnostic criteria/methods are gender neutral (Volkmar et al., 2021), the evidence that autism diagnostic processes need to include gender is one of the issues that needs to be disseminated more widely. Diagnostic measures have been shown to be adequate for identification within comprehensive evaluations, but the autism research community is strongly stressing the need to interpret behaviors within contexts (including cultural expectations for gender and possible biologically based sex differences). Standardized measures are not enough. It is also required that we gather detailed developmental histories to supplement when giving diagnostic impressions (Rosen et al., 2021).

> *Autistic girls mess up norms. We bust misconceptions about gender and autism. These are assets in spite of a world that thinks otherwise. Don't expect girls to labor under the burdens of wrong expectations. Instead, nurture possibility and difference.* Karen Lean (Ballou et al., 2021, p. 47).

It is not currently known what reference norms are most appropriate when assessing non-binary and transgender individuals, particularly those who have not received hormone treatment. One study suggests that early developmental history tends to align with assigned sex/gender (e.g., transgender autistic boys displayed early communication skills more similar to cisgender autistic girls—Strang et al., 2021). However, structural findings from the general transgender population suggest that transgender brains often show some characteristics less typical of their assigned gender (Cleveland Clinic, 2019). Information about if and when hormones were administered can possibly affect brain organization (early history of hormone exposure) and activation (current presence of hormone exposure). Differences in brain structures and various cognitive abilities are not yet definitively established in the scientific literature. See Trittschuh et al. (2018) for a summary.

Assessment Approaches

Barriers to identification detailed above for all nuanced types of autism are ample justification for broader interpretation of norms and cutoffs for standardized measures given gender contexts. Adjusting results (e.g., cutoffs and ranges) based on male samples, the need for comprehensive evaluations, additional time to gather additional interview and observational data, and more thorough exploration of each domain of function relevant to current difficulties is needed. This "weight of evidence" approach is more likely to reveal patterns of differences that indicate autistic traits and avenues for appropriate supports:

> Standardized behavioral diagnostic instruments with good psychometric properties, including caregiver interviews, questionnaires and clinician observation measures, are available and can improve reliability of diagnosis over time and across clinicians. However, the symptoms of autism spectrum disorder occur as dimensions without universally accepted cutoff scores for what would constitute a disorder. Thus, the diagnosis remains a clinical one, taking all available information into account, and is not solely dictated by the score on a particular questionnaire or observation measure. (DSM-5-TR: Autism Spectrum Disorder, APA, 2022)

We recommend carving out additional time for the assessment of these cases, although considerable pressure usually exists to complete the diagnosis as quickly as possible. The DSM-5-TR describes autism traits as possibly subtle within individual modes, but perhaps more observable in the individual's difficulty maintaining higher-level skills for sustained periods when under stress (2022). Each of the subsequent chapters provides more detail on the research and first-person experiences to guide your assessment planning and clinical decision-making.

Support Recommendations

The objective of this work is to promote earlier and appropriate identification of autism when it is more nuanced, especially in females. This is, in and of itself, obviously the most critical step toward supports. But what are the next steps? First, we have to decide if any of the more "typical" supports might be needed. Because the traits are nuanced and easily missed, there may be two hurdles to overcome in planning treatment and supports.

The first obstacle to overcome is that an autism diagnosis means that an individual needs to be "fixed" with a long list of "must have" treatment approaches. The idea of stepped care, detailed in the *Lancet Commission on the Future of Care and Clinical Research in Autism* (Lord et al., 2022), is a relevant framework to conceptualize a support plan that meets individual and family needs rather than a prescribed program approach. Not all individuals will need the standard "package" of applied behavior analysis (ABA), speech and language services, or social skills groups or individual therapy, for example. The benefit of a comprehensive evaluation is that it can pinpoint areas for support that might be missed in more cursory evaluations.

If behavior change or independent skill acquisition is needed, ABA may be helpful, but there are considerable concerns and controversies about ABA and ethics (see Chap. 13). Care should always be taken with vulnerable individuals (autistic, female, transgender, nonverbal, etc.) to not reinforce compliance with any and all requests. This is a significant safety issue that needs to be addressed in all treatment approaches (Catherine Flaherty in Grandin et al., 2019).

If conversational skills, more efficient expressive language, receptive language (understanding directions), or other language-related improvements are desired, then speech and language therapy can cover a wide range of desired supports. Social skills groups or interventions may need to be individualized, may need to be formal, or may be infinitely better if the person can just find a consistent social group that "gets" them and accepts their authentic selves to share common interests with. See Chap. 5.

It is likely, however, that many will benefit from executive function supports or coaching. See Chap. 7 for more information on the multiple ways executive function difficulties can be significantly problematic. Other chapters will outline specific supports for other areas commonly found to need support.

In Chap. 8, we explore the long list of diagnoses that females and others with nuanced autism experience before they finally arrive at their autism diagnosis. This does not mean that the various conditions they have previously been identified with don't exist. The traits, barriers, and difficulties do exist, but the neurology driving these differences is not in line with the way an allistic (not autistic) person may experience them. Autistic females are usually seeking help for a long time before they find the supports tailored to the way their brains work and their experiences.

This leads us to our second hurdle. How do you find the supports you need if the support systems are not well-informed about nuanced autism, commonly found in females, including gender-diverse people? If the treatment provider has also been the diagnostician for autism, the level of expertise related to their client's needs is likely to be higher to start with. If this is not the case, it is obviously going to take some effort on the part of parents or the autistic individual herself/themselves.

Step 1: Get a release of information so that your diagnostician can talk to your treatment provider and/or education team. This may provide some resources or at least illumination regarding how to adjust treatments and educational supports to get started.

Step 2: Address each of the areas needing support (e.g., executive function, anxiety, depression, suicidal thoughts and behaviors, sensory sensitivities, employment difficulties, reading comprehension, social communication, eating disorders, rigid thinking). Mainstream intervention approaches may be effective if the therapeutic partners understand the client's neurodiversity. We will make more suggestions in each chapter addressing each of these supports.

Step 3: Develop a personal social story to help the support team know what the person needs and how to work with them most effectively. Social stories are a helpful way to use visual media to teach new skills, especially for young children (Gray, 2015). As children get older, they may still benefit from social stories to teach new skills in social situations, with adaptations to respect age and interest. For most within the group we focus on here, however, you may need to flip the social story idea so that the individual learns how to communicate how they work and what they need in high-stakes settings such as family, relationships, and employment. This approach can improve social communication skills, self-awareness, self-advocacy, and acceptance of the authentic individual. See Chapter 13.

Step 4: Find or create a community of support and belonging. Because autism is so variable, this may be much more complicated than just connecting with the local autistic community. More efforts are likely to be needed. Two of the best-known and oft-cited models for building communities for autistic females are Girls Night Out (GNO) at University of Kansas and Felicity House in New York City. Other communities and specialty clinics are beginning to offer groups for females, but there may still be the issue of right fit for diverse individuals. Finally, secondary schools, colleges, and universities are ideal settings for the development of groups or communities for females in particular and are likely to have more individuals with a desire to connect in a group suited to their needs. See Chap. 13 for more ideas. Decreasing social isolation is widely held as a protective factor to reduce risk of suicide and bullying, which is compounded if the individual is autistic and gender variant. Relationships, school, and employment may be difficult, so supports, including group supports, should address specific needs in these settings as well (Strang et al., 2018).

In general, treatment approaches should be straightforward and make extensive use of visual means to illustrate abstract concepts. Clear language, simple concepts, and concrete presentations are likely to increase participation in treatment (Strang et al., 2016). Supporting executive function difficulties (which often requires significant family involvement) is also key to treatment participation and success at school and work (Strang et al., 2021).

Recommendations for the assessment of transgender individuals are also an important support. Trittschuh et al. (2018) make the following recommendations:

- Create a safe zone environment that is gender neutral and affirmative and incorporates safe signs.
- Ask about gender identity at intake to avoid misgendering.
- Ask how the person wants to be addressed.
- Explore how the individual has been treated regarding gender status.

- Screen for suicidal thoughts and behaviors.
- Select assessment measures with gender-neutral norms when available.
- If using gendered norms, consider both gendered scores.
- Use preferred names and pronouns and gender-affirmative language in reports.
- Carefully consider history in the interpretation of findings.
- During the feedback session, relax, reorient the person to current goals, remind the person of interview topics, ask permission to address gender, discuss normative difference of sex transparently, and include positive aspects of transition.

Finally, Strang et al. suggested developing a specialized consent plan for treatment and intervention, particularly for medical interventions and support. Presenting the benefits and risks in a concrete manner, appropriate for the person's cognitive and communication abilities, is important to assure fully informed consent. This is yet another reason for a comprehensive evaluation for autism as part of the broader assessment of gender variance (Strang et al., 2018). See Table 1.1 for a summary of strategies introduced in this chapter.

Table 1.1 At-a-glance summary—sex, gender, autism, assessment, and equity

Barriers to identification	Strategies to reduce barriers
Male bias	Consider subthreshold assessment results as possibly valid for female or nuanced autism. Within a comprehensive evaluation, weight of evidence can show patterns consistent with autism, even if they don't quite meet standardized cutoffs (e.g., autism measures and other data that are just below cutoff, but still signaling autistic traits)
Autistic genes in females	Explore family histories for evidence of autism, which may indicate a higher genetic load and greater likelihood for autistic traits
Different profiles and patterns	The patterns of traits may look different from traditional expectations; look for patterns of signals of neurodiversity to emerge in assessment data (e.g., lower special interests and behaviors, more sensory sensitivities, executive functions issues, mild language or motor issues)
Milder, less apparent differences	"Pink flags," (Duvall et al., 2021) should not be dismissed, especially if there are many of them
Comparisons to the wrong reference group(s)	Compare autistic females to neurotypical females to more accurately assess differences (autistic males are not a good comparison)
Parent perceptions and positive traits invalidating consideration of autism	Success and competence in some domains do not rule out autism. Look for patterns in positive traits that may suggest autism traits
Camouflaging behaviors	More than brief or casual observation, interview, and assessment will be necessary to see past masking behaviors that may be hard for the person to "turn off" even during assessment. Repeated assessment sessions over time are likely to illuminate differences in play, conversation, and interests
Clinician expertise	Seek consultation and updated research on females and nuanced autism. Comprehensive evaluations are typically needed to come to a clinical decision using weight of evidence rather than relying on definitive results on measures

(continued)

Table 1.1 (continued)

Barriers to identification	Strategies to reduce barriers
Gendered social expectations	Examine your own gender bias in social behavior, including appearance, interests, conversation, expectations, etc.
Transgender and non-binary 101	Create a safe and affirmative space and experience for transgender clients with respect for names, pronouns, and supports
Assessment approaches	Standardized measures will need to be supplemented substantially with interviews and observations. Adjust interviewing style to reduce open-ended questions, etc. particularly when screening for suicidality, eating disorders, etc.
Support recommendations	Individualized supports are required, with ongoing monitoring for developing needs and progress. Common techniques for supporting autistic students can also apply in therapy (e.g., visual supports, reducing sensory overload, video modeling, etc.)

References

American Psychiatric Association. (1980). *Diagnostic and statistical manual of mental disorders* (3rd ed.). Author.

American Psychiatric Association. (2013). *Diagnostic and statistical manual of mental disorders* (5th ed.). Author.

American Psychiatric Association. (2022). Diagnostic and statistical manual of mental disorders (5th, Text Rev ed.). Author.

Asperger, H. (1944). "'Autistic psychopathy' in childhood," in *Autism and Asperger syndrome*, edited by Uta Frith (Cambridge: Cambridge University Press, 1991), 37–92. Originally published as "Die 'Autistischen Psychopathen' im Kindesalter". *Archiv für Psychiatrie und Nervenkrankheiten, 117*, 76–136.

Attwood, T., Grandin, T., Bolic, T., Faherty, C., Iland, L., Myers, J. M., Snyder, R., Wagner, S., & Wrobel, M. (2006). *Asperger's and girls*. Future Horizons.

Ballou, E. P., da Vanport, S., & Onaiwu, M. G. (Eds.). (2021). *Sincerely, your autistic child*. Beacon Press.

Bargiela, S., Steward, R., & Mandy, W. (2016). The experiences of late-diagnosed women with autism spectrum conditions: An investigation of the female autism phenotype. *Journal of Autism and Developmental Disorders, 46*(10), 3281–3294. https://doi.org/10.1007/s10803-016-2872-8

Baron-Cohen, S. (2004). *The essential difference: Male and female brains and the truth about autism*. Basic Books.

Bejerot, S., Eriksson, J. M., Bonde, S., Carlström, K., Humble, M. B., & Eriksson, E. (2012). The Extreme Male Brain Revisited: Gender coherence in adults with autism spectrum disorder. *The British Journal of Psychiatry, 201*, 116–123. https://doi.org/10.1192/bjp.bp.111.097899

Bourson, L., & Prevost, C. (2022). Characteristics of restricted interests in girls with ASD compared to boys: a systematic review of the literature. *European Child & Adolescent Psychiatry*. https://doi.org/10.1007/s00787-022-01998-5. Epub ahead of print.

Brown, C. M., & Stokes, M. A. (2020). Intersection of eating disorders and the female profile of autism. *The Psychiatric Clinics of North America, 43*(4), 735–743. https://doi.org/10.1016/j.psc.2020.08.009

Charman, T., Young, G. S., Brian, J., Carter, A., Carver, L. J., Chawarska, K., Curtin, S., Dobkins, K., Elsabbagh, M., Georgiades, S., Hertz, P. I., Hutman, T., Iverson, J. M., Jones, E. J., Landa, R., Macari, S., Messinger, D. S., Nelson, C. A., Ozonoff, S., et al. (2017). Non-ASD outcomes at 36 months in siblings at familial risk for autism spectrum disorder (ASD): A Baby Siblings Research Consortium (BSRC) study. *Autism Research, 10*(1), 169–178. https://doi.org/10.1002/aur.1669

Child and Adolescent Health Measurement Initiative. (2022). *2019–2020 National Survey of Children's Health (NSCH) data query*. Data Resource Center for Child and Adolescent Health supported by the U.S. Department of Health and Human Services, Health Resources and Services Administration (HRSA), Maternal and Child Health Bureau (MCHB). www.child-healthdata.org

Cleveland Clinic. (2019, March 27). *Research on the transgender brain: What you should know; Expanding knowledge of the brain and gender identity.* Cleveland Clinic Health Essentials: Brain & Spine. https://health.clevelandclinic.org/research-on-the-transgender-brain-what-you-should-know/

Constantino, J. N., & Charman, T. (2016). Diagnosis of autism spectrum disorder: Reconciling the syndrome, its diverse origins, and variation in expression. *Lancet Neurology, 15*, 279–291. https://doi.org/10.1016/S1474-4422(15)00151-9

Cooper, K., Smith, L. G., & Russell, A. J. (2018). Gender identity in autism: Sex differences in social affiliation with gender groups. *Journal of Autism and Developmental Disorders, 48*(12), 3995–4006. https://doi.org/10.1007/s10803-018-3590-1

DaWalt, L. S., Taylor, J. L., Bishop, S., Hall, L. J., Steinbrenner, J. D., Kraemer, B., Hume, K. A., & Odom, S. L. (2020). Sex differences in social participation of high school students with autism spectrum disorder. *Autism Research, 13*(12), 2155–2163. https://doi.org/10.1002/aur.2348

de Marchena, A., & Miller, J. (2017). "Frank" presentations as a novel research construct and element of diagnostic decision-making in autism spectrum disorder. *Autism Research, 10*(4), 653–662. https://doi.org/10.1002/aur.1706

De Vries, A. L., Noens, I. L., Cohen-Kettenis, P. T., van Berckelaer-Onnes, I. A., & Doreleijers, T. A. (2010). Autism spectrum disorders in gender dysphoric children and adolescents. *Journal of Autism and Developmental Disorders, 40*(8), 930–936. https://doi.org/10.1007/s10803-010-0935-9

Duvall, S., Armstrong, K., Shahabuddin, A., Grantz, C., Fein, D., & Lord, C. (2021). A road map for identifying autism spectrum disorder: Recognizing and evaluating characteristics that should raise red or "pink" flags to guide accurate differential diagnosis. *The Clinical Neuropsychologist*, 1–36. Advance online publication. https://doi.org/10.1080/13854046.2021.1921276.

Eckerd, M. (2020). Detection and diagnosis of ASD in females. *Journal of Health Service Psychology, 46*(1), 37–47. https://doi.org/10.1007/s42843-020-00006-1

Fombonne, E. (2020). Camouflage and autism. *Journal of Child Psychology and Psychiatry, 61*(7), 735–738. https://doi.org/10.1111/jcpp.13296

Frazier, T. W., Georgiades, S., Bishop, S. L., & Hardan, A. Y. (2014). Behavioral and cognitive characteristics of females and males with autism in the Simons Simplex Collection. *Journal of the American Academy of Child and Adolescent Psychiatry, 53*(40.e1–3), 329. https://doi.org/10.1016/j.jaac.2013.12.004

George, R., & Stokes, M. A. (2018). Gender identity and sexual orientation in autism spectrum disorder. *Autism, 22*(8), 970–982. https://doi.org/10.1177/1362361317714587

Giarelli, E., Wiggins, L. D., Rice, C. E., Levy, S. E., Kirby, R. S., Pinto-Martin, J., & Mandell, D. (2010). Sex differences in the evaluation and diagnosis of autism spectrum disorders among children. *Disability and Health Journal, 3*(2), 107–116. https://doi.org/10.1016/j.dhjo.2009.07.001

Grandin, T., Attwood, T., Garnett, M., Faherty, C., Wagner, S., Iland, L., Wrobel, M., Bolick, T., Myers, J. M., & Snyder, R. (2019). *Autism and girls*. Future Horizons.

Gray, C. (2015). *The new social story book, revised and expanded 15th anniversary edition: Over 150 social stories that teach everyday social skills to children and adults with autism and their peers*. Future Horizons.

Griffin, A. (2016, September 12). *Gender identity issues and females on the spectrum. #ActuallyAutistic perspective, females and autism.* https://the-art-of-autism.com/gender-identity-issues-and-females-on-the-spectrum/

Hendrickx, S. (2015). *Women and girls with autism spectrum disorder: Understanding life experiences from early childhood to old age.* Jessica Kingsley.

Hull, L., Lai, M.-C., Baron-Cohen, S., Allison, C., Smith, P., Petrides, K. V., & Mandy, W. (2020). Gender differences in self-reported camouflaging in autistic and non-autistic adults. *Autism, 24*(2), 352–363. https://doi.org/10.1177/1362361319864804

Jack, A., Sullivan, C. A. W., Aylward, E., Bookheimer, S. Y., Dapretto, M., Gaab, N., Horn, J. D. V., Eilbott, J., Jacokes, Z., Torgerson, C. M., Bernier, R. A., Geschwind, D. H., McPartland, J. C., Nelson, C. A., Webb, S. J., Pelphrey, K. A., Gupta, A. R., Consortium, the G., Van Horn, J. D., & GENDAAR Consortium. (2021). A neurogenetic analysis of female autism. *Brain: A Journal of Neurology, 144*(6), 1911–1926. https://doi.org/10.1093/brain/awab064

Jamison, R., Bishop, S. L., Huerta, M., & Halladay, A. K. (2017). The clinician perspective on sex differences in autism spectrum disorders. *Autism, 21*(6), 772–784. https://doi.org/10.1177/1362361316681481

Janssen, A., Huang, H., & Duncan, C. (2016). Gender variance among youth with autism spectrum disorders: A retrospective chart review. *Transgender Health, 1*(1), 63–68. https://doi.org/10.1089/trgh.2015.0007

Jensen, C. M., Steinhausen, H. C., & Lauritsen, M. B. (2014). Time trends over 16 years in incidence-rates of autism spectrum disorders across the lifespan based on nationwide Danish register data. *Journal of Autism and Developmental Disorders, 44*(8), 1808–1818. https://doi.org/10.1007/s10803-014-2053-6

Kanfiszer, L., Davies, F., & Collins, S. (2017). "I was just so different": The experiences of women diagnosed with an autism spectrum disorder in adulthood in relation to gender and social relationships. *Autism, 21*, 661–669. https://doi.org/10.1177/1362361316687987

Kanner, L. (1943). Autistic disturbances of affective contact. *Nervous Child, 2*, 217–250. http://simonsfoundation.s3.amazonaws.com/share/071207-leo-kanner-autistic-affective-contact.pdf

Kim, Y. S., Leventhal, B. L., Koh, Y.-J., Fombonne, E., Laska, E., Lim, E.-C., Cheon, K.-A., Kim, S.-J., Kim, Y.-K., Lee, H. K., Song, D.-H., & Grinker, R. (2011). Prevalence of autism spectrum disorders in a total population sample. *The American Journal of Psychiatry, 168*, 904–912. https://doi.org/10.1176/appi.ajp.2011.10101532

Kirkovski, M., Enticott, P. G., & Fitzgerald, P. B. (2013). A review of the role of female gender in ASD. *Journal of Autism and Developmental Disorders, 43*, 2584–2603. https://doi.org/10.1007/s10803-013-1811-1

Kopp, S., & Gillberg, C. (1992). Girls with social deficits and learning problems: Autism, atypical Asperger syndrome or a variant of these conditions. *European Child & Adolescent Psychiatry, 1*, 89–99. https://doi.org/10.1007/BF02091791

Kreiser, N. L., & White, S. W. (2014). ASD in females: Are we overstating the gender difference in diagnosis? *Clinical Child and Family Psychology Review, 17*(1), 67–84. https://doi.org/10.1007/s10567-013-0148-9

Lai, M.-C. (2020). Editorial: Meaningfully Stratifying the Autism Spectra. *Journal of the American Academy of Child and Adolescent Psychiatry, 59*(12), 1324–1326. https://doi.org/10.1016/j.jaac.2020.08.002

Lai, M. C., & Szatmari, P. (2020). Sex and gender impacts on the behavioural presentation and recognition of autism. *Current Opinion in Psychiatry, 33*(2), 117–123. https://doi.org/10.1097/YCO.0000000000000575

Lawrence, K. E., Hernandez, L. M., Fuster, E., Padgaonkar, N. T., Patterson, G., Jung, J., Okada, N. J., Lowe, J. K., Hoekstra, J. N., Aylward, E., Gaab, N., Van Horn, J. D., Bernier, R. A., McPartland, J. C., Webb, S. J., Pelphrey, K. A., Green, S. A., Bookheimer, S. Y., et al. (2022). Impact of autism genetic risk on brain connectivity: A mechanism for the female protective effect. *Brain, 145*(1), 378–387. https://doi.org/10.1093/brain/awab204

Lord, C., Charman, T., Havdahl, A., Carbone, P., Anagnostou, E., Boyd, B., Carr, T., de Vries, P. J., Dissanayake, C., Divan, G., Freitag, C. M., Gotelli, M. M., Kasari, C., Knapp, M., Mundy, P., Plank, A., Scahill, L., Servili, C., Shattuck, P., et al. (2022). The Lancet commission on the future of care and clinical research in autism. *Lancet, 399*(10321), 271–334. https://doi.org/10.1016/S0140-6736(21)01541-5

Maenner, M. J., Warren, Z., Williams, A. R., Amoakohene, E., Bakian, A. V., Bilder, D. A., Durkin, M. S., Fitzgerald, R. T., Furnier, S. M., Hughes, M. M., Ladd-Acosta, C. M., McArther, D., Pas, E. T., Salinas, A., Vehorn, S., Williams, S., Esler, A., Grzybowski, A., Hall-Lande, J., et al. (2023). Prevalence and characteristics of autism spectrum disorder among children aged 8 years—Autism and Developmental Disabilities Monitoring Network, 11 sites, United States, 2020. *MMWR Surveillance Summaries, 72*(2), 1–14. https://doi.org/10.15585/mmwr.ss7202a1

Mattila, M.-L., Kielinen, M., Linna, S.-L., et al. (2011). Autism spectrum disorders according to DSM-IV-TR and comparison with DSM-5 draft criteria: An epidemiological study. *Journal of the American Academy of Child and Adolescent Psychiatry, 50*, 583–592.e11. https://doi.org/10.1016/j.jaac.2011.04.001

Miller, J. K. (Ed.). (2015). *Women from another planet? Our lives in the universe of autism.* AuthorHouse.

Mussey, J. L., Ginn, N. C., & Klinger, L. G. (2017). Are males and females with autism spectrum disorder more similar than we thought? *Autism: The International Journal of Research and Practice, 21*(6), 733–737. https://doi.org/10.1177/1362361316682621

Nerenberg, J. (2021). *Divergent mind: Thriving in a world that wasn't designed for you.* HarperOne.

Øien, R. A., Schjølberg, S., Volkmar, F. R., Shic, F., Cicchetti, D. V., Nordahl-Hansen, A., Stenberg, N., Hornig, M., Havdahl, A., Øyen, A.-S., Ventola, P., Susser, E. S., Eisemann, M. R., & Chawarska, K. (2018). Clinical features of children with autism who passed 18-month screening. *Pediatrics, 141*(6), 1–10. https://doi.org/10.1542/peds.2017-3596

O'Toole, J. C. (2018). *Autism in heels: The untold story of a female life on the spectrum.* Skyhorse Publishing.

Pierce, K., Gazestani, V. H., Bacon, E., Barnes, C. C., Cha, D., Nalabolu, S., Lopez, L., Moore, A., Pence-Stophaeros, S., & Courchesne, E. (2019). Evaluation of the diagnostic stability of the early autism spectrum disorder phenotype in the general population starting at 12 months. *JAMA Pediatrics, 173*(6), 578–587. https://doi.org/10.1001/jamapediatrics.2019.0624

Ratto, A. B., Kenworthy, L., Yerys, B. E., Bascom, J., Wieckowski, A. T., White, S. W., Wallace, G. L., Pugliese, C., Schultz, R. T., Ollendick, T. H., Scarpa, A., Seese, S., Register-Brown, K., Martin, A., & Anthony, L. G. (2018). What about the girls? Sex-based differences in autistic traits and adaptive skills. *Journal of Autism and Developmental Disorders, 48*(5), 1698–1711. https://doi.org/10.1007/s10803-017-3413-9

Rosen, N. E., Lord, C., & Volkmar, F. R. (2021). The Diagnosis of Autism: From Kanner to DSM-III to DSM-5 and Beyond. *Journal of Autism and Developmental Disorders, 51*, 4253–4270. https://doi.org/10.1007/s10803-021-04904-1

Russell, G., Steer, C., & Golding, J. (2011). Social and demographic factors that influence the diagnosis of autistic spectrum disorders. *Social Psychiatry and Psychiatric Epidemiology: The International Journal for Research in Social and Genetic Epidemiology and Mental Health Services, 46*(12), 1283–1293. https://doi.org/10.1007/s00127-010-0294-z

Rutherford, M., McKenzie, K., Johnson, T., Catchpole, C., O'Hare, A., McClure, I., Forsyth, K., McCartney, D., & Murray, A. (2016). Gender ratio in a clinical population sample, age of diagnosis and duration of assessment in children and adults with autism spectrum disorder. *Autism: The International Journal of Research and Practice, 20*(5), 628–634. https://doi.org/10.1177/1362361315617879

Sedgewick, F., Hill, V., & Pellicano, E. (2019). "It's different for girls": Gender differences in the friendships and conflict of autistic and neurotypical adolescents. *Autism: The International Journal of Research and Practice, 23*(5), 1119–1132. https://doi.org/10.1177/1362361318794930

Shattuck, P. T., Durkin, M., & Maenner, M. (2009). Timing of identification among children with an autism spectrum disorder: findings from a population-based surveillance study. *Journal of the American Academy of Child and Adolescent Psychiatry, 48*(5), 474–483. https://doi.org/10.1097/CHI.0b013e31819b3848

Shaw, K. A., Maenner, M. J., Bakian, A. V., Bilder, D. A., Durkin, M. S., Furnier, S. M., Hughes, M. M., Patrick, M., Pierce, K., Salinas, A., Shenouda, J., Vehorn, A., Warren, Z., Zahorodny,

W., Constantino, J., DiRienzo, M., Esler, A., Fitzgerald, R. T., Grzybowski, M. S., … Cogswell, M. E. (2021). Early identification of autism spectrum disorder among children aged 4 years—Autism and Developmental Disabilities Monitoring Network, 11 Sites, United States, 2018. *MMWR Surveillance Summaries, 70*(10), 1–14. https://doi.org/10.15585/mmwr.ss7010a1

Shaw, K. A., Bilder, D. A., McArthur, D., Williams, A. R., Amoakohene, E., Bakian, A. V., Durkin, M. S., Fitzgerald, R. T., Furnier, S. M., Hughes, M. M., Pas, E. T., Salinas, A., Warren, Z., Williams, S., Esler, A., Grzybowski, A., Ladd-Acosta, C. M., Patrick, M., Zahorodny, W., … Maenner, M. J. (2023). Early identification of autism spectrum disorder among children aged 4 years—Autism and Developmental Disabilities Monitoring Network, 11 sites, United States, 2020. *MMWR Surveillance Summaries, 72*(1), 1–15. https://doi.org/10.15585/mmwr.ss7201a1

Spack, N. P., Edwards-Leeper, L., Feldman, H. A., Leibowitz, S., Mandel, F., Diamond, D. A., & Vance, S. R. (2012). Children and adolescents with gender identity disorder referred to a pediatric medical center. *Pediatrics, 129*(3), 418–425. https://doi.org/10.1542/peds.2011-0907

Strang, J. F., Kenworthy, L., Dominska, A., Sokoloff, J., Kenealy, L. E., Berl, M., Walsh, K., Menvielle, E., Slesaransky-Poe, G., Kim, K. E., Luong-Tran, C., Meagher, H., & Wallace, G. L. (2014). Increased gender variance in autism spectrum disorders and attention deficit hyperactivity disorder. *Archives of Sexual Behavior, 43*(8), 1525–1533. https://doi.org/10.1007/s10508-014-0285-3

Strang, J. F., Meagher, H., Kenworthy, L., de Vries, A. L. C., Menvielle, E., Leibowitz, S., Janssen, A., Cohen-Kettenis, P., Shumer, D. E., Edwards-Leeper, L., Pleak, R. R., Spack, N., Karasic, D. H., Schreier, H., Balleur, A., Tishelman, A., Ehrensaft, D., Rodnan, L., Kuschner, E. S., … Anthony, L. G. (2016). Initial clinical guidelines for co-occurring autism spectrum disorder and gender dysphoria or incongruence in adolescents. *Journal of Clinical Child and Adolescent Psychology, 47*, 1–11. https://doi.org/10.1080/15374416.2016.1228462

Strang, J.F., Meagher, H., Kenworthy, L., . de Vries, A.L.C., Menvielle, E., Leibowitz, S., Janssen, A., Cohen-Kettenis, P., Shumer, D.E., Edwards-Leeper, L., Pleak, R.R., Spack, N., Karasic, D.H., Schreier, H., Balleur, A., Tishelman, A., Ehrensaft, D., Rodnan, L., Kuschner, E.S., … Anthony, L.G. (2018) Initial clinical guidelines for co-occurring autism spectrum disorder and gender dysphoria or incongruence in adolescents, *Journal of Clinical Child & Adolescent Psychology, 47*:1, 105-115, https://doi.org/10.1080/15374416.2016.1228462.

Strang, J. F., Klomp, S. E., Caplan, R., Griffin, A. D., Anthony, L. G., Harris, M. C., Graham, E. K., Knauss, M., & van der Miesen, A. I. R. (2019). Community-based participatory design for research that impacts the lives of transgender and/or gender-diverse autistic and/or neuro-diverse people. *Clinical Practice in Pediatric Psychology, 7*(4), 396. https://doi.org/10.1037/cpp0000310

Strang, J. F., Anthony, L. G., Song, A., Lai, M.-C., Knauss, M., Sadikova, E., Graham, E., Zaks, Z., Wimms, H., Willing, L., Call, D., Mancilla, M., Shakin, S., Vilain, E., Kim, D.-Y., Maisashvili, T., Khawaja, A., & Kenworthy, L. (2021). In addition to stigma: Cognitive and autism-related predictors of mental health in transgender adolescents. *Journal of Clinical Child & Adolescent Psychology*, 1–18. Published online. https://doi.org/10.1080/15374416.2021.1916940

Tang, J. W., Li, J. W., Baulderstone, D., & Jeyaseelan, D. (2021). Presenting age and features of females diagnosed with autism spectrum disorder. *Journal of Paediatrics & Child Health, 57*(8), 1182–1189. https://doi.org/10.1111/jpc.15417

Trittschuh, E. H., Parmenter, B. A., Clausell, E. R., Mariano, M. J., & Reger, M. A. (2018). Conducting neuropsychological assessment with transgender individuals. *The Clinical Neuropsychologist, 32*(8), 1393–1410. https://doi.org/10.1080/13854046.2018.1440632

Tsai, L., Stewart, M. A., & August, G. (1981). Implication of sex differences in the familial transmission of infantile autism. *Journal of Autism and Developmental Disorders, 11*, 165–173. https://doi.org/10.1007/BF01531682

Volkmar, F. R., Woodbury-Smith, M., Macari, S. L., & Øien, R. A. (2021). Seeing the forest and the trees: Disentangling autism phenotypes in the age of DSM-5. *Development and Psychopathology, 33*(2), 625–633. https://doi.org/10.1017/S0954579420002047

Walsh, R. J., Krabbendam, L., Dewinter, J., & Begeer, S. (2018). Brief report: Gender identity differences in autistic adults: Associations with perceptual and socio-cognitive profiles. *Journal of Autism and Developmental Disorders, 48*(12), 4070–4078. https://doi.org/10.1007/s10803-018-3702-y

Warrier, V., Greenberg, D. M., Wier, E., Buckingham, C., Smith, P., Lai, M.-C., Allison, C., & Baron-Cohen, S. (2020). Elevated rates of autism, other neurodevelopmental and psychiatric diagnoses, and autistic traits in transgender and gender-diverse individuals. *Nature Communications, 11*(1), 3959–3970. https://doi.org/10.1038/s41467-020-17794-1

whaletuuune. (2021, February 10). *Feeling subwoman because Of ASD?* [Online forum post] Wrong planet. https://wrongplanet.net/forums/viewtopic.php?t=394667

Wigdor, E., Weiner, D., Grove, J., Fu, J., Thompson, W., Carey, C., Baya, N., van der Merwe, C., Mortensen, P. B., Daly, M., Talkowski, M., Sanders, S., Bishop, S., Børglum, A., & Robinson, E. (2021). The female protective effect against autism spectrum disorder. *European Neuropsychopharmacology, 51*, e13–e14. https://doi.org/10.1016/j.euroneuro.2021.07.035

Willey, L. H. (2012). *Safety skills for Asperger women: How to save a perfectly good female life.* Jessica Kingsley Publishers.

Willey, L. H. (2014). *Pretending to be normal: Living with asperger's syndrome (Autism spectrum disorder) expanded edition.* Jessica Kingsley.

Wing, L. (1981). Sex ratios in early childhood autism and related conditions. *Psychiatry Research, 5*(2), 129–137. https://doi.org/10.1016/0165-1781(81)90043-3

Zeidan, J., Fombonne, E., Scorah, J., Ibrahim, A., Durkin, M. S., Saxena, S., Yusuf, A., Shih, A., & Elsabbagh, M. (2022). Global prevalence of autism: A systematic review update. *Autism Research: Official Journal of the International Society for Autism Research, 15*(5), 778–790. https://doi.org/10.1002/aur.2696

Chapter 2
Early Identification of Females with Autism: Comprehensive Evaluation

Early identification of autism is a universal goal, but complicated by the involvement of multiple systems, with family systems being primary, and both education and health care systems needing to coordinate efforts as gatekeepers. When all agree, the process can be fairly straightforward. In the case of nuanced autism in females, there may be widely differing and changing opinions, making the road to identification complicated, frustrating and often delayed.

> *For the parents of these children there is often not anything 'wrong' with their child that they can define or that requires medical assistance, but more a nagging sense of something being different that they can't quite put their finger on.* Hendrickx (2015, p. 49)

Early Identification Processes

Recent improvements in early identification rates (see Chap. 1) generally have not necessarily impacted the average age of comprehensive evaluation for females as of this writing. The Centers for Disease Control and Prevention (CDC) *Learn the Signs, Act Early* guidance on developmental milestones recently changed. Milestones listed are now those that are achieved by 75% of children at that particular age to reduce the chances of "wait and see" approaches when differences are noticed (CDC, 2022), but there are no mentions of gender differences. Overall efforts for early identification and more emphasis on *comprehensive* evaluation may result in the earlier identification of the more nuanced autism traits. Comprehensive evaluation is the key concept of each of the following chapters, beginning here with early childhood. The diagnostic characterization of autism clarifies that "Diagnoses are most valid and reliable when based on multiple sources of information, including clinician's observations, caregiver history, and, when possible, self-report" (American Psychiatric Association [APA], 2022, p. 60). Several years prior, the Board of Directors of the American Academy of Clinical Neuropsychology reinforced the multidimensional

T. P. Gabrielsen et al., *Assessment of Autism in Females and Nuanced Presentations*, https://doi.org/10.1007/978-3-031-33969-1_2

aspect of diagnosing nuanced autism, citing expertise needed in "intellectual and language functioning; comorbid neurodevelopmental, psychiatric and medical conditions and other aspects of functioning (e.g., eating, sleeping, maladaptive behaviors, motor skills, and psychosocial challenges); and diagnostic assessment processes that include interviews with collateral informants around complex medical conditions (Board of Directors, 2007)" (as cited in Duvall et al., 2021, p. 1173). According to recent scientific reviews and large dataset studies, measurable autistic traits change over time (Bourson & Prevost, 2022; Stroth et al., 2022), so we will be looking at the assessment of autism using a lifespan approach throughout this text.

Case Study—Ellie: Early Issues with Sleep, Feeding, Sensory Behaviors, and Attachment to an Object

Ellie is a 30-month-old sibling of a child with an existing autism diagnosis. Her parents have not seen the same type of language delay her older brother exhibited. She is, however, much pickier about eating, parents are seldom successful introducing new foods, and she has an extremely limited diet, which has been a concern for her pediatrician. She has difficulty going to sleep at night, requiring 1–2 hours with a parent in her room before she falls asleep. She often ends up in parents' bed before morning as well. She was observed to be carrying a plastic spoon with her on the day of the evaluation, and a recent photo portrait taken of her also included a plastic spoon in her hand. She is very sensitive to changes in light and sound and, to some extent, strangers. The evaluation took place in her home rather than the clinic because she was not able to calm down in the clinic (i.e., clinging to parent, screaming when clinicians were in the room). She was very cooperative in the home setting and was observed to be friendly and playing with blocks, singing throughout the evaluation, and toe-walking.

Autism Screener Performance for Females

One of the questions that can affect what we know about autism in the first few years of life for females is related to the performance of autism screeners in female toddlers and very young children. Later chapters will examine this for older children, but in the target years for early identification (before age 3), little is known about how well screeners perform by gender. Andersson et al. (2013) concluded that although no gender differences were found in screening children younger than 4 years old, either (1) prior studies showing differences had overestimated differences, or (2) there are young autistic girls who are not identified by current screening instruments.

Øien et al. (2018) examined screening records at age 18 months in Norway and found the false-negative result group to include differences in social communication and fine motor development compared to neurotypical peers. These differences were more pronounced in female toddlers than in males, but were not picked up on the screeners as positive for autism risk (in this case, the M-CHAT or Modified Checklist for Autism in Toddlers; Robins et al., 2001). In a large US community-based study by Carbone et al. (2020) and Guthrie et al. (2019), lower positive predictive values were found for female children using the M-CHAT and M-CHAT-R/F (Modified Checklist for Autism in Toddlers, Revised with Follow-Up; Robins et al., 2009, 2014).

Diagnostic Measure Performance for Females

My youngest has autism and although we had her evaluated a number of times… they would say 'Well, she is too affectionate to have autism' even though she had so many of the characteristics. We did not get her diagnosis until she was six. I really wish that there was a scale that was more tailored to females for diagnosing autism. (Mother of a 7-year-old girl with autism, diagnosed at age 6). (Nichols, 2009, p. 21)

Gender issues in diagnosis have been explored using common diagnostic measures with mixed results. A study of the Autism Diagnostic Interview-Revised (ADI-R; LeCouteur et al., 2003) found slight gender bias that may account for some underdiagnosis of girls (Beggiato et al., 2017). A study of the other most common diagnostic measure, the Autism Diagnostic Observation Schedule, Generic and 2nd Ed. (ADOS-G; Lord et al., 2000, and ADOS-2; Lord et al., 2012a, b), found no gender differences, but warned that on parent report measures, parental gender expectations may affect ratings (Kaat et al., 2021). Expert clinicians reported differences in core (70%) and associated (54%) autistic traits, but differences were most apparent in school age and adolescence, indicating fewer differences in very young children across genders (Jamison et al., 2017).

Barriers to Early Identification for Females

The first step is for professionals to understand that the profile shows itself differently in females than in males. You have to work a bit harder to find it, but it's there. And just because it's not too visible, doesn't mean it's not 'severe'. Increased access to diagnosis is the first step to enable women to get the validation and access to services that they need. (Hendrickx, 2015, p. 235)

Little is actually known in the scientific literature about barriers to earlier identification for females, particularly in the first years of life, when some suggest differences in autistic traits between genders may not yet have become apparent (Bourson & Prevost, 2022; Jamison et al., 2017; Stroth et al., 2022). The heterogeneity of autism in general is widely held as one barrier to identification in all genders, but as the above quotes illustrate, the variance in presentation among females and others with nuanced autism present more barriers than perhaps has been expected. Many hypotheses have been discussed, from a possible genetic female factor (also referred to as a "protective" factor in earlier research) (Jacquemont et al., 2014; Lawrence et al., 2022; Robinson et al., 2013; Wigdor et al., 2021) to the extreme male theory of autism (Baron-Cohen, 2002). One documented reason for delay in diagnosis is the presence of co-occurring attention deficit disorders.

"[The diagnosis] has helped us understand and empathize with her better. And it has shut up other members of the family who were convinced she was just 'difficult'!" (Hendrickx, 2015, p. 45)

Kentrou et al. (2019) found very young females with attention disorders or difficulties to be diagnosed with autism just over a year later than boys with attention difficulties (on average). Ros-Demarize et al. (2020) have also called for greater attention to social communication differences particular to females that may not be adequately captured in current screening measures, leading to delays in evaluation and diagnosis. More typical and less noticeable special interests and stimming behaviors have consistently been reported (Kaat et al., 2021; Lord et al., 2022). Another barrier is a confound with IQ—specifically that most historical autism research samples have included females with lower IQ levels and that in samples with higher IQ scores, the male-to-female ratio is even more disparate than the overall ratio. Children presenting with age-normative language, memory, cognitive, and social communication skills may also be missed for autism diagnosis (Halladay et al., 2015), despite the presence of other autistic traits. It is entirely possible that the most significant barrier to the early identification of autistic females and nuanced autism is that they are not likely to be screened or brought to the attention of professionals or specialists who might be able to identify autism in the early years.

Importance of Interviewing

As specialty centers have struggled to find ways to reduce their wait lists, it is tempting to shorten the amount of time in direct contact with families throughout the diagnostic process. Carefully consider interviewing as an important part of the process, however. Kim and Lord (2012b) also stressed the importance of interviewing.

> Because social difficulties are a common presenting concern across a myriad of diagnoses, a thorough diagnostic interview by a well-seasoned clinician will frequently unearth a number of pink flags, even if they are not part of the original reasons for referral, and sometimes even when the individual or informants downplay their relevance. The clinician's role is not only to recognize these features, but to systematically determine their true source or etiology to rule out or rule in a diagnosis of ASD. Both tasks can be complicated by a number of factors including comorbidities, similar presentations across multiple diagnoses (with differing etiologies), diagnostic overshadowing, and specific characteristics in the patient and/or system. Having a solid understanding of each of these features can help to ensure that the diagnostic conceptualization best captures the individual's symptom presentation, profile, and etiology. (Duvall et al., 2021, p. 1177)

Female-Sensitive Approaches to Early Identification

> A careful analysis of when a patient's social difficulties emerged and their intact skills relating to social reciprocity can therefore help to clarify the source of their current impairments. The *absence* of other pink and red flags in a patient's developmental history can also help with differential diagnosis. (Duvall et al., 2021, p. 1182)

Given the gaps in the literature, gender bias in samples, and various theories to explain why females are diagnosed less often and also probably later in life, how are we to proceed to obtain earlier diagnoses for females in particular and, along with them, children whose autistic traits are more nuanced than the unambiguous presentations of autism that are easier for community providers to diagnose? The answer to this question is twofold. Ultimately, it will likely take more clinical time to screen and evaluate autistic traits in females. In addition, more measures will probably need to be incorporated, as multiple sources of data are more likely to reveal patterns in traits (e.g., social communication, executive function, feeding, sensory, language differences rather than delays, uneven cognitive profile, mismatched adaptive skills) that have been observed in both scientific literature and first-person accounts of early childhood. Neither of these strategies are likely to be effective, however, if awareness of what nuanced autism looks like at all ages and in all genders is not achieved (Duvall et al., 2021; Hull et al., 2017). To begin to accomplish this paradigm shift, the voices of autistic individuals and their families are instructive. First-person accounts from women and girls with autism are helpful for families and clinicians working with autistic girls and women, primarily because they provide models of female autistic self-identity (Grandin & Scariano, 1996).

Context and Examples from First-Person Narratives

Eye contact was mentioned by parents of girls with autism as being noticeably different in infancy in their daughters...eye contact differences in individuals with autism can range from little or no eye contact through to staring. (Hendrickx, 2015, p. 53)

As a young toddler I would sometimes seek out physically stimulating activities or rough play with certain adults, such as rubbing up against them, rocking in their lap, seeking to have my back or my arms scratched or tickled, roughly playing with their hair or their hands, etc. (Hendrickx, 2015, p. 76)

I would definitely have liked to have been diagnosed earlier. I spent the first 13 years of my life thinking I was nothing but a freak (that mindset still sticks with me today), simply because I know that's how the world viewed me. Woman with autism (Hendrickx, 2015, p. 123)

Their anger did not make me love the texture any less, but it did teach me, early on, that what I perceive and love and what other people perceive and love, are two different and incompatible things. I learned to be a quiet, private child. Daina Krumins (Miller, 2015, p. 99)

When, from early childhood, you live out of sync with social norms and expectations, it's easy to feel as if you are alien, wrong, and bad. In such a situation, one would have to be catatonic not to be at least a little depressed. Jane Strauss (Ballou et al., 2021, p. 14)

Comprehensive Evaluations for Autism

In some cases, it may be appropriate to place less emphasis on ADOS-2 scores and cutoffs, and instead use the rich observations and clinical information obtained from the ADOS-2 to map onto the DSM-5 or ICD-11 diagnostic criteria in concert with information gathered from collateral sources and early history. (Duvall et al., 2021)

The Centers for Disease Control and Prevention's (CDC) Autism and Developmental Disabilities Monitoring studies (ADDM: Maenner et al., 2023) use the age of "comprehensive evaluation" as the time marker for when autism is identified in children. There is some movement in clinical specialty centers to *reduce* the number of measures used to establish a diagnosis of autism, primarily to reduce unnecessary wait time for children who need immediate intervention (de Marchena & Miller, 2017; Penner et al., 2018). For unambiguous presentations of autism, this may be very helpful in the short term. In the case of females and nuanced autism however, taking more time to examine possible patterns in data collected through evaluation may be crucial in arriving at an accurate diagnosis (Kanne & Bishop, 2020; Wieckowski et al., 2021). Immediate intervention is much less likely to be the most pressing goal in these situations. As we talk more about this goal, some definitions are useful.

Definitions and Descriptions

Early "Early" has multiple origins with similar meanings, but generally means by about age 3. The "Early Intervention" system in the United States (Part C of IDEA legislation [Individuals with Disabilities Education Act, 2004]) is responsible for finding children under the age of 3 years and providing necessary intervention to address any developmental delays. Age 3 is also the target age for comprehensive evaluation described in the CDC ADDM studies (Maenner et al., 2023). Age 3 is also a typical age for children to be exposed to systems outside of their family systems (e.g., preschool) for the first time without their parents, most likely the first of the transitions referred to in the current *Diagnostic and Statistical Manual of Mental Disorder*'s diagnostic criteria for autism spectrum disorder (DSM-5-TR; American Psychiatric Association [APA], 2022).

Identification This may be an educational classification or a medical/clinical diagnosis, obtained for the purpose of appropriate intervention to promote development.

Screening Measures

Because of the time invested by clinicians, parents, and individuals in a comprehensive evaluation, in most settings, the process begins with screening instruments to determine if an autism evaluation is appropriate for the referral question. Each of the following has a specific age range. Examples of screening instruments and considerations include:

- Infant Toddler Checklist (ITC; Wetherby & Prizant, 2002)
- Modified Checklist for Autism in Toddlers, Revised with Follow-Up (M-CHAT-R/F; Robins et al., 2009, 2014)
- Parent's Observation of Social Interactions (POSI; Perrin et al., 2010)
- Toddler Autism Symptom Interview (TASI; Coulter et al., 2021)

- Social Communication Questionnaire: 4+ years, with lower cutoffs for children 2–3 years (SCQ; Rutter et al., 2003; Corsello et al. 2013)
- Social Responsiveness Scales, 2nd Ed. Pre-school (SRS-2; Constantino & Gruber, 2012)

When screens are used with females, there is mixed evidence of their ability to identify female or nuanced autism as well as they can for males, likely due to sampling bias (Kaat et al., 2021). In the absence of female norms, consider a result near the clinical cutoff as being perhaps positive to adjust for unknown bias in cutoff scores (Koenig & Tsatsanis, 2005).

Comprehensive or Developmental Evaluation The CDC's ADDM studies describe a "comprehensive" or "developmental" evaluation as one incorporating more than screening measures and one conducted by a "qualified professional." No further description is available. In this text, we consider a comprehensive evaluation to measure multiple developmental domains, which may vary somewhat by referral questions and availability of qualified professionals. We describe possible components of a comprehensive evaluation below. Please note that measures for each of these domains may not necessarily be needed, but gathering data or evidence in each domain by some means is important at every age.

Cognitive or Developmental In children younger than 6 years, cognitive assessment results are generally considered to be not as predictive of later abilities as assessments conducted for ages 6 and older. Measures of cognitive abilities in younger children can also be called developmental measures.

Examples of measures according to setting and available trained personnel include:

- Ages and Stages Questionnaire, 3rd Ed. (ASQ-3; Squires & Bricker, 2009).
- Bayley Scales of Infant and Toddler Development, 4th Ed. (Bayley-4; Bayley & Aylward, 2019).
- Developmental Assessment of Young Children, 2nd Ed. (DAY-C-2; Voress et al., 2012).
- Developmental Indicators for the Assessment of Learning, 4th Ed. (DIAL-4; Mardell & Goldenberg, 2011).
- Differential Ability Scales, 2nd Ed. (DAS-II; Elliott, 2007).
- Kaufman Assessment Battery for Children, 2nd Ed., Normative Update (KABC-2-NU; Kaufman & Kaufman, 2018).
- Mullen Scales of Early Learning (MSEL; Mullen, 1995).
- Stanford-Binet Scales of Intelligence, 5th Ed. (SB-V; Roid, 2003).
- Woodcock-Johnson-IV Tests of Cognitive Abilities (WJ-IV Cog; Schrank et al., 2014a).
- Wechsler Preschool and Primary Scales of Intelligence-IV (WPPSI-IV; Wechsler, 2012).

In the case of nuanced autism like that found in many autistic females, cognitive results are likely to be within the average range or higher, yet there may be variability among or within subtests. Processing speed and working memory are indexes most frequently cited as lower than other scores, with subtle difficulties in language also mentioned (Wechsler, 2012). Interpretation of subtest differences is not typically reliable or helpful, but in this case, the presence of variability, particularly significant variability within cognitive profiles, is one of the autism criteria indicated on the Childhood Autism Rating Scales, 2nd Ed., High Functioning (CARS-2-HF: Schopler et al., 2010):

> Regarding the specifier "with or without accompanying intellectual impairment," understanding the (often uneven) intellectual profile of a child or adult with autism spectrum disorder is necessary for interpreting diagnostic features. Separate estimates of verbal and nonverbal skill are necessary (e.g., using untimed nonverbal tests to assess potential strengths in individuals with limited language). DSM-5-TR (APA, 2022)

Adaptive At all ages, adaptive skills measures describe the level of independence reached in everyday living, compared to same-age peers. Usually measured by parent or caregiver report, communication, socialization, daily living skills, and motor skills may be evaluated. Although cognitive abilities are likely to be measured in the average range (including verbal abilities), there are often striking differences between cognitive and adaptive abilities, also captured in the rating scales of the CARS-2-HF (Schopler et al., 2010). Adaptive questionnaires are helpful, but if time allows, an interview format can provide more information about what the child is like in a familiar and comfortable environment, particularly for children who are already incorporating imitation, masking, or camouflaging behaviors for social acceptance. Comparison of Teacher and Parent versions of adaptive measures may show different levels of independence in different settings. Examples of adaptive measures include:

- Vineland Adaptive Behavior Scales, 3rd Ed. (Interview available) (Vineland-3; Sparrow et al., 2016).
- Adaptive Behavior Assessment System, 3rd Ed. (ABAS-3; Harrison & Oakland, 2015a, b).
- Although less detailed, adaptive abilities are part of the following developmental instruments as well:
  - Adaptive Behavior Scales, Bayley Scales of Infant and Toddler Development, 4th Ed. (Bayley-4; Bayley & Aylward (2019).
  - Adaptive Items—Developmental Indicators for the Assessment of Learning, 4th Ed. (DIAL-4; Mardell & Goldenberg, 2011).
  - Conners Early Childhood (Conners-EC; Conners, 2009).
  - Developmental Assessment of Young Children, 2nd Ed. (DAYC-2; Voress et al., 2012).
- Social-emotional broad-band screeners also have subscales related to adaptive abilities that may or may not capture differences when autism is more nuanced.
  - Adaptive Behavior Items, Ages and Stages Questionnaire: Social-Emotional 2nd Ed. (ASQ:SE2; Squires et al., 2015).
  - Adaptive Behavior Scale, Behavior Assessment System for Children, 3rd Ed. (BASC-3; Reynolds & Kamphaus, 2015).

Adaptive skill assessment can provide starting points for intervention, but in the case of female or nuanced autism, it can also illustrate that a child with well-developed cognitive abilities in some areas may still be developmentally different from same-age peers in terms of gaining independence in adaptive skills. Neglecting to assess adaptive skills may be one reason children with higher cognitive and language skills are missed. Adaptive measures also assess the ability to follow directions as part of communication skills, which is important for autism identification, but not apparent in cognitive measures alone. Follow-up with speech and language assessment may be indicated if receptive and/or expressive communication skills are rated lower than expected.

Social/Emotional Generally measured by parent, caregiver, and/or teacher report, questionnaires may also be completed by older individuals themselves. Domains measured vary, but often include attention, aggression, anxiety, depression, attention, social skills, atypicality, functional communication, etc. Examples of social/emotional assessment for this young age range can include:

- Ages and Stages Questionnaire: Social-Emotional 2nd Ed. (ASQ:SE2; Squires et al., 2015)
- Conners Early Childhood (Conners EC; Conners, 2009) *(G = gendered norms available)*
- Behavior Assessment System for Children, third Ed. (BASC-3; Reynolds & Kamphaus, 2015) *(G)*
- Preschool Pediatric Symptom Checklist (PPSC) of the Survey of Well-Being in Young Children (SWYC; Perrin et al., 2010).
- Social Responsiveness Scales, 2nd Ed. Preschool Version (SRS-2; Constantino & Gruber, 2012)
- Infant Toddler Social Emotional Assessment (ITSEA; Briggs-Gowan & Carter, 1998) *(G)*
- Brief Infant Toddler Social Emotional Assessment (BITSEA; Briggs-Gowan et al., 2004)
- Child Behavior Checklist (CBCL; Achenbach & Rescorla, 2001) *(G)* *(not to be used as a screener for autism;* Havdahl et al., 2016).

As social reciprocity and communication are central to autism diagnostic criteria, gathering data regarding perceptions of social abilities may reveal slight differences, particularly if both parents and teachers are asked to complete questionnaires. Social withdrawal, social motivation, and emotional lability may be captured in these measures to establish differences between autistic females and female peers, as some of these questionnaires also provide gendered norms for scoring. The DSM-5-TR warns that social communication differences may be difficult to notice; Criterion A deficits in social communication may be more subtle when an individual has better overall communication skills in some ways and does not have intellectual impairments (APA, 2022).

Executive Function Even very small children have developmental milestones related to executive function. In addition to skills related to goal-directed behaviors, the ability to be flexible (as opposed to rigid) in the face of dynamic changes in the environment is an important part of executive functioning. Inhibitory control and working memory are also evident in early years. Most commonly measured by questionnaires, direct observational measures may also become part of the assessment for older children adolescents and adults. Examples of executive function assessment include:

- Behavior Rating Inventory of Executive Function, Preschool (BRIEF-P; Gioia et al., 2003) *(G)*
- Comprehensive Executive Function Inventory (CEFI; Naglieri & Goldstein, 2013)
- NEPSY-II (Korkman et al., 2007) *Executive Function Scale.*
- Leiter International Performance Scale, 3rd Ed. (Leiter-3; Roid et al., 2013) *Nonverbal Stroop Tests*

There have been mixed findings in executive function research (please see Chap. 7 for a more detailed discussion), which may reflect the differences between standardized, directly administered measures, which do not necessarily match results from questionnaires and interviews. One advantage of questionnaire measures is that gendered norms exist for most.

Academic or Achievement Beginning with pre-literacy skills, academic skills related to written language and number systems are typically measured directly either by standardized measures, by curriculum-based measures for school-aged children, or by parent observation. In very young children, this may be difficult to assess, but in 3–6-year-olds, some measurement of skills is possible, by standardized measures and/or curriculum-based measures and data from multi-tiered systems of support in kindergarten. Examples of academic or achievement measures include:

- Woodcock-Johnson-IV Tests of Achievement (WJ-IV Ach; Schrank et al., 2014b)
- Differential Ability Scales, 2nd Ed. (DAS-II; Elliott, 2007) *School Readiness Subtests*
- Kaufman Test of Educational Achievement, 3rd Ed. (KTEA-2; Kaufman & Kaufman, 2014) *4–6-year-old battery*
- Informal assessment (see Lonigan et al. 2011)
- Language assessment (see Chap. 3)

It is possible that even very young children (with nuanced autism or autistic females) may be reading at young ages and have intense interests in reading (Gould & Ashton-Smith, 2011). Comprehension may not necessarily match the reading level, however (Åsberg et al., 2010). See Chap. 7 for more about reading.

Broad and Narrow Screeners Parent and caregiver questionnaires may assess broadly (such as social-emotional above) or narrowly (e.g., feeding, sleep, anxiety, depression, theory of mind). Broad screeners may provide a signal to prompt more refined measurement of narrow skills in these areas, typically by questionnaire. At this young age, most screening instruments are broad. Narrow-band screeners are almost exclusively autism measures at this age; see Autism Specific Measures for Very Young Children.

Sensory Although direct assessment is possible, parent or caregiver report (and for older individuals with appropriate reading levels, self-report) of sensory sensitivities can be gathered by interview and/or sensory questionnaires which measure the pervasiveness and severity of either avoidance or seeking behaviors related to taste, touch, smell, sound, or sight of any sensory input. See Chap. 4 for more details.

Sensory Profile, 2nd Ed. (SP-2; Dunn, 2014) *Infant, Toddler, and Child Versions.*

Special or Intense Interests and Stimming Behaviors (Aka Restricted and Repetitive Behaviors and Interests) One of the more noticeable features of autism (typically) is a strong tendency toward intense interests that involve a great deal of an individual's time and energy and, for those with verbal language, conversation. Also referred to as restricted and repetitive behaviors and interests (RRBIs), it is now more acceptable to many self-advocates to refer to these as special or intense interests, passions, etc. to describe a range of interests they feel strongly about. In the DSM-5-TR, autism Criterion B criteria (differences in intensity of interests and behaviors) may be less obvious if the interests are closer to age-typical norms (APA, 2022). See Chap. 5 for a more detailed discussion of how RRBIs are different and noticed less often in females and those with nuanced autism.

Language Even for individuals with no verbal language, communication using symbolic systems (e.g., sign language, gestures, or unique vocalizations) may be assessed by speech and language pathologists. Although predominantly assessed by direct observation, parent or caregiver questionnaires may also be used to capture communication strategies used in familiar environments. For narrow-band measures related to language, please see Chap. 3. "Since receptive language may lag behind expressive language development in autism spectrum disorder, receptive and expressive language skills should be considered separately" (APA, 2022).

Developmental History The DSM-5-TR diagnostic criteria for autism require that traits have their origins in early childhood, but acknowledge that differences may not be as apparent until social demands exceed capacities and/or differences may be masked by strategies learned over time (APA, 2022). Obtaining information about early childhood can be easy to overlook, but may be critical to case conceptualization. Note that *deficits or delays* may not be reported, but *traits* are the focus of obtaining a developmental history. Examples of specific developmental history measures include the following:

- Structured Developmental History (BASC-3; Reynolds & Kamphaus, 2015).
- Autism Diagnostic Interview-Revised (ADI-R; LeCouteur et al., 2003).
- Parent interview regarding early development—refer to CDC developmental milestones by nearest age (CDC, 2022).
- Ages and Stages Questionnaire, 3rd Ed. (ASQ-3; Squires, & Bricker, 2009) *for very young children.*

Within this young age range, development (including autism) is still unfolding. The focus of the assessment of early development is to ask about anything parents may have noticed regarding developmental milestones, social development, play interests, language, etc. in broad terms. For females and others with nuanced autism, it is possible that parents have adapted their lifestyles to avoid meltdowns due to sensory sensitivities or executive function difficulties related to challenges transitioning or rigidity. Listen in interviews for hints that this may have happened to enable you to get more details. Examples of such hints might be the following: "So, we just don't go [someplace like restaurant, stadium, mall, etc.] anymore," "We have to be careful to …," and "She doesn't like [x], so we [eliminated it]." *Specifically ask about sleep and feeding issues.* Listen for evidence of long bedtime routines, sleeping in parent's bed, limited variety of foods accepted, etc. See Chap. 4 for specific assessment planning related to sleep and feeding.

Autism Specific Measures for Very Young Children Screening instruments and observational measures with outcomes that indicate autism or not autism, level of evidence for autism, cutoffs, etc. are obviously helpful and needed, but a more indepth interpretation for females and nuanced autism questions is needed. These measures can include parent or caregiver report, teacher report, self-report, and direct observation. A variety of measures are listed, with varying levels of training required.

- Autism Diagnostic Observation Schedule, 2nd Ed. (ADOS-2; Lord et al., 2012a, b).
- Autism Diagnostic Interview-Revised (ADI-R; LeCouteur et al., 2003) *with published algorithms for children younger than 4* (see Kim & Lord, 2012a; Kim et al. 2013).
- Childhood Autism Rating Scales, 2nd Ed., Standard Version (CARS-2-ST; Schopler et al., 2010).
- Screening Tool for Autism in Toddlers and Young Children (STAT; Stone et al., 2000, 2004).
- Rapid Interactive Screening Test for Autism in Toddlers (RITA-T; Choueiri & Wagner, 2015).
- TELE-ASD-PEDS (Corona et al., 2020; Wagner et al., 2021).
- Naturalistic Observation Diagnostic Assessment (NODA; Smith et al., 2017).
- Brief Observation of Symptoms of Autism (BOSA; Dow et al., 2021; Lord et al., 2020).

None of these measures have gendered norms, and some have been found to under-identify females in certain domains at certain ages (Wang et al., 2017). They have been found to be adequate and helpful (Kaat et al., 2021), but clinician expertise is important for correct interpretation of results (Jamison et al., 2017). The importance of consideration of more than one autism-specific measure was illustrated by Mussey et al. (2017) as they found slightly higher scores on the CARS than the ADOS in females and also by Greene et al., who found a relatively high rate of false positives on the ADOS alone. Females in this sample (which was predominantly white, male, and slightly low average cognitive abilities) were *less* likely to be false positives (Greene et al., 2022). Specific items on the ADI-R which have been identified as showing significant differences across genders are the variety of facial expressions used to communicate, pretend play, special interests, and unusual preoccupations (Beggiato et al., 2017).

A more extensive list of measures that can be used (and domains to be assessed) can be found in the *Lancet Commission on the Future of Care and Clinical Research in Autism* (Lord et al., 2022). Measures listed here are available for general use. Measures listed in the Lancet article also include some that are available for research only.

Key Concepts for Early Identification (Ages 6 and Younger)

Existing assessment and screening tools are not well-normed for females in particular and may not be as sensitive to nuanced autism traits. However, the research on young children shows fewer differences in terms of measurable traits between genders than at older ages, making early childhood one of the best opportunities for observing autistic traits—if children have opportunities for screening and evaluation. Comprehensive evaluation for these referrals (and referring even if screening measure scores are just below cutoff) is key to early and accurate identification. Instead of expecting clearly significant results in one or two measures, look for consistent patterns of variable or different development across multiple domains. Extra time taken to gather more evidence (including parent and teacher/other caregiver interviews, if available) will present a clearer diagnostic picture. As mentioned in the DSM-5-TR autism spectrum disorder criteria:

> The range of developmental deficits or differences varies from very specific limitations of learning or control of executive functions to global impairments of social skills or intellectual ability. Once thought to be categorically defined, more recent dimensional approaches to measurement of the symptoms demonstrate a range of severity, often without a very clear boundary with typical development. (APA, 2022)

Supports and Recommendations – Including First Person Narratives

> *What some people find frustrating, however, is that frequently specialist knowledge stops at the point of diagnosis (Eaton, 2012), leaving individuals and families without significant follow-up support or expertise from then onwards. (Hendrickx, 2015, p. 46)*

> *Formalized processes can begin and appropriate support plans can be implemented. The diagnosis is the key to progress for the individual and their family, and the benefits extend beyond the 'medical' explanation....Psychologically, the family or individual now know what they are facing, so they can move on and deal with it. (Hendrickx, 2015, p. 43)*

> *One of the best things about tapping into the resources that Autistic adults provide is that, unlike the experts, they don't insist that there is one way to learn and progress. They don't insist that rigid inflexible regimens be followed until a child is broken. Instead they seem to,*

almost universally, support the value of respecting individual needs. Beth Ryan (Ballou et al., 2021. p. 195)

Let's revisit the case of Ellie in terms of recommendations for supports.

Safety

At Ellie's young age, elopement and subsequent harm (e.g., drowning; Guan & Li, 2017) are the most significant safety issues. Awareness of the increased risk for children with autism is indicated. Resources for preventing elopement are available in toolkits, webinars, and resource guides online at no cost. Offerings are always being updated, but safety, crisis, and elopement topics are typically found on websites such as the Organization for Autism Research, etc., your local Family to Family Network, etc. Consultation with a behavior specialist could also benefit Ellie's family and teachers to reduce any elopement behaviors.

Speech and Language

Ellie's language is more advanced than her brother's, but speech and language assessment are important to identify any subtle differences in language development, including social reciprocity. Speech and language treatment and intervention can be considered based on the results of assessment.

Emotional and Behavioral Regulation

Assessment of sensory and language issues can help parents and teachers plan strategies for mitigating and teaching coping strategies. At Ellie's young age, not many manualized curricula are available, but increasing communication skills and mitigating sensory input can reduce the intensity and frequency of meltdowns. In addition to speech and language therapy, consultation with autism specialists can be helpful, and occupational therapists can assist with sensory intervention as needed. Early intervention agencies can provide some of these services, as can local outpatient clinics.

Social Reciprocity

For oldest and only children, taking turns is a skill that may take more practice and coaching than for children who have older siblings. If Ellie is participating in other therapies, coordinate care across providers (with appropriate releases of information) so that routines and rules used in one setting are consistent across others. The back and forth of therapy routines can then be extended to naturalistic play scenarios.

Attending Skills

When Ellie is comfortable, she is friendly and happy and participates in novel activities. Eye contact may or may not be necessary from a therapeutic standpoint, so consideration of her individual needs should be the guiding principle in providing her supports. Supports to help her learn independence skills are available in a wide range of options to suit Ellie's particular needs.

Sensorimotor

Ellie has some toe-walking behavior, very restricted feeding behaviors, and other sensory sensitivities that are already presenting some barriers to her physical and social development. This area of intervention will need to be addressed using an interdisciplinary approach. Sensory issues are typically addressed by occupational therapists according to particular need. If Ellie's toe-walking begins to affect or restrict the growth of her tendons, the multidisciplinary team, including medical specialists, may recommend restorative or preventative measures.

Pre-literacy

Little is mentioned about Ellie's pre-literacy skills, but she is fast approaching preschool age or transition across systems from Early Intervention to Special Education Preschool through her local school district or preferred school. These therapeutic settings involve basic pre-literacy activities around which social skills and language development are practiced. If Ellie is not qualified for special education services, neighborhood or regular preschools may be able to meet these needs for her, with some preparation and support.

Feeding

In Ellie's case, feeding is the most concerning of her present symptoms or traits. Benefits of appropriate feeding interventions can have a dramatic impact on Ellie's quality of life and health. Some speech and language pathologists may be specialized in feeding intervention, as are some other autism specialists. Consultation with the pediatrician (to rule out physiological causes) and nutritionist rounds out the interdisciplinary approach for improving Ellie's feeding behaviors. Parents will need professional support to ensure that interventions are not distressing, are suited to the child and the family, and support Ellie's nutritional needs and that gains are generalized across settings. Local feeding clinics may be available for consultation or outpatient treatment. Online toolkits and readily available books on feeding and eating disorders in autism can be helpful to both parents and clinicians. See Chap. 4 for more on feeding.

Sleep

Ellie's sleep difficulties are not likely to be sustainable for her or her family. Her long bedtime routines and night wakings are disruptive to her and her parents' sleep. Sleep specialists, if available, are ideal for consultation regarding strategies to improve sleep, starting with bedtime. Online toolkits and several specific books, based on decades of research in behavioral sleep medicine, have specifically focused on the higher prevalence of sleep disorder and disruption in autism, much of which can be treated to benefit the individual and family.

Adaptive Skills

Toilet training is the most frequent target for adaptive skill development in young children, and although autism traits may be nuanced, delays in toilet training completion are still found across the autism spectrum. Online toolkits and several books specifically addressing the sensory and behavioral needs of autistic children are readily available for reference, consultation, and intervention. Ellie's mother has not yet begun toilet training her, as her focus has been on the evaluation of her other issues, and her older brother took several years to complete toilet training with the support of a behavior specialist.

Play

Modeling flexible, spontaneous play with Ellie or even video modeling of new play activities may be helpful in expanding her play horizons. Language is critical for play with others, so encourage all play partners to talk, narrate play scenarios, ask questions out loud, etc. while they play to encourage socially reciprocal language patterns as well. See Table 2.1 for a summary of assessment strategies.

Table 2.1 At-a-glance summary—early identification (infant and toddler through kindergarten age)

Domain	Focus and considerations	Assessment choices and age ranges
Initial screening	Establishing initial concerns to guide assessment—*Screening results for females and nuanced autism may be borderline or slightly below-cutoff scores, so evaluations may still be warranted*	Level 1 screeners (can be used universally): *Infant Toddler Checklist* *(**ITC**): 0–24 mos. *Modified Checklist for Autism in Toddlers, Revised with Follow-Up* *(**M-CHAT-R/F**): 16–30 mos. *Parent's Observation of Social Interactions* *(**POSI**): 18–34 mos. Level 2 screeners (indicators for more comprehensive evaluation): *Toddler Autism Symptom Interview (40 min.)* *(**TASI**): 12–36 mos. *Social Responsiveness Scales, 2nd Ed. Preschool* *(**SRS-2**): 2.5–4.5 years *Social Communication Questionnaire—Current and Lifetime* *(**SCQ**) age 4 and older, with adjustment of cutoffs down to age 2 (see Corsello et al. 2013).
Autism specific	Adjust cutoffs to reflect typically lower scores in females	Observational assessments *Autism Diagnostic Observation Schedule, 2nd Ed.* *(**ADOS-2**): 12 mos. and older *Childhood Autism Rating Scales, 2nd Ed. Standard Version* *(**CARS-2-ST**): ages 2–57 years Screening questionnaires, interviews, and observations *Autism Diagnostic Interview, Revised* *(**ADI-R**): 4+ yrs, toddler scoring algorithms now available (Kim & Lord, 2012a, b; Kim et al. 2013) *Rapid Interactive Screening Test for Autism in Toddlers* *(**RITA-T**): 18–36 mos. *Social Communication Questionnaire* *(**SCQ**—**Current or Lifetime**): >4 yrs or 2–3 with adjusted cutoffs *Screening Tool for Autism in Toddlers and Young Children*™ (**STAT**): 24–36 mos. *Toddler Autism Symptom Interview* *(**TASI**): 12–36 mos. Telehealth Options for Observational Measures **TELE-ASD-PEDS**: 16–36 mos. *Naturalistic Observation Diagnostic Assessment* (**NODA**): 18 mos.–6 years *Brief Observation of Symptoms of Autism* (**BOSA**): any age (likely 12 mos. and up)

(continued)

Table 2.1 (continued)

Domain	Focus and considerations	Assessment choices and age ranges
Cognitive or developmental	Many with nuanced autism have uneven cognitive profiles, possibly all within the average range or higher. Processing speed may be lower or higher than other abilities. Consider language ability and attention level when choosing a measure	Ages and Stages Questionnaires *(**ASQ-3**): 1 mo. to 66 mos. *The Bayley Scales of Infant and Toddler Development, 4th Ed.* (**Bayley-4**): 16 days–42 months *Differential Ability Scales, 2nd Ed.* *(**DAS-II**): 30 mos.–17:11 *(extended norms available to age 19) *Developmental Assessment of Young Children, 2nd Ed.* (**DAYC 2**): birth–5:11 *Developmental Indicators for the Assessment of Learning, 4th Ed.* *(**DIAL-4**): 2:6–5:11 *Mullen Scales of Early Learning* (**Mullen**): birth–5:8 *Stanford-Binet Scales of Intelligence, 5th Ed.* (**SB-V**): 2–85+ years *Woodcock-Johnson-IV Tests of Cognitive Abilities* *(**WJ-IV Cog**): 2–90+ *Wechsler Preschool and Primary Scales of Intelligence* *(**WPPSI-IV**): 2:6–7:7
Language	Gaps, idiosyncratic language, prosody	Please see Chap. 3 for a detailed discussion of the assessment of language
Adaptive	Discrepancy with other domains	*Vineland Adaptive Behavior Scales, 3rd Ed.* *(**VABS-3**): birth to 90+ *Adaptive Behavior Assessment System, 3rd Ed.* *(**ABAS-3**): birth to 89:11 *Conners Early Childhood* (**Conners EC**): 2–6 years (**G**) *Adaptive Skills Index, Behavior Assessment System for Children* (**BASC-3**): 2–21 or 25 years for self-report (**G for ages 12–18 only**)
Pre-literacy skills	Precocity may be present	**Parent interview** *Woodcock-Johnson-IV Tests of Achievement* *(**WJ-IV Ach**): 2–90+ years
Executive function	Difficulties with cognitive flexibility (rigidity), inhibitory control, and working memory	*Behavior Rating Inventory of Executive Function* *(**BRIEF-P**): 2:0–5:11; ***BRIEF-2** for **5–18** (**G**) *Comprehensive Executive Function Inventory* *(**CEFI**): 5–18 years One *NEPSY-II subtest of executive function avail. for 3–4-year-olds*, **NEPSY-II**: 3:0–4:11 and 5:0–16:11 *Leiter-3 Nonverbal Stroop Tests* (**Leiter-3**): 3–75+

Play	Pretend play may be observed, but look for rehearsed or repetitive storylines or actions, differences in collaborative play, invitations to play, ability to join group play, and parallel play	*Observation (ADOS-2, CARS-2-ST scoring) Home video and interview Please see Chap. 5 for a detailed discussion of the assessment of play
Sensory	Sensitivities are likely but also watch for sensory seeking behaviors; cover all seven sensory systems	*Sensory Profile, 2nd Ed. **SP2 Infant Toddler:** 7–35 mos. **SP2 Child:** 3:0-14:11 **SP2 School:** 3:0-14:11 **SP2 Short:** 3:0-14:11 Please see Chap. 4 for more details on sensory assessment
Narrow band Social reciprocity	Eye contact differences may not be evident	Observation Video from parents Interview *Autism Diagnostic Observation Schedule, 2nd Ed.* *ADOS-2: 12 mos. + *Social Reciprocity Scales, 2nd Ed. Preschool Version* *(**SRS-2**): 2.5–4.5 years *NEPSY-II Social Perception Index: 3:0–16:11
Feeding	Sensory sensitivities and/or highly selective eating beyond developmental expectations	Food diary Meal observation See Chap. 4 for feeding assessment options
Sleep	Difficulty transitioning to sleep	Parent interview See Chap. 4 for sleep screening instruments
Developmental history	Differences, not necessarily deficits in early development	*Structured Developmental History, Behavior Assessment System for Children* *(**SDH, BASC-3**): 2–21 years or older

(continued)

Table 2.1 (continued)

Domain	Focus and considerations	Assessment choices and age ranges
Broad band Social/emotional	Differences in social behaviors including social approaches that are passive, repeatedly not successful, atypicality, social withdrawal, etc.	Ages and Stages Questionnaire: Social Emotional, 2nd Ed. *(ASQ:SE2): 1–72 mos. (refer if a girl's score is near cutoff, but below, per Squires et al. 2015) Conners Early Childhood *(Conners): 2–6 years (G) -Behavior Assessment System for Children, 3rd Ed. *(BASC-3): 2–21 or 25 years for self-report (G) Preschool Pediatric Symptom Checklist (Survey of Well-Being in Children) *(PPSC-SWYC): 18–65 mos. Social Responsiveness Scales, 2nd Ed. Preschool Version *(SRS-2 Preschool): 2.5–4.5 years Infant Toddler Social Emotional Assessment *(ITSEA): 1–3 years (G) Brief Infant Toddler Social Emotional Assessment *(BITSEA): 1–3 years Child Behavior Checklist for Ages 1.5–5 *(CBCL/1.5–5): 1.5–5 yrs (G)
Special interests and stimming behaviors	Special interests may be fairly typical in terms of topic, but more intense than usual	Interview Autism Diagnostic Observation Schedule, 2nd Ed. ADOS-2: 12 mos. + Childhood Autism Rating Scales, 2nd Ed. Standard Version *(CARS-2-ST): ages 2–57 years
Medical	Hearing and other possible medical conditions to explain traits observed	Hearing and vision screening through pediatrician or early intervention, surveillance (healthcare provider interview) for GI issues, motor development delays, metabolic or genetic concerns

Please see the "References" section at the end of this chapter for additional information on measures.

Not all measures and processes listed are available in all settings or appropriate for all cases. Qualification levels apply. Multiple measures in a single domain are not necessary. Some measures can provide data in multiple domains. This is meant to provide a relatively quick reference for assessment planning and implementation, not an endorsement of any particular measure as "best." See above for details. Emphasis here is on readily available, commonly used measures, but similar measures may also be useful.

Measures available in languages other than English are marked with *. Measures with gendered norms are marked with (G). Measures not requiring spoken responses include "nonverbal" in their title or domain title

For more information about these and other developmental screeners, please see Compendium of Screeners from Birth to 5: Watch Me Thrive! (US Dept. of Health and Human Services, 2014)

References

Achenbach, T. M., & Rescorla, L. A. (2001). *Manual for the ASEBA school-age forms & profiles*. University of Vermont, Research Center for Children, Youth, & Families.

American Psychiatric Association. (2022). *Diagnostic and statistical manual of mental disorders* (5th, Text revision ed.). Author.

Andersson, G. W., Gillberg, C., & Miniscalco, C. (2013). Pre-school children with suspected autism spectrum disorders: Do girls and boys have the same profiles? *Research in Developmental Disabilities, 34*(1), 413–422. https://doi.org/10.1016/j.ridd.2012.08.025

Åsberg, J., Kopp, S., Berg-Kelly, K., & Gillberg, C. (2010). Reading comprehension, word decoding and spelling in girls with autism spectrum disorders (ASD) or attention-deficit/hyperactivity disorder (AD/HD): Performance and predictors. *International Journal of Language & Communication Disorders, 45*(1), 61–71. https://doi.org/10.3109/13682820902745438

Ballou, E. P., da Vanport, S., & Onaiwu, M. G. (Eds.). (2021). *Sincerely, your autistic child*. Beacon Press.

Baron-Cohen, S. (2002). The extreme male brain theory of autism. *Trends in Cognitive Sciences, 6*, 248–254. https://doi.org/10.1016/s1364-6613(02)01904-6

Bayley, N., & Aylward, G. P. (2019). *The Bayley scales of infant and toddler development* (Technical manual) (4th ed.).

Beggiato, A., Peyre, H., Maruani, A., Scheid, I., Rastam, M., Amsellem, F., Gillberg, C. I., Leboyer, M., Bourgeron, T., Gillberg, C., & Delorme, R. (2017). Gender differences in autism spectrum disorders: Divergence among specific core symptoms. *Autism Research, 10*(4), 680–689. https://doi.org/10.1002/aur.1715

Board of Directors. (2007). American Academy of clinical neuropsychology (AACN) practice guidelines for neuropsychological assessment and consultation. *The Clinical Neuropsychologist, 21*(2), 209–231. https://doi.org/10.1080/13825580601025932

Bourson, L., & Prevost, C. (2022). Characteristics of restricted interests in girls with ASD compared to boys: A systematic review of the literature. *European Child & Adolescent Psychiatry*. https://doi.org/10.1007/s00787-022-01998-5. Epub ahead of print.

Briggs-Gowan, M. J., & Carter, A. S. (1998). *Infant toddler social emotional assessment*. MAPI Research Trust. https://eprovide.mapi-trust.org/instruments/infant-toddler-social-emotional-assessment

Briggs-Gowan, M. J., Irwin, J. R., Wachtel, K., Carter, A. S., & Cicchetti, D. V. (2004). *Brief infant toddler social emotional assessment*. MAPI Research Trust. https://eprovide.mapi-trust.org/instruments/brief-infant-toddler-social-emotional-assessment

Carbone, P. S., Campbell, K., Wilkes, J., Stoddard, G. J., Huynh, K., Young, P. C., & Gabrielsen, T. P. (2020). Primary care autism screening and later autism diagnosis. *Pediatrics, 146*(2), e20192314. https://doi.org/10.1542/peds.2019-2314

Centers for Disease Control. (2022). *Developmental milestones*. https://www.cdc.gov/ncbddd/actearly/milestones/index.html.

Choueiri, R., & Wagner, S. (2015). A new interactive screening test for autism spectrum disorders in toddlers. *Journal of Pediatrics, 167*, 460–466. https://doi.org/10.1016/j.jpeds.2015.05.029

Conners, C.K. (2009). Conners early childhood. Technical manual .

Constantino, J., & Gruber, C. P. (2012). *Social responsiveness scale* (2nd ed.). Western Psychological Services.

Corsello, C. M., Akshoomoff, N., & Stahmer, A. C. (2013). Diagnosis of autism spectrum disorders in 2-year-olds: a study of community practice. *Journal of Child Psychology and Psychiatry, and Allied Disciplines, 54*(2), 178–185. https://doi.org/10.1111/j.1469-7610.2012.02607.x

Corona, L., Hine, J., Nicholson, A., Stone, C., Swanson, A., Wade, J., et al. (2020). *TELE-ASD-PEDS: A telemedicine-based ASD evaluation tool for toddlers and young children*. Vanderbilt University Medical Center. https://vkc.vumc.org/vkc/triad/tele-asd-peds

Coulter, K., Barton, M., Boorstein, H., Cordeaux, C., Dumont-Mathieu, T., Haisley, L., Herlihy, L., Jashar, D., Robins, D., Stone, W., & Fein, D. (2021). The Toddler Autism Symptom Inventory

(TASI): Use in diagnostic evaluations of toddlers. *Autism: International Journal of Research and Practice.* https://doi.org/10.1177/13623613211021699

de Marchena, A., & Miller, J. (2017). "Frank" presentations as a novel research construct and element of diagnostic decision-making in autism spectrum disorder. *Autism Research, 10*(4), 653–662. https://doi.org/10.1002/aur.1706

Dow, D., Holbrook, A., Toolan, C., McDonald, N., Sterrett, K., Rosen, N., Kim, S. H., & Lord, C. (2021). The Brief Observation of Symptoms of Autism (BOSA): Development of a new adapted assessment measure for remote telehealth administration through COVID-19 and beyond. *Journal of Autism and Developmental Disorders*, 1–12. https://doi.org/10.1007/s10803-021-05395-w. Epub ahead of print.

Dunn, W. (2014). *Sensory profile 2.* Pearson.

Duvall, S., Armstrong, K., Shahabuddin, A., Grantz, C., Fein, D., & Lord, C. (2021). A road map for identifying autism spectrum disorder: Recognizing and evaluating characteristics that should raise red or "pink" flags to guide accurate differential diagnosis. *The Clinical Neuropsychologist*, 1–36. Advance online publication. https://doi.org/10.1080/13854046.2021.1921276.

Eaton, L. (2012). Under the radar and behind the scenes: The perspectives of mothers with daughters on the autism spectrum. *Good Autism Practice (GAP), 13*(2), 9–17.

Elliott, C. D. (2007). *The differential ability scales* (Technical Manual) (2nd ed.).

Gioia, G. A., Espy, K. A., & Isquith, P. (2003). *Behavior rating inventory of executive function – Preschool version.* PARinc.

Gould, J., & Ashton-Smith, J. (2011). Missed diagnosis or misdiagnosis? Girls and women on the autism spectrum. *Good Autism Practice (GAP), 12*(1), 34–41. https://www.ingentaconnect.com/content/bild/gap/2011/00000012/00000001/art00005

Grandin, T., & Scariano, M. M. (1996). *Emergence: Labeled autistic.* Warner Books.

Greene, R. K., Vasile, I., Bradbury, K. R., Olsen, A., & Duvall, S. W. (2022). Autism Diagnostic Observation Schedule (ADOS-2) elevations in a clinical sample of children and adolescents who do not have autism: Phenotypic profiles of false positives. *The Clinical Neuropsychologist, 36*(5), 943–959. https://doi.org/10.1080/13854046.2021.1942220

Guan, J., & Li, G. (2017). Characteristics of unintentional drowning deaths in children with autism spectrum disorder. *Injury Epidemiology, 4*(32). https://doi.org/10.1186/s40621-017-0129-4

Guthrie, W., Wallis, K., Bennett, A., Brooks, E., Dudley, J., Gerdes, M., Pandey, J., Levy, S. E., Schultz, R. T., & Miller, J. S. (2019). Accuracy of autism screening in a large pediatric network. *Pediatrics, 144*(4), e20183963. https://doi.org/10.1542/peds.2018-3963. PMID: 31562252.

Halladay, A. K., Bishop, S., Constantino, J. N., Daniels, A. M., Koenig, K., Palmer, K., Messinger, D., Pelphrey, K., Sanders, S. J., Singer, A. T., Taylor, J. L., & Szatmari, P. (2015). Sex and gender differences in autism spectrum disorder: Summarizing evidence gaps and identifying emerging areas of priority. *Molecular Autism, 6*(1), 1–5. https://doi.org/10.1186/s13229-015-0019-y

Harrison, P., & Oakland, T. (2015a). *Adaptive behavior assessment system* (3rd ed.). Western Psychological Services.

Harrison, P., & Oakland, T. (2015b). *Adaptive behavior assessment system* (Technical manual) (3rd ed.).

Havdahl, K. A., Hus Bal, V., Huerta, M., Pickles, A., Øyen, A.-S., Stoltenberg, C., Lord, C., & Bishop, S. L. (2016). Multidimensional influences on autism symptom measures: Implications for use in etiological research. *Journal of the American Academy of Child & Adolescent Psychiatry, 55*(12), 1054–1063. https://doi.org/10.1016/j.jaac.2016.09.490

Hendrickx, S. (2015). *Women and girls with autism spectrum disorder: Understanding life experiences from early childhood to old age.* Jessica Kingsley.

Hull, L., Mandy, W., & Petrides, K. V. (2017). Behavioural and cognitive sex/gender differences in autism spectrum condition and typically developing males and females. *Autism, 21*(6), 706–727. https://doi.org/10.1177/1362361316669087

Individuals With Disabilities Education Act, 20 U.S.C. § 1400. (2004). https://sites.ed.gov/idea/

Jacquemont, S., Coe, B. P., Hersch, M., Duyzend, M. H., Krumm, N., Bergmann, S., Beckmann, J. S., Rosenfeld, J. A., & Eichler, E. E. (2014). A higher mutational burden in females supports a "female protective model" in neurodevelopmental disorders. *American Journal of Human Genetics, 94*, 415–425. https://doi.org/10.1016/j.ajhg.2014.02.001

Jamison, R., Bishop, S. L., Huerta, M., & Halladay, A. K. (2017). The clinician perspective on sex differences in autism spectrum disorders. *Autism, 21*(6), 772–784. https://doi.org/10.1177/1362361316681481

Kaat, A. J., Shui, A. M., Ghods, S. S., Farmer, C. A., Esler, A. N., Thurm, A., Georgiades, S., Kanne, S. M., Lord, C., Kim, Y. S., & Bishop, S. L. (2021). Sex differences in scores on standardized measures of autism symptoms: A multisite integrative data analysis. *Journal of Child Psychology and Psychiatry, 62*, 97–106. https://doi.org/10.1111/jcpp.13242

Kanne, S. M., & Bishop, S. L. (2020). Editorial perspective: The autism waitlist crisis and remembering what families need. *Journal of Child Psychology and Psychiatry., 62*(2), 140–142. https://doi.org/10.1111/jcpp.13254

Kaufman, A. S., & Kaufman, N. L. (2014). *Kaufman test of educational achievement* (3rd ed.). Pearson.

Kaufman, A. S., & Kaufman, N. L. (2018). *Kaufman assessment battery for children* (Normative update) (2nd ed.). Pearson.

Kentrou, V., de Veld, D. M., Mataw, K. J., & Begeer, S. (2019). Delayed autism spectrum disorder recognition in children and adolescents previously diagnosed with attention-deficit/hyperactivity disorder. *Autism: The International Journal of Research and Practice, 23*(4), 1065–1072. https://doi.org/10.1177/1362361318785171

Kim, S. H., & Lord, C. (2012a). New autism diagnostic interview-revised algorithms for toddlers and Young Preschoolers from 12 to 47 months of age. *Journal of Autism and Developmental Disorders, 42*, 82–93. https://doi.org/10.1007/s10803-011-1213-1

Kim, S. H., & Lord, C. (2012b). Combining information from multiple sources for the diagnosis of autism spectrum disorders for toddlers and young preschoolers from 12 to 47 months of age. *Journal of Child Psychology and Psychiatry, 53*, 143–151. https://doi.org/10.1111/j.1469-7610.2011.02458.x

Kim, S. H., Thurm, A., Shumway, S., & Lord, C. (2013). Multisite study of new autism diagnostic interview-revised (ADI-R) algorithms for toddlers and young preschoolers. *Journal of Autism and Developmental Disorders, 43*(7), 1527–1538. https://doi.org/10.1007/s10803-012-1696-4

Koenig, K., & Tsatsanis, K. (2005). Pervasive developmental disorders in girls. In *Handbook of behavioral and emotional problems in girls*. Springer. https://doi.org/10.1007/0-306-48674-1_7

Korkman, M., Kirk, U., & Kemp, S. (2007). *NEPSY* (2nd ed.). Pearson.

Lawrence, K. E., Hernandez, L. M., Fuster, E., Padgaonkar, N. T., Patterson, G., Jung, J., Okada, N. J., Lowe, J. K., Hoekstra, J. N., Jack, A., Aylward, E., Gaab, N., Van Horn, J. D., Bernier, R. A., McPartland, J. C., Webb, S. J., Pelphrey, K. A., Green, S. A., Bookheimer, S. Y., et al. (2022). Impact of autism genetic risk on brain connectivity: A mechanism for the female protective effect. *Brain, 145*(1), 378–387. https://doi.org/10.1093/brain/awab204

LeCouteur, A., Lord, C., & Rutter, M. (2003). *Autism diagnostic interview-revised*. Western Psychological.

Lonigan, C. J., Allan, N. P., & Lerner, M. D. (2011). Assessment of preschool early literacy skills: Linking children's educational needs with empirically supported instructional activities. *Psychology in the Schools, 48*(5), 488–501. https://doi.org/10.1002/pits.20569

Lord, C., Risi, S., Lambrecht, L., et al. (2000). The Autism Diagnostic Observation Schedule—Generic: A standard measure of social and communication deficits associated with the spectrum of autism. *Journal of Autism and Developmental Disorders, 30*, 205–223. https://doi.org/10.1023/A:1005592401947

Lord, C., Rutter, M., Di Lavore, P. C., Risi, S., Gotham, K., & Bishop, S. L. (2012a). *Autism Diagnostic Observation Schedule* (Modules 1–4) (2nd ed.). Western Psychological Services.

Lord, C., Luyster, R. J., Gotham, K., & Guthrie, W. (2012b). *Autism Diagnostic Observation Schedule* (Toddler module) (2nd ed.). Western Psychological Services

Maenner, M.J., Warren, Z., Williams, A.R., Amoakohene, E., Bakian, A.V., Bilder, D.A., Durkin, M.S., Fitzgerald, R.T., Furnier, S.M., Hughes, M.M., Ladd-Acosta, C.M., McArther, D., Pas, E.T., Salinas, A., Vehorn, S., Williams, S., Esler, A., Grzybowski, A., Hall-Lande, J. . . . & Shaw, K.A. (2023) Prevalence and Characteristics of Autism Spectrum Disorder Among Children Aged 8 Years — Autism and Developmental Disabilities Monitoring Network, 11 Sites, United States, 2020. MMWR Surveill Summ 72(No. SS-2):1–14. https://doi.org/10.15585/mmwr. ss7202a1

Mardell, C., & Goldenberg, D. S. (2011). *Developmental indicators for assessment of learning* (4th ed.). Pearson.

Miller, J. K. (Ed.). (2015). *Women from another planet? Our lives in the universe of autism.* AuthorHouse.

Mullen, E. M. (1995). *Mullen scales of early learning manual.* Pearson.

Mussey, J. L., Ginn, N. C., & Klinger, L. G. (2017). Are males and females with autism spectrum disorder more similar than we thought? *Autism: The International Journal of Research and Practice, 21*(6), 733–737. https://doi.org/10.1177/1362361316682621

Naglieri, J. A., & Goldstein, S. (2013). *Comprehensive Executive Function Inventory.* Multi Health Systems.

Nichols, S. (2009). *Girls growing up on the autism spectrum: What parents and professionals should know about the pre-teen and teenage years.* Jessica Kingsley.

Øien, R. A., Schjølberg, S., Volkmar, F. R., Shic, F., Cicchetti, D. V., Nordahl-Hansen, A., et al. (2018). Clinical features of children with autism who passed 18-month screening. *Pediatrics, 141*(6). https://doi.org/10.1542/peds.2017-3596

Penner, M., Anagnostou, E., & Ungar, W. J. (2018). Practice patterns and determinants of wait time for autism spectrum disorder diagnosis in Canada. *Molecular Autism, 9,* 16. https://doi. org/10.1186/s13229-018-0201-0

Perrin, E. C., Sheldrick, C., Visco, Z., & Mattern, K. (2010). *Parent's Observation of Social Interactions in Survey of Well-being in Young Children* (User's manual). Tufts Medical Center. https://www.tuftschildrenshospital.org/the-survey-of-wellbeing-of-young-children/ parts-of-the-swyc/posi

Reynolds, C. R., & Kamphaus, R. W. (2015). *Behavior assessment system for children* (3rd ed.). Pearson.

Robins, D., Fein, D., Barton, M., & Green, J. (2001). The Modified Checklist for Autism in Toddlers (M-CHAT): An initial investigation in the early detection of autism and pervasive developmental disorders. *Journal of Autism and Developmental Disorders, 31*(2), 131–144. https://doi.org/10.1023/a:1010738829569

Robins, D. L., Fein, D. A., & Barton, M. L. (2009). *The Modified Checklist for Autism in Toddlers, Revised, with Follow-up (M-CHAT-R/F).* Self-Published. www.mchatscreen.com

Robins, D. L., Casagrande, K., Barton, M., Chen, C.-M. A., Dumont-Mathieu, T., & Fein, D. (2014). Validation of the The Modified Checklist for Autism in Toddlers, Revised, with Follow-up (M-CHAT-R/F). *Pediatrics, 133*(1), 37–45. https://doi.org/10.1542/peds.2013-1813

Robinson, E. B., Lichtenstein, P., Anckarsater, H., Happé, F., & Ronald, A. (2013). Examining and interpreting the female protective effect against autistic behavior. *Proceedings of the National Academy of Sciences of the United States of America, 110,* 5258–5262. https://doi.org/10.1073/ pnas.1211070110

Roid, G. H. (2003). *Stanford Binet Intelligence Scales* (Technical manual) (5th ed.). Pro-ed Inc.

Roid, G. H., Miller, L. J., Pomplun, M., & Koch, C. (2013). *Leiter International Performance Scale* (3rd ed.). Stoelting Co.

Ros-Demarize, R., Bradley, C., Kanne, S. M., Warren, Z., Boan, A., Lajonchere, C., Park, J., & Carpenter, L. A. (2020). ASD symptoms in toddlers and preschoolers: An examination of sex differences. *Autism Research, 13*(1), 157–166. https://doi.org/10.1002/aur.2241

Rutter, M., Bailey, A., & Lord, C. (2003). *The Social Communication Questionnaire (SCQ): Technical manual.* Western Psychological Services.

Schopler, E., Van Gourgondien, M. E., Wellmand, G. J., & Love, S. R. (2010). *The Childhood Autism Rating Scales* (2nd ed.). Western Psychological Services.

Schrank, F. A., McGrew, K. S., & Mather, N. (2014a). *Woodcock-Johnson-IV: Tests of Cognitive Abilities*. Riverside.

Schrank, F. A., Mather, N., & McGrew, K. S. (2014b). *Woodcock-Johnson-IV: Tests of Achievement*. Riverside.

Smith, C. J., Rozga, A., Matthews, N., Oberleitner, R., Nazneen, N., & Abowd, G. (2017). Investigating the accuracy of a novel telehealth diagnostic approach for autism spectrum disorder. *Psychological Assessment, 29*(3), 245–252. https://doi.org/10.1037/pas0000317

Sparrow, S. S., Cichetti, D. V., & Saulnier, C. A. (2016). *Vineland adaptive scales* (3rd ed.). Pearson.

Squires, J. & Bricker, D. (2009). *Ages & Stages Questionnaires(R), Third Edition*. Brookes Publishing.

Squires, J., Bricker, D., & Twombly, E. (2015). *Ages & Stages Questionnaires®: Social-emotional* (2nd ed.). Paul H. Brookes Publishing.

Stone, W. L., Coonrod, E. E., & Ousley, O. Y. (2000). Screening Tool for Autism in Two-year-olds (STAT): Development and preliminary data. *Journal of Autism and Developmental Disorders, 30*, 607–612.

Stone, W. L., Coonrod, E. E., Turner, L. M., & Pozdol, S. L. (2004). Psychometric properties of the STAT for early autism screening. *Journal of Autism and Developmental Disorders, 34*, 691–701. https://doi.org/10.1007/s10803-004-5289-8. (The STAT is available through Vanderbilt University http://stat.vueinnovations.com/licensing)

Stroth, S., Tauscher, J., Wolff, N., et al. (2022). Phenotypic differences between female and male individuals with suspicion of autism spectrum disorder. *Molecular Autism, 13*(11), https://doi.org/10.1186/s13229-022-00491-9.

US Department of Health and Human Services. (2014). *A compendium of screening measures for young children*. https://www2.ed.gov/about/inits/list/watch-me-thrive/files/screening-compendium-march2014.pdf

Voress, J. K., Maddox, T., & Hammill, D. D. (2012). *Developmental Assessment of Young Children* (2nd ed.). Pro-ed, Inc.

Wagner, L., Corona, L. L., Weitlauf, A. S., March, K. L., Berman, A. F., Broderick, N. A., Francis, S., Hine, J., Nicholson, A., Stone, C., & Warren, Z. (2021). Use of the TELE-ASD-PEDS for autism evaluations in response to COVID-19: Preliminary outcomes and clinician acceptability. *Journal of Autism and Developmental Disorders, 51*, 3063–3072. https://doi.org/10.1007/s10803-020-04767-y

Wang, S., Deng, H., You, C., et al. (2017). Sex differences in diagnosis and clinical phenotypes of Chinese children with autism spectrum disorder. *Neuroscience Bulletin, 33*, 153–160. https://doi.org/10.1007/s12264-017-0102-9

Wechsler, D. (2012). *Wechsler Preschool and Primary Scales of Intelligence* (Technical manual) (4th ed.). Pearson.

Wetherby, A., & Prizant, B. (2002). *Communication and Symbolic Behavior Scales Developmental Profile*—First normed edition. Brookes.

White, E. I., Wallace, G. L., Bascom, J., Armour, A. C., Register-Brown, K., Popal, H. S., et al. (2017). Sex differences in parent-reported executive functioning and adaptive behavior in children and young adults with autism spectrum disorder. *Autism Research, 10*(10), 1653–1662. https://doi.org/10.1002/aur.1811

Wieckowski, A. T., de Marchena, A., Algur, Y., Nichols, L., Fernandes, S., Thomas, R. P., McClure, L. A., Dufek, S., Fein, D., Adamson, L. B., Stahmer, A., & Robins, D. L. (2021). The first five minutes: Initial impressions during autism spectrum disorder diagnostic evaluations in young children. *Autism Research, 14*(9), 1923–1934. https://doi.org/10.1002/aur.2536

Wigdor, E., Weiner, D., Grove, J., Fu, J., Thompson, W., Carey, C., Baya, N., van der Merwe, C., Mortensen, P. B., Daly, M., Talkowski, M., Sanders, S., Bishop, S., Børglum, A., & Robinson, E. (2021). The female protective effect against autism spectrum disorder. *European Neuropsychopharmacology, 51*, e13–e14. https://doi.org/10.1016/j.euroneuro.2021.07.035

Chapter 3
Communication and Language Assessment in Females with Autism

Speech and language assessment needs are not limited to young children as part of a comprehensive evaluation. Social or pragmatic language, receptive language, and sometimes even expressive language issues may present barriers to success for autistic individuals even when autism has not yet been suspected. We have outlined domains to focus on for assessment, types of measures that can be useful, first-person accounts of language difficulties, and a discussion of possible supports for communication and language needs across the lifespan, with a strong focus on early years aligned with our goal of earlier identification and support.

Communication and language are sometimes oversimplified when it comes to detecting early signs of autism. If a child has spoken language, often their communication skills are summarized as "typical," which may disguise some of the more nuanced language and communication differences that are strong signals of autistic traits. Closer consideration of language and communication skills, even at early ages and in children with spoken language may be the key to picking up on early signs of autism in many children who are currently missed until possibly adulthood.

> *She has difficulty with idiom, sarcasm, tone of voice, multiple and complex instructions. This becomes increasingly evident as her peers begin to understand these language usages. It was less obvious when she was younger as very few of the children had these skills. (Parent of girl with autism).* Hendrickx (2015, p. 56)

Case Study—Naya: Limited Verbal Sharing, Dysfluency, and Pragmatic Differences

Although parents of 7-year-old Naya noted that she developed language skills at an expected age, they are noticing some differences in the ways she uses her words as compared to how her older sister, Reva, communicated at the same age. While Reva was excited to share things about her school day and regaled her parents with stories

© The Author(s), under exclusive license to Springer Nature Switzerland AG 2023
T. P. Gabrielsen et al., *Assessment of Autism in Females and Nuanced Presentations*, https://doi.org/10.1007/978-3-031-33969-1_3

about her friends and teachers, Naya struggles to respond to her parents' questions and often just doesn't reply. When she does speak, her parents aren't always able to understand what Naya is referring to, as she "starts in the middle of her own thoughts." Naya also repeats the final syllables in many words. For example, she might say, "I was thinking-ing about-out it." Her parents have noticed that this is more prevalent when Naya seems eager to talk or when she is nervous, and it can be difficult to understand her at those times. Naya's family, including Reva, integrate nuanced and specific facial expressions, hand gestures, and head movements with their speech, but Naya doesn't seem to use or understand this type of communication despite having been exposed to it all her life. Parents are most concerned with Naya's safety, as she tends to share personal details (e.g., home address, family members' names) or make unexpected comments to strangers (e.g., commenting on their appearance).

Early Female Performance on Language Assessment

As stated earlier, autism assessments were created with a typical male presentation in mind. Language assessment is typically non-gendered and therefore provides an opportunity to describe difficulties that autism assessments might overlook. One study found the average age of diagnosis in girls to be 8 years of age (Eaton, 2012). Quality language assessments, with a focus on social-emotional development, can help to identify girls at earlier ages.

Late language development is common in autistic children. Toddlers and preschoolers with autism are often referred for assessment due to concerns regarding delayed speech and language. Many children with autism will exhibit significant delays in speech acquisition, producing first words at age 24 months (12 months delayed) and first phrases at 48 months (18–24 months delayed) (Eigsti & Schuh, 2017). Parents are understandably concerned about their child's lack of communication. Girls with autism are more likely than their male counterparts to have typical or above-average development of speech. Parents will comment that the child used big words earlier than expected and might be referred to as "little professor." Their expressive language is developing typically or precociously, but their understanding and response to language are less adept.

> "*Consider language processing limitations—just because she is highly articulate (her words) doesn't mean that she can comprehend what you require (your words).*" (Hendrickx, 2015, p. 115)

Barriers to Early Identification

Females who present with age-expected cognitive and language abilities may escape notice by clinicians. Unexpected behaviors are often attributed to a reason other than autism, such as anxiety or ADHD. Behaviors like making eye contact, showing interest in people, and pretend play are things that many young children with nuanced autism can do. Attention to the quality and quantity of the behaviors is important in order to improve early identification:

> The only gender difference found in our very young community-based sample of children with autism was in their social communication difficulties, where females exhibited more difficulties than males with autism. (Lawson et al., 2018)

Parents rated their female autistic child more critically than parents of a male autistic child, despite no difference being identified by clinicians using the Autism Diagnostic Observation Schedule (ADOS). It was suggested that this could be the result of an interpretation bias by parents who may expect "more socially desired behavior from their daughters than their sons," (Sturrock et al., 2020). With this in mind, it is very important that those completing speech and language evaluations be aware of the need to include assessment of social and emotional development in addition to speech and receptive and expressive language. Speech and language pathologists need to become accustomed to talking about concern for autism and to open discussions with parents about the need for further assessment.

To improve early identification, the simplest adjustment we recommend to a quality speech and language assessment is to include a social-emotional rating scale. This one addition improves the identification of children with delayed social-emotional development and enhances referrals for further autism assessment. There are a variety of rating scales to choose from that should be part of a typical speech and language testing protocol:

- *Communication and Symbolic Behavior Scales Developmental Profile Infant/ Toddler Checklist* (CSBS DP ITC): 6-24 months (Wetherby & Prizant, 2002).
- *Bayley Scales of Infant and Toddler Development, 4th Ed. Social-Emotional Questionnaire* (Bayley-4 SEQ): 16 days–42 months (Bayley & Aylward, 2019).
- *Clinical Evaluation of Language Fundamentals-Preschool, 3rd Ed. Descriptive Pragmatic Profile* (CELF-P3 DPP): 3–6 years (Wiig et al., 2020).
- *-Clinical Evaluation of Language Fundamentals, 5th Ed. Pragmatic Profile* (CELF-5 PP): 5–21 years (Wiig et al., 2013)
- *-Children's Communication Checklist, 2nd Ed.* (CCC-2): 4–18 years (Bishop, 2006).

The CELF-P3 (Wiig et al., 2020) also includes a Pragmatic Activities subtest which provides criterion-based information about the manner, relevance, quality, and quantity of the verbal communication.

Diagnostic Measurement Performance

The *Communication and Symbolic Behavior Scales Developmental Profile Behavior Sample* (CSBS DP) (Wetherby & Prizant, 2002) is an assessment instrument created for children between the developmental ages of 6 and 24 months. The CSBS DP is helpful in determining if a child has delays in social communication, expressive language/speech, and symbolic functioning, i.e., language understanding and use of objects. Situations are designed to entice the child to communicate, and strategies are designed to encourage spontaneous behavior and interactions.

The *Preschool Language Scales, 5th Ed. (PLS-5)* (Zimmerman et al., 2011), assesses social cognition as part of the early developmental test items. It is important that practitioners understand the purpose of these items and consider them carefully when scoring.

- Searching to find a person who is talking.
- Interrupting an activity when you call her name.
- Looking at things the caregiver points to and names.
- Following routine, familiar directions with gestures.
- Following commands with gestures.
- Taking multiple turns vocalizing.
- Playing simple games with another with eye contact.
- Using a representational gesture (e.g., waving bye-bye, clapping hands, dancing to music).
- Using eye contact while participating in a play routine with another person for at least 1 min.
- Initiating a turn-based social routine.
- Using gestures along with vocalizations to request objects.
- Demonstrating joint attention.
- Using words more often than gestures to communicate.
- Using words for a variety of pragmatic functions (e.g., request objects or actions, label objects or actions, request repetition, request assistance, answer yes/no questions with a word, use a word to get attention).

When scoring the PLS-5, it is important to consider the discrepancy of the scores. Comparing scores for auditory comprehension and expressive communication can often indicate a cause for the difference. When the score for expressive communication is significantly lower than auditory comprehension, the discrepancy indicates concern for delayed speech sound acquisition, indicating the child should be referred for further testing of dysarthria or childhood apraxia of speech. When the auditory comprehension score is clinically less than the expressive communication score, this discrepancy indicates the difference is caused by delayed social-emotional development and indicates the child should be referred for an autism evaluation.

The receptive-expressive split is not universal, but it can persist throughout development and often presents in receptive and expressive vocabulary assessment differences as well.

> If children with autism present with an expressive over receptive language advantage, it may hold potential to support differential diagnosis of autism from other developmental diagnoses. (Mitchell et al.,2011)

Narrative Language Assessment

One way to evaluate pragmatic language is through storytelling or narratives. In a narrative, the speaker describes a story or an event with the goal of having the listener understand what is happening. When a parent asks "What happened at school today?", they are asking for a short narrative about what the child experienced during the school day. Many multiple-choice quizzes that students take are analyzing whether or not they understood the reading of a narrative. Understanding and telling stories engage the speaker and listener in a complex cognitive-linguistic task embedded in social context. A narrative language assessment provides "an index of pragmatic discourse impairments that traditional tests of language may not capture" (Conlon et al., 2019, p. 1939).

The CELF-P3 (Wiig et al., 2020) includes a narrative measure called the Connected Speech Sample (CSS). The child retells a story read aloud by the clinician. The CSS assesses the child's ability to create a narrative that is organized, is linguistically complex, and uses age-normative story grammar.

Although adolescents with autism scored within the normal range of expressive and receptive language, their performance on narrative tasks revealed difficulties with both structural language and the ability to answer comprehension questions. It should be noted that both teachers and parents rated the pragmatic language skills of the young people with autism as significantly lower than those of the typically developing group but parents were more likely than teachers to additionally identify difficulties in speech and syntax (King & Palikara, 2018).

A standardized evaluation of narrative language is the *Test of Narrative Language, 2nd Ed.* (TNL-2): 5 years–15:11 (Gillam & Pearson, 2017). The TNL-2 provides standardized scores for both narrative comprehension and retell abilities.

Pragmatic Language

First-Person Narratives

I had no slang at all. Neat was a synonym for tidy, period. My brain had zero capacity for picking up the kid slang around me, and I often had no idea what my peers were saying to one another. In my speech, I fit the AS little professor stereotype. Jane Meyerding (Miller, 2015, p. 187).

As a young child, I never babbled but spoke with purpose using minimal words to express a need or thought. (Cohen, 2017, p. 14)

Many of the women and girls who participated in this book were precocious early talkers, often with extensive vocabularies. (Hendrickx, 2015, p. 105)

I understood their language,.... but, I never came to hear what they were really saying. I never understood their vernacular. Suffice to say that, at that point, I was unable to read between the lines. Subtext and innuendo may as well have been birds flying by my window.

It was frustrating being unable to break into the thought processes of my peers but I was more upset when I came to discern I never learned from one experience to the next. (Willey, 2014, p. 59).

Pragmatics and discourse serve as the most "socially motivated" domains of language, in that "they require the speaker to be aware of and respond to the social status, knowledge, interest, motivation, and other qualities of the listener; these skills exhibit a long trajectory of development in most children, with an asymptote at approximately five years of age" (Eigsti et al., 2011, p. 683).

Pragmatic language is like a trail of social breadcrumbs that involve picking up on social clues and cues that infer meaning. Difficulty with pragmatics can have devastating consequences, as they are important for successful everyday interactions, such as developing friendships and learning in school. Skills established and honed in the school years lay the foundation for personal success and satisfaction as an adult, both at work and in establishing personal relationships. Some evidence suggests that "pragmatic skills may be more important for females than for males, as girls' friendships and social activities often occur within smaller, more intimate groups than boys' and are characterized by expectations for conversations that focus on interpersonal relationships" (Conlon et al., 2019, p. 1938)

Evaluation of Pragmatic Language

Pragmatic language deficits are among the core challenges of autism, and it is important that language assessments include an evaluation of pragmatic competence and not be limited to the formal, structural aspects of language. As a group, those with nuanced autism tend to demonstrate strong language skills, but a weakness in pragmatics. As a result, they often fail to qualify for speech-language services since they score well on formal language assessments. A variety of assessment strategies should be used, including direct assessment, naturalistic observation, and interviewing significant others, including parents and educators who are valuable sources of information.

The Formulated Sentences subtest of the *Clinical Evaluation of Language Fundamentals, 5th Ed. Pragmatic Profile* (CELF-5 PP): 5–21 years (Wiig et al., 2013), requires that the stimulus word be used appropriately in a grammatically correct sentence and the sentence needs to be pragmatically applicable. Since pragmatic awareness is part of the scoring for this subtest, it can help determine the need for further pragmatic evaluation.

The *Test of Pragmatic Language, 2nd Ed.* (TOPL-2): 6 years–18:11 (Phelps-Terasaki & Phelps-Gunn, 2007), is a valid and reliable measure of pragmatic language and assists in identifying strengths and areas that need support or training. This assessment requires average language ability to understand and participate in the testing items.

Other standardized measures of pragmatic language include:

- *Clinical Evaluation of Language Fundamentals, 5th Ed. Metalinguistics* (**CELF-5 Metalinguistics**): 9 years–21:11 (Wiig & Secord, 2014).
- *Social Emotional Evaluation* (**SEE**): 6 years to 12:11 (Wiig, 2008).
- *Social Language Development Test-Elementary: Normative Update* (**SLDT-E:NU**): 6 years–11:11 (Bowers et al., 2016).
- *Social Language Development Test-Adolescent: Normative Update* (**SLDT-A: NU**): 12 years–17:11 (Bowers et al., 2017).

Prosody

Prosody, an important component of pragmatic language skills, refers to the "melody of the voice." Important components of prosody include pitch, or the frequency of speech; amplitude or intensity; and rhythm and duration. Individuals with ASD, including those with strong verbal skills, consistently show differences in prosody, including reduced/monotone prosody, unusual stress patterns, and differences in the quality of the voice (Eigsti & Schuh, 2017).

"It's not what you say, but how you say it." This common saying elucidates how critical speech prosody—the melody and timing of speech—is to effectively communicate affect and intention. Unfortunately, many verbal individuals with autism have deficits in both discerning a speaker's intent and producing appropriate prosody, which are detrimental to social functioning (Bone et al., 2016).

Prosody can significantly affect intelligibility when it is unusual. It is a perceptual piece of information that should be observed and considered as a part of a quality speech and language evaluation. Prosodic differences that should be considered include:

- Exaggerated intonation.
- Syllable-timed stress patterns.
- Long pauses.
- Monotone.
- Unusual voice quality.
- Idiosyncratic stress patterns at the sentence level.
- Precise articulation of speech sounds.

Parents will often say things like "she talks with an accent" or "he talks in sentences, but it's easier to understand him when he says words."

Fluency and Autism

Fluency refers to the smooth flow of speech, and disfluency is often referred to as stuttering or stammering. A fluency disorder is defined by the American Speech and Hearing Association as *an interruption in the flow of speaking characterized by atypical rate, rhythm, and disfluencies (e.g., repetitions of sounds, syllables, words, and phrases; sound prolongations; and blocks), which may also be accompanied by excessive tension, speaking avoidance, struggle behaviors, and secondary mannerisms.*

Typical disfluencies are considered to occur during the production of the first sound of a word, "l-l-l-l-like this." Recent research by Sisskin found that people with autism demonstrate disfluencies that occur in the middle or at the end of the word. These disfluencies can significantly affect the intelligibility and smoothness of speech. The following are examples of atypical disfluencies:

Types of disfluencies considered atypical:

- MWB: mid-word break [be-come].
- MWR: mid-word repetition [be-e-come].
- BSI: sound insertion (in-word or between-words) [be-uh-come].
- FSR: final sound (or syllable) repetition [become-m-m] [become-ome-ome].
- FSP: final sound prolongation [become-mmm].

These types of disfluencies occur predominantly in people with autism and those with high degree of ADHD. (Sisskin, 2014).

Supports and Recommendations

Language services for those with autism need to include particular attention to the social communicative functions of language (e.g., turn taking, perspective shifting, understanding of inferences) as well as to the nonverbal skills needed to communicate and regulate interaction (e.g., gestures, facial expressions, and body language).

Considering Social Skills

When working on social cognition skills, it is important to be intentional in planning goals and interventions. A meta-analysis of group social skills interventions for autistic youth (Gates et al., 2017) suggested that these interventions led to large increases in social knowledge, but little to no increase in the actual use of expected social skills. It can be more discouraging than helpful when an intervention simply increases awareness of problems without providing suitable solutions. In addition, social skills training often attempts to teach "one-size-fits-all" strategies for fitting in and/or obtaining approval, without consideration for whether these are appropriate goals for the context.

That said, autistic people can often benefit from well-timed and well-tailored support in perspective taking. One area of focus is effectively communicating their intentions; for example, if they want to show support for a grieving friend, then they may benefit from learning scripts and/or nonverbal behaviors that will be readily understood. Learning to interpret body language and indirect communication can help them understand social situations and make informed choices. Safety skills are particularly vital. However, they should not be taught rote responses to others' cues. While it may be helpful to learn about the ways that compromising and conforming can help them to achieve their goals, it is equally important to learn about the benefits of standing up for their own views and accepting the consequences of others' disapproval.

Improving a person's social thinking begins with improving self-awareness. Sensory processing difficulties can contribute to difficulty in this area, for example, having difficulty recognizing one's own anxiety due to lack of body awareness. Autistic individuals may have also received many messages that caused them to doubt their own perception, such as "This food isn't spicy, you're making a big deal about nothing." Only as individuals gain awareness of their own thoughts, emotions, and intentions can they become increasingly aware of the thoughts, emotions, intentions, and actions of others.

It is important to identify specific goals and support needs rather than attempting to approximate typical development across the board. Oftentimes, an unconventional approach may be more suitable for achieving those goals. For example, a client who is distressed by eye contact can be taught to self-advocate by saying "It's hard for me to look at you and listen at the same time." If the goal is to indicate that they are paying attention, they can use more comfortable strategies such as nodding and saying "Uh-huh." It can also be very helpful to explicitly describe and discuss behaviors enacted by NT individuals to gain understanding of why those behaviors occur as a way to inform the autistic individual's possible responses. For example, understanding that a specific group of girls in the class might push each other while engaging in teasing behaviors might help an autistic girl better conceptualize their behaviors, including when pushing is likely to happen and when it is not. This type of explicit explanation is most successful when it is paired with an actual observation rather than an assumption that all people behave similarly (e.g., not all girls engage in pushing or teasing behaviors). Social Stories™ (described later in this chapter) and Comic Strip Conversations, created by Carol Gray (2015), are tools that can help illustrate these concepts.

Project ImPACT

Early intervention models are generally centered around communication and language development. There are many ways to do this. One example of an approach that includes clinicians and parents and is readily available is Project ImPACT (ages 18 months–8 years; Ingersoll & Dvortcsak, 2010). The curriculum teaches parents ways to enhance children's social engagement, communication, imitation, and play skills, within meaningful activities and daily routines (Barber et al., 2020).

Augmentative and Alternative Communication (AAC)

AAC is defined as "an area of clinical practice that supplements or compensates for impairments in speech-language production and/or comprehension, including spoken and written modes of communication." If the child's well-being is impacted by expressive language difficulties, it is recommended that she participate in trials of AAC, including high-tech AAC. Even verbally fluent individuals often benefit from AAC (augmentative and alternative communication), especially when under stress. Strategies such as text-to-speech apps and pointing at pre-written responses can be developed informally by the family, and if more support is needed, then an SLP can conduct a formal assessment.

AAC systems need to include (1) access to high-frequency core words; (2) quick and easy access to words or images for common wants and needs easily accessible, e.g., on the front of the refrigerator; (3) access to the alphabet for literacy; (4) the ability to participate in communication functions beyond requesting; and (5) access to a robust vocabulary in order to meet communication needs as expressive language skills grow.

AAC Sample Core Word list:
1. Again
2. All done
3. Away
4. Big
5. Do
6. Down
7. Get
8. Go
9. Help
10. Here
11. I
12. In
13. It
14. Like
15. Little
16. Mine
17. More
18. My
19. Off
20. On
21. Out
22. Put
23. Some
24. Stop
25. That
26. There

27. Up
28. Want
29. What
30. You

AAC Recommendations

- Continue to support your child's oral communication as one component of her whole communication system, as her use of oral language is at times effective.
- Support your child in using her speech output device during meaningful, functional activities such as playing a game or reading a book.
- Support her in using the speech output device across all school settings (i.e., the child should carry the device to every activity throughout the school day).
- Provide immediate, specific praise for attempts to communicate with the speech output device.
- Whenever the child uses her speech output device, even if unintentionally or her message is unclear, interpret and respond as if it were meaningful communication. This allows the child to learn the cause and effect of communication when using the speech output device.
- Promote a "total communication" approach, meaning you accept everything from written responses/signs/oral speech/communication produced via the speech output device, etc. Honor all effective communication. For example, if modeling on the child's device results in him responding with intelligible communication apart from the AAC system, honor and praise the communication. Always remember: If his message was comprehensible, it is unnecessary to request that they demonstrate it via another mode of communication. In the example above, it would be unnecessary to request that the child repeat the message using his AAC system, though you may follow his message with a model on the AAC device without further expectation.
- Prioritize core vocabulary (see list) when modeling on the child's AAC device during every activity throughout the school day.
- Ensure that the communication device is accessible to the child at all times.
- Aided language stimulation (Communication partner teaches symbol meaning and models language by combining his/her own verbal output with the selection of vocabulary on the AAC system. In other words, the communication partner simultaneously selects vocabulary on the AAC system and speaks).
- Provide the child with a low-tech/backup AAC system (created by the speech-language pathologist) for use when the speech output device is temporarily unavailable.
- Important figures in the autistic person's life can also use strategies to support the child's receptive communication, such as adding a "please reply" icon to their text message if the child has difficulty inferring when a response is expected.

Social Stories™ (3–22 Years)

Social Stories™ were created by Carol Gray in 1991. Social Stories™ are short descriptions of a particular situation, event, or activity, which include specific information about what to expect in that situation and why (Gray, 2015).

Social Stories™ can be used in the following ways:

- Develop self-care skills (e.g., how to clean teeth, wash hands, or get dressed), social skills (e.g., sharing, asking for help, saying thank you, interrupting), and academic abilities.
- Help the child to understand how others might behave or respond in a particular situation.
- Help others understand the perspective of a neurodiverse person and why they may respond or behave in a particular way.
- Help the child to cope with changes to routine and unexpected or distressing events (e.g., absence of teacher, moving house, thunderstorms).
- Provide positive feedback to the child about an area of strength or achievement in order to develop self-esteem.
- As a behavioral strategy (e.g., what to do when angry, how to cope with obsessions).

How do Social Stories™ help?

- Social Stories™ present information in a literal, "concrete" way, which may improve a person's understanding of a previously difficult or ambiguous situation or activity. The presentation and content can be adapted to meet different people's needs.
- They can help with sequencing (what comes next in a series of activities) and executive functioning (planning and organizing).
- By providing information about what might happen in a particular situation and some guidelines for behavior, you can increase structure in the child's life and thereby reduce anxiety.

Example of a Social Story™
Playdate

I am having a playdate.
   It's okay to be worried about the playdate.
   My mom or dad will help me get ready.
   I can put some of my favorite toys in a safe place if I am worried about them breaking or being played with.
   When my friend arrives I can meet her at the door and say, "Hi."
   First, my mom or dad will go over the schedule with us.
   When my friend is at my house, she will have an idea about how she wants to play with things.
   I can use my words to say if I want to play a certain way or to ask her to stop.
   If I get frustrated by something my friend is doing, I can take a deep breath and go tell mom/dad that I need a break.

After the play date, my friend will go home. When she goes home, I can say, "Thank you for playing" and ask to have another playdate soon.

Social Flowcharts (5 and Up)

Flowcharts are diagrams that give a step-by-step approach when learning a new skill. There are a variety of flowcharts available online. You can enter a search for flowcharts on a variety of social skills. teacherspayteachers.com has a variety of options, and a Google search can help you find them as well. You can also create your own using paper and pen or find a template online.

Video Modeling (VM) (2–14 Years)

VM is an intervention that uses video recording to provide a visual model of the targeted behavior or skill. VM is often combined with prompting and reinforcement in order to maximize the child's ability to learn what she has seen. Research has shown that it does not matter if she is watching herself or someone else in the video. The outcome is the same (Bellini & Akullian, 2007).

Types of video modeling include:

- Basic video modeling: recording someone besides the child engaging in the target behavior or skill (i.e., models). The child then views the video at a later time.
- Video self-modeling: record the child displaying the target skill or behavior and watch later.
- Point-of-view video modeling: the target behavior or skill is recorded from the perspective of the child.
- Video prompting: breaking the skill into steps and recording each step with incorporated pauses during which the child attempts the step before viewing subsequent steps. Video prompting may be done with either the child or someone else acting as a model.

VM has been found to be effective in changing many behaviors. However, the behavior or skill must be observable. Examples of observable behaviors include

- Sharing.
- Initiating conversation or requesting.
- Responding to question.
- Playing with others.
- Completing tasks such as washing hands or brushing teeth.
- Exhibiting challenging behaviors or aggression (hitting, biting, scratching, pushing).

Once you have decided the behavior or skill that you want to address, you may need to break the task into smaller steps. For example, washing hands could be broken down into smaller skills to facilitate learning.

Steps/Skills for Washing Hands:

- Step 1 Turn on water.
- Step 2 Wet hand.
- Step 3 Apply soap.
- Step 4 Rub hands together.
- Step 5 Rinse hands.
- Step 6 Dry hands.

Consider using a script. A script tells the model what they need to say or do during the taping process. Scripted responses or verbal behavior may be used to increase the likelihood of video recording appropriately modeled behavior. Scripts should be developed before the video taping process and can be rehearsed a few times prior to the actual recording. Scripted statements are best if they are simple, often consisting of two- or three-word phrases, i.e., "my turn," "clean up," and "bed time."

Videos can range in length depending on the skill or behavior targeted. An ideal length is approximately 2–3 min. Once the video is recorded, take a moment to review what has been recorded. The video may need to be edited to remove any errors, particularly removing prompts or added cues (beyond naturally occurring cues). Voice-overs may be used to further support the video and increase the child's comprehension. Voice-overs might include narration of the steps (e.g., "I wait in line. I use a spoon to take the food I want to eat.") or to describe the target behavior (e.g., child picking up toys).

When the child is viewing the video, consider limiting distractions during video watching and setting up the materials that will be needed for performing the skill immediately following the video. Incorporate the showing of the video into her routine or schedule, for example, if using the video to improve eating, show the video just prior to snack or a meal. If the video shows her washing his hands after using the bathroom, the video should be shown before entering the bathroom.

Once the child is consistently using the target behavior, fade the use of the VM. Fading the video allows her to independently use and maintain the target behavior and allows her to use his newly acquired skill in new situations. You don't want her to become dependent on the video. Use one of the following procedures when fading videos:

- Delaying start or premature stop: By delaying the start of the video or ending it before it is over, less of the video is shown. When the amount of the video is gradually decreased, the child sees less of the video modeling. This procedure is maintained if she continues to use the target behavior successfully. At a certain point, the video can be stopped entirely. Once she can perform the new skill independently, a new video can be made of her actively performing the task successfully (video self-modeling). This video self-modeling is often reinforcing.

- Error correction: This procedure can be used if she continues to make mistakes with certain parts of the target behavior or skill. Only the particular scene where the mistake has been occurring is played for her to re-watch and practice. In the washing hands example, if she correctly performs all the steps except drying them once she is done, then the section of the video that shows drying hands would be the only piece shown. You can also allow her to continue watching the video and point out specific skills that she may have difficulty mastering. Using the washing hands example, you may say "look at how they are drying their hands" when it is demonstrated in the video.

For further information visit the following website: https://asdtoddler.fpg.unc. edu/video-modeling.html. The IRIS Center Video Collection provides some examples. https://www.youtube.com/watch?v=GS9IFwuM_G8.

Treatments for Atypical Disfluency (Sisskin, 2014)

- Identification: Increase the child's awareness of her disfluencies so that she can learn to identify them.
- Self-Monitoring: Mindful attention to disfluencies and developing the ability to self-monitor in the structured therapy setting.
- Pausing/Phrasing: Smoothing out the message by using appropriate pausing, phrasing, and breathing.
- Cancellation: Teach her to stop, pause, reverse, and start over.

Return to the Case Study

Naya's parents effectively used Social Stories™ to help Naya practice safe communication with strangers. With Naya's input on wording and pictures to include, they created a story that described ways Naya could interact with unfamiliar people without sharing personal details. They also collaborated with Naya to create a story that helped her see what types of observational comments she should refrain from sharing in the moment but might want to share personally with parents later. To reinforce these stories, Naya had fun creating videos that brought these stories to life while providing a visual model for how to engage in safe interactions with others. To help increase Naya's verbal intelligibility and minimize dysfluencies, Naya's speech therapist worked with her on pausing and mindfully attending to the words she was saying. Naya's sister and parents reinforced this practice at home. Naya's speech therapist also taught her things to say when she wasn't sure how to answer a question. For example, if her parents asked Naya how school was and Naya didn't have an immediate response, she could say something like "Let me think about that" or "I'm not sure what to say" to allow her additional time to think. Naya's parents and sister also tried to clarify their nonverbal communication by putting in words things they were saying with their gestures and body movements (e.g., agreement/disagreement, emotional responses) while also explicitly sharing with Naya what their nonverbal communication meant (e.g., "this facial expression means that I am feeling x way") (Table 3.1 provides a summary of assessment strategies for communication and language).

Table 3.1 At-a-glance summary of communication and language assessment

Domain	Focus	Assessment planning
Early social communication and language	Norm-referenced measure	*Communication and Symbolic Behavior Scales developmental Profile Behavior Sample* **(CSBS DP):** 6–24 months *Preschool Language Scales, 5th Ed.* **(PLS-5):** Birth–7:11
Early social communication and language	Standardized rating scale for the examiner, parent, or teacher or a combination of	*Communication and Symbolic Behavior Scales Developmental Profile Infant/ Toddler Checklist* (CSBS DP ITC): 6–24 months
Language	Standardized receptive and expressive language assessment	*Preschool Language Scales, 5th Ed.* **(PLS-5):** Birth–7:11 *Bayley Scales of Infant and Toddler Development, 4th Ed.* **(Bayley-4):** 16 days–42 months *Clinical Evaluation of Language Fundamentals-Preschool, 3rd Ed.* **(CELF-P3):** 3–6 years *Clinical Evaluation of Language Fundamentals, 5th Ed.* **(CELF-5):** 5–21 years *Oral and Written Language Scales, 2nd Ed.* **(OWLS-2):** 5–21 years *Test of Language Development-Primary, 5th Ed.* **(TOLD-P:5)** 4 years–8:11 *Test of Language Development-Intermediate, 5th Ed.* **(TOLD-I:5):** 8 years–17:11 **Telehealth options:** **Q-global** (Pearson, 2023a) *Clinical Evaluation of Language Fundamentals-Preschool, 3rd Ed.* **(CELF-P3):** 3–6 years *Clinical Evaluation of Language Fundamentals, 5th Ed.* **(CELF-5):** 5–21 years **Q-interactive** (Pearson, 2023b) *Clinical Evaluation of Language Fundamentals-Preschool, 3rd Ed.* **(CELF-P3):** 3–6 years *Clinical Evaluation of Language Fundamentals, 5th Ed.* **(CELF-5):** 5–21 years

(continued)

Table 3.1 (continued)

Domain	Focus	Assessment planning
Bilingual language	Standardized receptive and expressive language assessment for Spanish-speaking children	*Preschool Language Scales, 5th Ed. Spanish* (**PLS-5 Spanish**): Birth–7:11 *Clinical Evaluation of Language fundamentals Spanish, 4th Ed.* (**CELF-4 Spanish**): 5–21 years *Clinical Evaluation of Language Fundamentals Preschool-2 Spanish* (**CELF P-2 Spanish**): 3 years to 6:11 <u>**Telehealth options:**</u> **Q-global** (Pearson, 2023a) *Clinical Evaluation of Language Fundamentals Spanish, 4th Ed.* (**CELF-4 Spanish**): 5–21 years *Clinical Evaluation of Language Fundamentals Preschool-2 Spanish* (**CELF P-2 Spanish**): 3 years to 6:11
Narrative language	Norm-referenced test	*Test of Narrative Language, 2nd Ed.* (**TNL-2**): 5 years–15:11
Pragmatic	Standardized rating scale for the examiner, parent, or teacher or a combination of	*Bayley Scales of Infant and Toddler Development, 4th Ed. Social-Emotional Questionnaire* (**Bayley-4 SEQ**): 16 days–42 months *Clinical Evaluation of Language Fundamentals-Preschool, 3rd Ed. Descriptive Pragmatic Profile* (**CELF-P3 DPP**): 3–6 years *Clinical Evaluation of Language Fundamentals, 5th Ed. Pragmatic Profile* (**CELF-5 PP**): 5–21 years *Children's Communication Checklist, 2nd Ed.* (**CCC-2**):4–18 years
Pragmatic	Standardized pragmatic language assessment	*Test of Pragmatic Language, 2nd Ed.* (**TOPL-2**): 6 years–18:11 *Clinical Evaluation of Language Fundamentals, 5th Ed. Metalinguistics* (**CELF-5 Metalinguistics**): 9 years–21:11 *Social Emotional Evaluation* (**SEE**): 6 years to 12:11 *Social Language Development Test-Elementary: Normative Update* (**SLDT-E:NU**): 6 years–11:11 *Social Language Development Test-Adolescent: Normative Update* (**SLDT-A: NU**): 12 years–17:11

References

Barber, A. B., Swineford, L., Cook, C., & Belew, A. (2020). Effects of Project ImPACT parent-mediated intervention on the spoken language of young children with autism spectrum disorder. *Perspectives of the ASHA Special Interest Groups*, 1–9. https://doi.org/10.1044/2020_PERSP-20-10005

Bayley, N., & Aylward, G. P. (2019). *The Bayley Scales of Infant and Toddler Development, 4th Ed. Technical manual*. Pearson.

Bellini, S., & Akullian, J. (2007). A meta-analysis of video modeling and video self- modeling interventions for children and adolescents with autism spectrum disorders. *Exceptional Children, 73*, 264–287. https://doi.org/10.1177/001440290707300301

Bishop, D. (2006). *Children's Communication Checklist-2*. Pearson.

Bone, D., Bishop, S., Gupta, R., Lee, S., & Narayanan, S. S. (2016). Acoustic-prosodic and turn-taking features in interactions with children with neurodevelopmental disorders. *Proc. Interspeech, 2016*, 1185–1189. https://doi.org/10.21437/Interspeech.2016-1073

Bowers, L., Huisingh, R., & LoGiudice, C. (2016). *Social Language Development Test–Elementary: Normative update*. Pro-Ed.

Bowers, L., Huisingh, R., & LoGiudice, C. (2017). *Social Language Development Test–Adolescent: Normative update*. Pro-Ed.

Cohen, T. (2017). *Six-word lessons on female Asperger syndrome: 100 lessons to understand and support girls and women with Asperger's*. Pacelli Publishing.

Conlon, O., Volden, J., Smith, I. M., et al. (2019). Gender differences in pragmatic communication in school-aged children with *autism spectrum disorder* (ASD). *Journal of Autism and Developmental Disorders, 49*, 1937–1948. https://doi.org/10.1007/s10803-018-03873-2

Eaton, L. (2012). Under the radar and behind the scenes: The perspectives of mothers with daughters on the autism spectrum. *Good Autism Practice (GAP), 13*(2), 9–17.

Eigsti, I. M., de Marchena, A. B., Schuh, J. M., & Kelley, E. (2011). Language acquisition in autism spectrum disorders: A developmental review. *Research in Autism Spectrum Disorders, 5*(2), 681–691. https://doi.org/10.1016/j.rasd.2010.09.001

Eigsti, I.-M., & Schuh, J. M. (2017). Language acquisition in ASD: Beyond standardized language measures. In L. R. Naigles (Ed.), *Innovative investigations of language in autism spectrum disorder* (pp. 183–200). Walter de Gruyter GmbH; American Psychological Association. https://doi.org/10.1037/15964-010

Gates, J. A., Kang, E., & Lerner, M. D. (2017). Efficacy of group social skills interventions for youth with autism spectrum disorder: A systematic review and meta-analysis. *Clinical Psychology Review, 52*, 164–181.

Gilliam, R. B., & Pearson, N. A. (2017). *Test of Narrative Language, Second Edition*. Western Psychological Services.

Gray, C. (2015). *The new social story book, revised and expanded 15th anniversary edition: Over 150 social stories that teach everyday social skills to children and adults with autism and their peers*. Future Horizons.

Hendrickx, S. (2015). *Women and girls with autism spectrum disorder: Understanding life experiences from early childhood to old age*. Jessica Kingsley.

Ingersoll, B., & Dvortcsak, A. (2010). *Teaching social communication to children with autism: A practitioner's guide to parent training*. The Guilford Press.

King, D., & Palikara, O. (2018). Assessing language skills in adolescents with autism spectrum disorder. *Child Language Teaching and Therapy, 34*(2), 101–113. https://doi.org/10.1177/0265659018780968

Lawson, L. P., Joshi, R., Barbaro, J., et al. (2018). Gender differences during toddlerhood in autism spectrum disorder: A prospective community-based longitudinal follow-up study. *Journal of Autism and Developmental Disorders, 48*, 2619–2628. https://doi.org/10.1007/s10803-018-3516-y

NCS Pearson, Inc. (2023a). *Q-global™ web-based administration, scoring, and reporting*. Author. https://qglobal.pearsonclinical.com/

NCS Pearson, Inc. (2023b). *Q-interactive Assess App*. Author. https://qiactive.com/

Miller, J. K. (Ed.). (2015). *Women from another planet? Our lives in the universe of autism*. AuthorHouse.

Mitchell, S., Oram Cardy, J., & Zwaigenbaum, L. (2011). Differentiating autism spectrum disorder from other developmental delays in the first two years of life. *Developmental Disabilities Research Reviews, 17*(2), 130–140. https://doi.org/10.1002/ddrr.1107

Phelps-Terasaki, D., & Phelps-Gunn, T. (2007). *Test of Pragmatic Language, Second Edition*. Western Psychological Services.

Sisskin, V., & Wasilus, S. (2014). Lost in the literature, but not the caseload: Working with atypical disfluency from theory to practice. *Seminars in Speech and Language, 35*(2), 144–152. https://doi.org/10.1055/s-0034-1371757. Epub Apr 29.

Sturrock, A., Marsden, A., Adams, C., & Freed, J. (2020). Observational and reported measures of language and pragmatics in young people with autism: A comparison of respondent data and gender profiles. *Journal of Autism and Developmental Disorders, 50*(3), 812–830. https://doi.org/10.1007/s10803-019-04288-3

Wetherby, A., & Prizant, B. (2002). *Communication and Symbolic Behavior Scales Developmental Profile—First normed edition*. Baltimore.

Wiig, E. H. (2008). *Social Emotional Evaluation*. Western Psychological Services.

Wiig, E.H., Secord, W.A., Semel, E. (2013) *Clinical Evaluation of Language Fundamentals, Fifth Edition*. Pearson.

Wiig, E. H., & Secord, W. A. (2014). *Clinical Evaluation of Language Fundamentals, Fifth Edition. Metalinguistics*. Pearson.

Wiig, E. H., Secord, W. A., & Semel, E. (2020). *Clinical Evaluation of Language Fundamentals, Preschool-3*. Pearson.

Willey, L. H. (2014). *Pretending to be normal: Living with Asperger's syndrome (autism spectrum disorder) expanded edition*. Jessica Kingsley.

Zimmerman, I. L., Steiner, V. G., & Pond, R. E. (2011). *Preschool Language Scales, Fifth Edition*. Pearson.

Chapter 4
Assessment for Sleep, Feeding, Sensory Issues, and Motor Skills in Females with Autism

Introduction

Sensory sensitivities and aversions are possibly one of the more overlooked autistic traits at any age. In young children they may seem to be an oddity or quirkiness. In adults, they are easily dismissed as irrelevant to possible mental health issues—perhaps because it seems to have a biological underpinning. In the first-person literature, sensory issues (primarily sensitivities) are pervasive in the daily lives of women and have a significant impact on quality of life. Sleep, eating and motor skills issues are similarly often pushed to the side as not part of the current issues someone may be seeking help for. This may also be to a lack of awareness of ways to capture or measure the significance of these issues. It may also be that clinicians neglect to ask about these issues.

> *I have major problems with light [...] I do not like unexpected touch and will flinch, push away or go rigid when others touch me [...] Smells make me retch, quiet noises like leaves rustling or birds tweeting engulf my brain. However, I do feel blessed because although the unpleasant stuff is heightened, so is the good stuff. Certain music makes my brain dance [...] I feel very attached and deeply moved by the beauty of nature too. Woman with autism*
> (Hendrickx, 2015, p. 134)

Case Study—Jill: Selective Eating; Sensitivities to Food Textures, Sound, and Light; Resists Motor Activities; and Very Light Sleeper

Jill is a 9-year-old girl who enjoys reading graphic novels, watching anime, and drawing fan art of her favorite characters. Although her parents have tried to engage her in various sports, Jill struggles with body coordination, and she

© The Author(s), under exclusive license to Springer Nature Switzerland AG 2023
T. P. Gabrielsen et al., *Assessment of Autism in Females and Nuanced Presentations*, https://doi.org/10.1007/978-3-031-33969-1_4

strongly dislikes team-based sports. Jill's parents describe her as an extremely "picky" eater. She refuses to try unfamiliar foods, and she has a strong resistance to foods with strong flavors or smells, soft or chewy textures, and bright colors. She will gag or throw up if forced to eat such foods. Jill has always struggled with lunchtime at school. The overwhelming sounds and smells of the cafeteria can induce intense emotional reactions. Jill has difficulty getting to sleep in the presence of any light or sound, and she wakes frequently through the night. Even when attempts are made to keep the room quiet and dark, Jill complains that her mind is filled with sounds and images that keep her awake. When she was younger, she would often enter her parents' bedroom at all hours of the night, saying that she couldn't sleep.

In the newest version of the *Diagnostic and Statistical Manual of Mental Disorders*, 5th Ed., Text Revision (DSM-5-TR; American Psychiatric Association [APA], 2022), more information is given about specifiers in an autism diagnosis, including that conditions that have long been considered "just part of" autism can and should be listed as additional diagnoses to guide treatment planning and intervention to improve outcomes. Feeding and sleep disorders are specifically listed as examples, as are attention-deficit/hyperactivity disorder (ADHD), anxiety, and depression. Weir et al. (2021) found that even into adulthood, autistic individuals, particularly females, have difficulty developing healthy eating, exercise, and sleep practices, which have inevitable effects on quality of life. If these issues can be addressed more effectively earlier in life, the possibility of improved quality of life and lifespan may be possible.

Sleep

First Person Narratives

> Our sensitivity to sound as well as touch strongly affects our sleep habits and many of us can't catch 40 winks without earplugs and noiseless, heavy blankets. Because we have minds like recorders, even hearing a song before bed means it might play over and over again, robbing us of our rest. We have to limit what we take in and we must be selective. A lot of these triggers, perhaps all of them, exist only in relation to our lack of control over them. (Simone, 2010, p. 37)

> My fear system is always on the alert for danger....Volume has nothing to do with the fear factor; the association with a possible threat does. Human voices are associated with a possible threat....A plane could land on the hotel and I wouldn't wake up. But people talking in the next room? Forget it. I might as well turn on the light and read, because I know I'm not going to go to sleep until they go to sleep. (Grandin & Panek, 2013, p. 32)

> I want to talk a bit about routine. My most dominant emotion is stress. I deal with my stress best by planning every single thing that goes on with my life. If I don't, I often forget to do

things, as big as attend meetings to as little as forgetting to eat or sleep. I feel I need structure for control in my life and also to remember all of the things most humans can't forget. If I don't plan when to eat, sleep and go to the bathroom, I won't. I have always had so much to do that it always feels like I don't have enough time to do anything. Doing anything is hard, but having it planned out is less hard. @paigelayle (2021)

Sleep problems associated with autism may be one of the least debated, but also possibly the least understood, features. Sleep issues significantly impact quality of life even into adulthood (McLean et al., 2021) and are a top priority for parents (McConachie et al., 2018). Specific causes for sleep problems related to autism are not known, and there may be multiple reasons for gender differences in sleep. One theory is that genetic differences alter circadian rhythms (Tye et al., 2019), suggesting that genetics related to gender may be important considerations.

The associations with sleep differ somewhat across studies, but there are consistent findings indicating more sleep problems associated with anxiety and depression in autistic females (Hartley & Sikora, 2009; Horiuchi et al., 2014). One intriguing line of research is looking at sleep problems in childhood that continue into adulthood, with additional focus on menopause (Croen et al., 2015; Mosely et al., 2020; Nicolaidis et al., 2014). See Chaps. 9 and 12 for more details on lifelong effects of sleep problems and Chap. 8 about anxiety. While overall prevalence rates are consistently reported to be high (Bauman, 2010; Hyman et al., 2020; Lai et al., 2019), thanks to large datasets, such as SPARK (Simons Foundation Powering Autism Research for Knowledge), differences by gender are beginning to be better understood. Sleep problems in this very large SPARK dataset (20% female) include overall strong associations with severity of behavioral problems. Females had more special interests and stimming behaviors correlated with sleep problems (Saré & Smith, 2020). This may not be true of all females, however, especially those with less significant repetitive behaviors who nevertheless have sleep problems. Asking specific (not open-ended) questions about sleep in detail can provide valuable information for treatment and supports.

Feeding/Eating

First Person Narratives

At this young age, it may be difficult to distinguish typical child phases and fads from something more complex and indicative of autistic-type behaviours, and as a standalone behaviour, this would not be in any way conclusive. Combined with other indicators, however, the child's behaviour around food can add weight to a potential diagnosis. (Hendrickx, 2015, p. 69)

I wasn't just being a picky eater (for example, I wouldn't eat if different foods touched each other), but that I was incapable of eating certain foods....Once my sensory issues were considered, things just became better for me. Mallory Cruz (Ballou et al., 2021, p. 158)

Please see Chap. 10 for more details about eating disorders in adolescents and adults. The focus of this section is on feeding disorders in younger children. A recent systematic review found the prevalence of feeding/eating disorders to include 51–89% of autistic children (Page et al., 2021). The odds of a feeding disorder in autistic children are as high as five times that of neurotypical children (Sharp et al., 2013). There are no studies found in that review, however, without the traditional male bias (4:1 ratios, male/female). This is surprising, given the much higher prevalence of subsequent eating disorders in autistic females. Sharp and colleagues took the further step of looking at nutritional intake and found significantly lower intake of both calcium and protein in the studies, both of which have long-term health implications unique to females in terms of maternal health and possible risk of injury in advanced age. One study found emotion-linked food approach behaviors to be more common in girls than boys in an autistic population, but not in neurotypical children, despite general population studies showing adult females present with more emotional eating than adult males. These behaviors included both overeating and undereating, with overeating more common in females (Wallace et al., 2021). Emotional eating was described as eating behaviors in the presence of heightened, especially negative, emotions. Stress was cited as a particularly relevant factor. Gastrointestinal difficulties that may lead to feeding disorders were reported in 9–90% of autistic children across studies (Buie et al., 2010). Both overeating and undereating were shown to be more prevalent in autistic girls than autistic boys, suggesting that feeding disorders may be a part of a female autism phenotype (van't Hof et al., 2020). Unfortunately, multiple and significant health concerns are reported for severe feeding disorders (Bourne et al., 2022).

Most autism population studies of feeding and eating disorders in childhood (independent of gender) focus on selective intake of food, which is a feeding problem, as well as problematic mealtime behaviors that may or may not restrict eating. Prevalence rates as high as 72% of autistic children with selective food intake have been reported. Possible reasons for feeding difficulties can include sensory sensitivity, which can involve visual presentation as well as taste and smell (Hubbard et al., 2014; Mayes & Zickgraf, 2019; Nadon et al., 2011; Nisticò et al., 2022), limited food preferences, and neophobia or fear of trying new foods (Baraskewich et al., 2021). Gut discomfort related to constipation or other gut disorders can also contribute to food selectivity. Rituals and idiosyncratic eating behaviors were also reported as impacting feeding (Bourne et al., 2022; Mayes & Zickgraf, 2019). In several studies, use of some nutritional supplementation was found to have some positive behavioral effect according to parent report (Narsizi et al., 2021).

While conventional wisdom may suggest that lower IQ and adaptive skills are associated with increased feeding problems (Postorino et al. 2015), most recent studies have not found cognitive performance to be associated with feeding issues, and few have found lower adaptive skills to be correlated (Bitsika & Sharpley, 2018;

Mayes & Zickgraf, 2019). Transition difficulties, rigidity, and restrictive and repetitive behaviors have been correlated with feeding difficulties, however (Postorino et al., 2015; Wallace et al., 2021). Some suggest that autism exacerbates feeding and eating disorders, but might not actually be the origin (Inoue et al., 2021). Conventional wisdom may also suggest that nutritional deficiencies would be associated with lower BMI, but one study found the opposite to be true—higher BMI was found to be associated with more nutritional deficiencies (Shmaya et al., 2015).

About two-thirds of feeding problems decline over time, even by age 6. Trajectories of feeding disorders have been characterized as less severe and stable (27%), moderate and declining over time (39%), severe and declining (27%), and very severe and stable (8%) (Peverill et al., 2019). Severely selective intake *not* associated with body image or fear of weight gain is now identified in the DSM-5-TR and the Interntional Statistical Classification of Diseases and Related Health Problems, 11th Revision (ICD-11), as avoidant/restrictive food intake disorder (ARFID; APA, 2022). There is considerable debate over whether ARFID is a feeding disorder (as described above) or an eating disorder (described below). Feeding problems unique to autism also overlap considerably with ARFID, with sensory issues (primarily texture) as the most cited association (Bourne et al., 2022). Pica (eating things that are not food) and rumination behaviors (regurgitating food with or without vomiting) may also be considered feeding disorders, but they are fairly obvious traits that usually bring attention to the child's differences, prompting early evaluation.

Eating disorders (cognitive concerns related to weight, shape, and/or body image) are seldom studied in autistic children. Baraskewich et al. (2021) conducted a scoping review, and although eating disorder studies were small in number compared to feeding disorder, preliminary evidence suggests higher risk for autistic people to develop eating problems compared to persons without autism. See Chap. 10 for more on eating disorders.

Sensory

First Person Narratives

> *In my world, there is non-stop sensory bombardment (touch, sound, light, taste). Every social encounter requires constand decoding and then selection of an appropriate response. I have preprogrammed/learned behaviors for church, meals, restaurants, casual, semi-casual, format situations. With these programs as a cover-up, I am able to accomplish much that is considered normal, successful, desirable. But this is a shell, and within it I'm bombarded and puzzled. Knowing I'm Aspie has encouraged me to choose a shell that is more selective and also harder. -Toni Sano* (Miller et al., 2015, p. 295)

> *Generally, I just wish that adults, who in this case were strangers, would've asked me why I was crying, or at least told my mother to ask me. I think that it would have been easier for me to learn how best to cope with sensory issues if adults would have asked me questions instead of making constant assumptions. – Dusya Lyubovskaya* (Ballou et al., 2021, p. 37)

My body fights it with its own output, and it is exhausting. I grow tired from trying to handle the sensory input from my environment; it might be a knot in my stomach, heavy breathing, or distracting my senses otherwise. Getting to explain this made more sense to an outsider than just having these feelings in a random moment. – Haley Moss (Ballou et al., 2021, p. 80)

Sensory sensitivities underlie many of the difficulties encountered in daily life of up to 90% of children with autism, including sensory issues affecting sleep and feeding (Page et al., 2021; Taylor et al., 2020). Sex and gender differences have been found across different aspects of sensory sensitivity that should be assessed specifically to guide supports. Autistic females (on average) show considerably more sensory sensitivity than autistic males and neurotypical children in areas such as hearing/sound, balance, motion, light, and touch (Eckerd, 2020; Gesi et al., 2021; Osorio et al., 2021). Sensory traits do not fade over time but persist into adulthood more commonly with autistic females than autistic males. Because females also tend to have better socio-communication abilities, their positive traits may overshadow some of the sensory issues that may be affecting their quality of life (Lai et al., 2011). Tsuji et al. found sensory sensitivities persisting into adulthood to be associated with more internalizing disorders which may also overshadow identification (2022). Although one of the more consistent traits reported throughout the first-person narratives, sensory sensitivities may be one of the least apparent or least recognized autistic traits in nuanced cases. Gesi et al. (2021) found higher sensory issues in females than males who were misdiagnosed (not correctly identified with autism), consistent with other reports of female sensory sensitivity not being believed or being misinterpreted.

Sensory issues (sometimes referred to as sensory overload) nevertheless are a primary trait that can interfere with daily function and social interaction. When asked to name the main barriers to school inclusion for autistic girls, sensory overwhelm/overload was listed as something that isolates autistic girls or makes it so they aren't able to be successful (or sometimes even attend school) (Sproston et al., 2017). Miller et al. found, even into adulthood, autistic females reported the need to suppress sensory sensitivities in order to camouflage, mask, or "pass" as typical, which eventually takes a toll on the individual (2021).

Sensory sensitivities can have detrimental effects on not just comfort but performance across settings. Sensory seeking is also a significant issue. They have been found to affect focus and attention in academic settings (Mallory & Keehn, 2021).

"The sensory issues are just, it's the most difficult thing in the world and it's so distressing and it really does make a difference between I think um having life quality or not for me – FF18." (Milner et al., 2019, p. 2397). *"Scratching, picking, rubbing and plucking hairs all featured as typical sensory behaviours. Many of these are not regarded as particularly unusual per se, but it is their intensity and frequency that demonstrate a difference."* (Hendrickx, 2015, p. 133)

Please see Chap. 9 for more about sensory sensitivities related to pregnancy, childbirth, breastfeeding, parenting, and menopause and Chap. 12 regarding sexuality.

Marcia Eckerd, an experienced autism clinician, describes sensory issues in females as something that the person is acutely aware of, but their defensive behaviors are not interpreted correctly by others. A sensory crisis or even avoidance episode may look like defiance, perhaps because the person is not explaining the problem well. She/they may also try to explain the sensitivity, but it is less likely to be believed, as it is unexpected (Eckerd, 2020). It is also possible that general autism assessment measures might not capture sensory sensitivities in females, as their individual or unique sensitivity may not be asked about (Øien et al., 2018b). Sensory screening is specifically recommended in the most recent American Academy of Pediatrics (AAP) guidelines for the identification, evaluation, and management of children with autism (Hyman et al., 2020). Finally, more readily recognized sensory differences have been found in addition to proprioception and vestibular issues, so if one is present, assess for the others (Tang et al., 2021).

Misophonia is a condition in which individuals experience intense anger and disgust when they are confronted with sounds made by other human beings. In particular, sounds like chewing, lip smacking, or breathing may cause intense anger (Schröder et al., 2019).

For those who struggle with misophonia, the distraction is immediate, and the fury can be overwhelming. The reaction to the stimulus leads to perseverative thoughts, and it becomes increasingly difficult to pay attention.

Having misophonia can be isolating since many social interactions are rife with human sounds. Avoiding places like movie theaters, restaurants, or in-person classes limits opportunities for social interaction.

For people with misophonia, identifying personal situations where they know they will be triggered can be helpful. For example, if your partner enjoys slurping their cereal at breakfast, it is probably best to eat breakfast at a different time and instead take a shower or go outside and pull weeds. Noise-canceling headphones, white noise, and calming sounds can be helpful.

Motor Skills

Kopp and Gillberg (1992) described mild motor delays present in a small sample of young girls whose diagnoses were delayed until after age 6. From that early finding to the present, Craig et al. (2020) generated a hypothesis that motor skills might be the core feature for sex differences in autism. In a relatively small but gender-balanced sample of 2–7-year-olds, fine motor skills were predictive of social impairment in males, but that did not hold true for females, who exhibited better social skills in this study. This suggested that female fine motor skills were not necessarily correlated with social skills. Messinger et al. (2015) cast some doubt on this hypothesis, finding sex differences to be consistent across autistic and neurotypical groups, but measurement methods and targets vary significantly across studies. These two examples represent the wide range of findings regarding motor skills in females—results are not consistent across different methodologies and samples. Samples with low representation of females show no differences or better fine motor skills in females (Mandy et al., 2012).

Consensus is further clouded by varied definitions of motor skills and bias in reporting. Frazier et al. (2014) found delayed gross motor coordination in females, but indicated the possibility of gender expectation bias in raters. Some studies included gestures as motor skills (Rynkiewicz et al., 2016); others analyzed repetitive motor skills (de Marchena & Miller, 2017), while still others considered "clumsiness" (Matheis et al., 2019), and in yet others, brain areas associated with motor function were measured and compared with distinct differences attributed to sex (Jack et al., 2021). Analysis of large datasets to allow for matched controls and gender balance in the samples showed gray matter differences in motor areas of the brain to be not only different in females but associated with social areas and restricted and repetitive behaviors (RRB) areas (Supekar & Menon, 2015). In a study of false-negative results on parent-reported autism screens, the "missed" females had more pronounced motor skill differences at age 18 months than their male peers (Øien et al., 2018a). Carter et al. (2007) found similarly less-developed motor skills in female toddlers. As Craig et al. (2020) suggested, motor skills may be one of the more important areas to focus on in assessment.

Although definitive conclusions may be obscured in a wide range of studies, some common themes arise. Special interests and stimming behaviors (also referred to as restricted and repetitive behaviors) are commonly associated with motor skills, but other correlations were found with social behaviors. Predictive factors were not consistent across studies related to motor skills, but the frequent associations with other skills and functions illustrate the importance of focusing on motor skills as interconnected with other autistic traits. Also, physical activity levels (dependent on motor skills) are associated with sleep, behavior, depression, anxiety, and constipation. In the majority of studies, motor skills differed between genders; therefore, expectations of motor abilities or deficits derived from predominantly male samples should not be expected to apply to females in the same ways.

Assessment Planning for Sleep, Feeding, Sensory Issues, and Motor Skills

Each of the topics in this chapter is easy to overlook in assessment, as they are not well-covered in typical comprehensive evaluation measures. They are also not specifically mentioned in the diagnostic criteria with the exception of sensory issues as one of the optional criteria in the DSM-5-TR (APA, 2022). Each of these issues is likely to be interconnected, as has been shown above. Assessment practices and measures tend not to be interconnected, so assessment planning needs to connect these areas, yet not extend the assessment process unnecessarily.

Interviews

A good intake interview is a low-cost way to include the assessment of these issues which are more likely to be found in females and/or the nuanced type of autism. Adding some questions to your standard intake process can guide further assessment of severity and characteristics of the issues and how much they impact quality of life. Open-ended questions (e.g., "How is her/your sleep?") may yield valuable information, but be sure to follow up with a more closed response question, especially if you are interviewing the client/student themselves (e.g., "What time did you go to sleep last night?" and, then, "When did you wake up?"). This specific type of question (applied across all of these domains) can be easier to answer and may be less vulnerable to responder bias.

Observations

Observations may not yield much information for sleep or feeding differences, but sensory interests are likely to appear on some measures, and it is possible you may observe sensory seeking or avoidant behaviors throughout your assessment processes. Adaptive and general development measures often have a motor domain, but some do not have normative ranges beyond early elementary years. Overall developmental measures are not designed to do much more than screen, however, and may not be sensitive enough to pick up on a motor delay, increasing the need for observation. Motor issues are the characteristic you may have multiple opportunities to observe throughout your assessment process if you are aware of them and provide multiple activities that may elicit gross and fine motor skills. If scores *or* observations suggest a need for more detailed assessment, physical therapists or occupational therapists should be consulted.

Gross Motor:

- Meet the client in the waiting room or classroom, and notice their gait as they walk with you to the exam room.
- If possible, take breaks that include walking or more active physical activities (including running for children).
- If you have stairs in your setting, find an excuse to go up and down to observe gross motor (e.g., on a break).
- Choose an exam room with enough floor space to observe gait if possible, or include motor assessment (see below) in hallways, gyms, or outdoors in your setting.
- Toss a ball, beanbag, or other object (e.g., small bag of snacks) during assessment.
- Ask that a similar object be tossed to you at some point.

Fine Motor:

- Cognitive and developmental measures often provide opportunities for writing or coloring—note the pencil/crayon grip and control in drawing, writing, or coloring tasks.
- Provide a quick break with coloring or drawing materials (including the ADOS-2 "Break" materials; Lord et al., 2012a, b).
- Small snack bags are opportunities to observe fine motor skill (opening and accessing).
- Peeling stickers/placing stickers on a page can also show fine motor skills.

Interpreting Standardized Measures for Females

Gendered norms are possible in some measures, but not common. Check the manual of developmental and adaptive measures for separate norms by gender. If not, be careful about the interpretation of skills, and note that gendered norms were not available. Females may be more or less advanced than male peers in some areas at some developmental stages, but any differences in sleep, feedings, sensory, or motor domains, regardless of normative samples, should be noted and addressed in recommendations.

Additional Measures to Inform the Assessment Process

If you are in an interdisciplinary setting and any of these issues are reported, observed, or suspected, consult with related professionals (physical therapists and occupational therapists for motor; speech and pediatrics for feeding; pediatrics and sleep medicine for sleep; and occupational therapists for sensory issues) for additional assessment resources. If consultation and/or diagnostic support from these professionals cannot be accomplished within the timeframe of your assessment, consider a recommendation for additional evaluation from these professionals. They may also be able to guide you to questionnaires or measures that are within your training to inform the diagnosis and possible treatment options. See Table 4.1 for some commonly used measures and practices in each of the domains.

Supports and Recommendations

Because sleep, feeding, sensory, and motor/physical activity are often interconnected, the most effective treatment modalities are interdisciplinary. Because these are characteristics that are most often seen at home, parent/family-led intervention plans are also most likely to be successful (Bourne et al., 2022).

Sleep

The Lancet Commission on the Future of Care and Clinical Research in Autism (Lord et al., 2022) reported that parent education, sleep hygiene, and development of independence are the first-line interventions, followed by melatonin if help is still needed. Not all countries support the use of sleep medications.

- For severe sleep issues, consult with healthcare providers about sleep specialist care, including possibly a sleep study.
- Consultation with a sleep specialist can also improve long-term sleep problems. See https://www.behavioralsleep.org/ for providers, helps, and more information.
- Sleep toolkits are available from autism organizations, and several well-researched books on sleep issues and autism are readily available.
- Sleep hygiene practices are also easily available from multiple sources, but many are aimed at adult sleep hygiene, which may not be helpful for insomnia of childhood.
- Physical activity during the day also improves multiple aspects of sleep (Tse et al., 2019).

Feeding/Eating

- Rule out physiological causes of feeding disorder through medical evaluation (e.g., oral/motor or swallowing problems, delayed gastric emptying, gastro-esophageal reflux disease (GERD) current or by history, genetic disorders, allergies, failure to thrive, etc.).
- Rule out chronic constipation or other causes of gut discomfort (may require medical rule out—simple questioning may not be sufficient).
- Appropriate treatment specialists vary by age, type of feeding/eating disorder, and availability in your area. Online treatment options are becoming more available even if providers are not within feasible distance.
- Feeding clinicians often focus on children. Anxiety-reducing and/or sensory approaches are the more common types of interventions. Avoidant/restrictive food intake disorder (ARFID) may be the diagnosis for children or adults who restrict either variety or volume of food intake such that their nutrition is insufficient for maintaining growth or weight. Look for feeding or feeding and swallowing clinics in your area. Professionals in this area include autism professionals, speech and language pathologists, nutritionists, psychologists, and occupational therapists.
- Treatment for anxiety is often indicated in cases of ARFID.
- Eating disorders are often associated with older children, adolescents, and adults with anorexia nervosa and bulimia as common diagnoses. Diagnostic criteria for

these conditions, however, all revolve around perceptions of weight and/or body image, which may or may not be present in autistic clients. This may result in ineffective treatment approaches if autism is not identified to inform behavior change strategies and thinking patterns.

- Pica is a distinct eating disorder characterized by eating non-food items that is sometimes associated with autism. Treatment is typically provided by autism specialists, but often healthcare providers are also involved to test for or intervene in subsequent adverse events. Pica can occur in adults or children over the age of 2.
- Mealtimes are typically social events, which further complicates feeding and eating problems. Attention to social eating behaviors can be included in treatment approaches to increase enjoyment of meals (e.g., Kuschner et al., 2007).
- It is also important to evaluate nutritional deficiencies that may be associated with eating/feeding disorders. Nutritionists and healthcare providers need to be involved to help determine the severity of the problem and appropriate treatments.

Sensory Issues (Recommendations Primarily from Mallory and Keehn, 2021)

- Sensory accommodations in academic and classroom environments (as well as work environments) can help autistic individuals and other students.
- Sound-dampening strategies can include wall and floor materials that absorb sound or noise-dampening earphones/earbuds or earplugs when no instruction is being given. Quiet places for test-taking are recommended.
- Changing lighting conditions or adapting by blocking light can reduce distraction (including the *sound* of fluorescent lighting). Although caps/hats with bills are prohibited in some schools, that is one example of reducing light distraction on an individual basis. Natural light sources are generally better tolerated.
- Reduce visual stimuli on the walls if necessary, but relevant visual helps should remain.
- Consider reducing other sources of sensory input (i.e., changing proximity to vents, windows, doors, odors, echoing).
- Allow for alternate seating options if sitting in a standard chair is excessively difficult.
- Teach the use of a personal social story—explaining to teachers, professors, and employers "I work best when …" to advocate for adaptations when needed. No explanation or disclosure of diagnosis is required, and the focus is on self-advocacy. See Chapter 13 for more about personal social stories.

Motor

- Consider referral for gross motor (often physical therapists) or fine motor (often occupational therapists) assessment and intervention. Improving motor skills can reduce social isolation and improve function, health, and self-concept.
- Increased moderate to vigorous physical activity levels can positively impact overall health, sleep, digestion, social participation, and quality of life.
- Normalize motor differences in physical education (PE) classes to avoid the possibility of bullying and shaming. This can include asking for additional skill development practice from PE teachers and/or different PE class settings or groupings. Physical therapists in schools can assist in multiple ways.
- Allow for alternate paths to PE credit in schools or fitness programs in adults. Reducing embarrassment about differences can increase lifelong enjoyment of physical activity and health. Online, private, or out-of-the-ordinary physical activities may be better suited than general PE or fitness offerings. Martial arts (e.g., Phung & Goldberg, 2019), yoga (Semple, 2018), and other individual activities that also include social interaction can be considered (e.g., horseback riding, dance, table tennis, golf, aquatics, and weight training).

Return to the Case Study

In Jill's case, it will be important for her parents to help her find a variety of nutritional options that don't trigger sensory reactions. Empowering her with the knowledge and self-advocacy skills to make well-rounded choices that fit with her sensory needs will go a long way toward developing healthy eating habits. Jill's sensory differences also impact her beyond her food choices. They impact her opportunities to participate in physical, social, and academic activities. Jill's parents and teachers can support Jill by helping to adjust her environment, when appropriate, to minimize the distraction and discomfort sensory differences can cause. They can also work with Jill to come up with strategies that help her cope with unwanted sensory input in settings where it isn't feasible to make changes. While it may make sense to allow Jill to sit with a few others in a quieter space during lunch, for example, it may not be possible to reduce the noise level of discussion in a group project in the classroom. It's important that Jill's parents and teachers involve Jill in these discussions to the extent that she would like to be involved, because she is the only person who can decide what is truly working for her. Jill's motor development may benefit from participation in non-competitive, individualized sports or low-stakes motor activities (e.g., taking a walk outside, playing hopscotch for fun), which can improve sleep, eating, and overall well-being. Jill's parents are unable to keep her room completely free of sensory input, so finding other ways to support healthy sleep is necessary. Consulting with a provider who specializes in autism and sleep in children can help Jill's parents discover other strategies to support healthy sleep.

Table 4.1 At-a-glance summary for sleep, feeding, sensory, and motor assessment

Domain	Focus	Assessment planning
Sleep	Ask about details of sleep Time of sleep onset Time of waking Quality of sleep Regularity of sleep Routines and supports necessary for sleep Barriers to sleep Changes in sleep in lifetime (or persistent sleep patterns) For 2–4-year-olds, difficulty settling to sleep at bedtime, nighttime awakenings, restlessness during sleep, and daytime tiredness distinguished autistic from typically developing children (Hatch et al., 2021)	Consult with a healthcare provider about the assessment of medical causes for sleep difficulties Interview using closed-ended questions (e.g., "what time did you go to sleep last night?" instead of "how is your sleep?") Sleep diary https://www.nhlbi.nih.gov/resources/sleep-diary *Pediatric Sleep Questionnaire* (**PSQ**): ages 2–18 (Chervin et al., 2000) *Children's Sleep Habits Questionnaire* (**CSHQ**): ages 4–10 (Owens et al., 2000); see Hatch et al. (2021) for ages 2–4 *Children's Sleep Habits Questionnaire-ASD* (**CSHQ-ASD**): ages 4–10 (Katz et al., 2018) *Sleep Disturbance Scale for Children* (**SDSC**): ages 6–15 (Bruni et al., 1996; see Romeo et al. (2021) for children under 3) *Pediatric Daytime Sleepiness Scale* (**PDSS**): ages 11–15 (Drake et al., 2003) *Pittsburgh Sleep Quality Index* (**PSQI**): adults (Buysse et al., 1989) *Insomnia Severity Index* (**ISI**): adults (Bastien et al., 2001)
Sleep impairment	Effects of sleep irregularity on everyday performance	*Epworth Sleepiness Scale*, Child and Adolescent and Adult Versions (Johns, 2021; see Packard et al. (2021) for gender and racial differences)
Feeding	Ask about variety and volume Ask where children are on the growth chart (World Health Organization charts for under 2 years, CDC charts for 2 and up)	**Consult with a healthcare provider to assess medical reasons for gut discomfort** Interview Feeding diary https://www.cdc.gov/healthyweight/pdf/food_diary_cdc.pdf Children's eating behavior questionnaire https://www.ucl.ac.uk/epidemiology-health-care/sites/epidemiology-health-care/files/cebqwithscore.pdf all

Eating disorder or avoidant/restrictive food intake disorder (ARFID) (see Chap. 10 for more on eating disorders in adults and adolescents)	Avoid focusing on indicators such as body image or body mass index for diagnosis, which may not be good indicators for someone with autism Think both ways—Does this autistic person also have a feeding disorder? Also, if you have a client with a feeding disorder, is it possible they may have autism?	Eating Disorder Examination – Questionnaire *EDE-Q exist and are available online. See Chap. 10* *Children's Eating Disorder Examination-Questionnaire* (**ChEDE-Q8**): ages 7–18 (best for ages 8–14) (Kliem et al., 2017)
Sensory	Sensory interests are highlighted in most first-person reports; may be "mainstream" in terms of the interest, but more intense than neurotypical sensory interests	**Interview:** Ask specifically about sensory issues Observation: Watch for signs of sensitivity in assessment sessions *Sensory profile 2 (SP-2):* Birth to 14:11 *SP2 infant toddler:* 7–35 Mos. *SP2 child:* 3:0-14:11 *SP2 school:* 3:0-14:11 *SP2 short:* 3:0-14:11 Spanish avail. *Adult/Adolescent Sensory profile:* 15+ (Dunn, 2002, 2014)
Fine motor—Early development	Fine motor delays may be mild, but fairly easy to measure at this age	*Beery-Buktenica Visual Motor Integration, 6th Ed.* (**VMI**): 2:0–99:11 (Beery et al., 2010) *Mullen Scales of Early Learning* (**MSEL:** Fine Motor subtest): birth–68 months (Mullen, 1995) *Bayley Scales of Infant and Toddler Development, 4th Ed.* (**Bayley-4**) 16 days–42 months (Fine Motor subtest) (Bayley & Aylward, 2019)

(continued)

Table 4.1 (continued)

Domain	Focus	Assessment planning
Fine motor—School age through adulthood	Fine motor delays may be evident in writing difficulties, self-care routines, etc. and may be more evident to the individual than the observer. Fine motor difficulties may be a source of stress and possibly low self-esteem for some individuals.	*Beery-Buktenica Visual Motor Integration, 6th Ed.* (**VMI**): 2:0–99:11 (Beery et al., 2010) Writing samples and observations **Keep in mind that screening measures may not be sensitive to all motor issues and an assessment by a physical therapist or occupational therapist may still be needed if motor issues are observed or reported, but are not coming up on screening or general developmental measures**
Gross motor	Development and skill levels vary widely by opportunity, so examination of opportunities available for skill development may be warranted if concerns are reported	*Mullen Scales of Early Learning* (**MSEL**: Gross Motor subtest): birth–68 months (Mullen, 1995) *Bayley Scales of Infant and Toddler Development, 4th Ed.* (**Bayley-4**): 16 days–42 months (Gross Motor subtest) (Bayley & Aylward, 2019) *Vineland Adaptive Behavior Scales, 3rd Ed.* (**Vineland-3**) comprehensive interview or parent report (birth–age 7 norms avail.) (Sparrow et al., 2016) **Observations and parent and teacher reports** *In-depth evaluations are through occupational or physical therapists*

Please see the "References" section in this chapter for additional information on measures.

Not all measures and processes listed are available in all settings or appropriate for all cases. Qualification levels apply. Multiple measures in a single domain are not necessary. Some measures can provide data in multiple domains. This is meant to provide a relatively quick reference for assessment planning and implementation, not an endorsement of any particular measure as "best." Emphasis here is on readily available, commonly used measures, but similar measures may also be useful.

References

American Psychiatric Association (2022). Diagnostic and statistical manual of mental disorders, Fifth Ed., Text revision.

@paigelayle (2/6/21) Instagram https://www.instagram.com/p/CK9rkLJpGqg/

Bauman, M. L. (2010). Medical comorbidities in autism: Challenges to diagnosis and treatment. *Neurotherapeutics, 7*(3), 320–327. https://doi.org/10.1016/j.nurt.2010.06.001

Ballou, E. P., da Vanport, S., & Onaiwu, M. G. (Eds.). (2021). *Sincerely, your autistic child.* Beacon Press.

Baraskewich, J., con Raonson, K.M, McCrimmon, A., & McMorrise, C. A. (2021). Feeding and eating problems in children and adolescents with autism: A scoping review. *Autism, 25*(6), 1505–1519. https://doi.org/10.1177/1362361321995631

Bastien, C. H., Vallières, A., & Morin, C. M. (2001). Validation of the Insomnia Severity Index as an outcome measure for insomnia research. *Sleep Medicine, 2*(4), 297–307. https://doi.org/10.1016/s1389-9457(00)00065-4

Bayley, N., & Aylward, G. (2019). *Bayley Scales of Infant and Toddler Development.* Pearson.

Beery, K.E., Butkenica, N.A., Beery, N.A. (2010) *Beery-Buktenica Developmental Test of Visual-Motor Integration, Sixth Edition.* Western Psychological Services.

Bitsika, V., & Sharpley, C. F. (2018). Using parent-and self-reports to evaluate eating disturbances in young girls with autism spectrum disorder. *International Journal of Developmental Neuroscience, 65*, 91–98. https://doi.org/10.1016/j.ijdevneu.2017.11.002

Bourne, L., Mandy, W., & Bryant-Waugh, R. (2022). Avoidant/restrictive food intake disorder and severe food selectivity in children and young people with autism: A scoping review. *Developmental Medicine and Child Neurology, 64*(6), 691–700. https://doi.org/10.1111/dmcn.15139

Bruni, O., Ottaviano, S., Guidetti, V., Romoli, M., Innocenzi, M., Cortesi, F., & Giannotti, F. (1996). The Sleep Disturbance Scale for Children (SDSC). Construction and validation of an instrument to evaluate sleep disturbances in childhood and adolescence. *Journal of Sleep Research, 5*(4), 251–261. https://doi.org/10.1111/j.1365-2869.1996.00251.x

Buie, T., Campbell, D. B., Fuchs, G. J., 3rd, Furuta, G. T., Levy, J., Vandewater, J., Whitaker, A. H., Atkins, D., Bauman, M. L., Beaudet, A. L., Carr, E. G., Gershon, M. D., Hyman, S. L., Jirapinyo, P., Jyonouchi, H., Kooros, K., Kushak, R., Levitt, P., Levy, S. E., et al. (2010). Evaluation, diagnosis, and treatment of gastrointestinal disorders in individuals with ASDs: A consensus report. *Pediatrics, 125*, S1–S18. https://doi.org/10.1542/peds.2009-1878C

Buysse, D. J., Reynolds, C. F. I. I. I., Monk, T. H., Berman, S. R., & Kupfer, D. J. (1989). The Pittsburgh Sleep Quality Index: A new instrument for psychiatric practice and research. *Psychiatry Research, 28*, 193213. https://doi.org/10.1016/0165-1781(89)90047-4

Carter, A. S., Black, D. O., Tewani, S., Connolly, C. E., Kadlec, M. B., & Tager-Flusberg, H. (2007). Sex differences in toddlers with autism spectrum disorders. *Journal of Autism and Developmental Disorders, 37*(1), 86–97. https://doi.org/10.1007/s10803-006-0331-7

Chervin, R. D., Hedger, K., & Dillon, J.e., Pituch, K.J. (2000). Pediatric Sleep Questionnaire (PSQ): Validity and reliability of scales for sleep-disordered breathing, snoring, sleepiness, and behavioral problems. *Sleep Medicine, 1*(1), 21–32. https://doi.org/10.1016/s1389-9457(99)00009-x

Craig, F., Crippa, A., De Giacomo, A., Ruggiero, M., Rizzato, V., Lorenzo, A., Fanizza, I., Margari, L., & Trabacca, A. (2020). Differences in developmental functioning profiles between male and female preschoolers children with autism spectrum disorder. *Autism Research, 13*(9), 1537–1547. https://doi.org/10.1002/aur.2305

Croen, L. A., Zerbo, O., Qian, Y., Massolo, M. L., Rich, S., Sidney, S., & Kripke, C. (2015). The health status of adults on the autism spectrum. *Autism, 19*(7), 814–823. https://doi.org/10.1177/1362361315577517

de Marchena, A., & Miller, J. (2017). "Frank" presentations as a novel research construct and element of diagnostic decision-making in autism spectrum disorder. *Autism Research, 10*(4), 653–662. https://doi.org/10.1002/aur.1706

Drake, C., Nickel, C., Burduvali, E., Roth, T., Jefferson, C., & Pietro, B. (2003). *The Pediatric Daytime Sleepiness Scale* (PDSS): Sleep habits and school outcomes in middle-school children. *Sleep, 26*(4), 455–458. https://doi.org/10.1093/sleep/26.4.455

Dunn, W. (2014). *Sensory Profile 2.* Pearson.

Dunn, W. (2002). *Adult/adolescent Sensory Profile.* Pearson.

Eckerd, M. (2020). Detection and diagnosis of ASD in females. *Journal of Health Service Psychology, 46*(1), 37–47. https://doi.org/10.1007/s42843-020-00006-1

Fairburn, C., Cooper, Z., & O'Conner, M. (2014). Eating Disorder Examination. Edition 17.0D https://www.corc.uk.net/media/1951/ede_170d.pdf

Frazier, T. W., Georgiades, S., Bishop, S. L., & Hardan, A. Y. (2014). Behavioral and cognitive characteristics of females and males with autism in the Simons Simplex Collection. *Journal of the American Academy of Child & Adolescent Psychiatry, 53*(3), 329–340. https://doi.org/10.1016/j.jaac.2013.12.004

Gesi, C., Migliarese, G., Torriero, S., Capellazzi, M., Omboni, A. C., Cerveri, G., & Mencacci, C. (2021). Gender differences in misdiagnosis and delayed diagnosis among adults with autism spectrum disorder with no language or intellectual disability. *Brain Sciences, 11*(7), 912. https://doi.org/10.3390/brainsci11070912

Grandin, T., & Panek, R. (2013). *The autistic brain: Helping different kinds of minds succeed.* Mariner Books.

Hartley, S. L., & Sikora, D. M. (2009). Sex differences in autism spectrum disorder: An examination of developmental functioning, autistic symptoms, and coexisting behavior problems in toddlers. *Journal of Autism and Developmental Disorders, 39*(12), 1715. https://doi.org/10.1007/s10803-009-0810-8

Hatch, B., Nordahl, C. W., Schwichtenberg, A. J., Ozonoff, S., & Miller, M. (2021). Factor structure of the Children's Sleep Habits Questionnaire in young children with and without autism. *Journal of Autism and Developmental Disorders, 51*(9), 3126–3137. https://doi.org/10.1007/s10803-020-04752-5

Hendrickx, S. (2015). *Women and girls with autism spectrum disorder: Understanding life experiences from early childhood to old age.* Jessica Kingsley.

Horiuchi, F., Oka, Y., Uno, H., Kawabe, K., Okada, F., Saito, I., & Ueno, S. I. (2014). Age-and sex-related emotional and behavioral problems in children with autism spectrum disorders: Comparison with control children. *Psychiatry and Clinical Neurosciences, 68*, 542–550. https://doi.org/10.1111/psc.12164

Hubbard, K. L., Anderson, S. E., Curtin, C., Must, A., & Bandini, L. G. (2014). A comparison of food refusal related to characteristics of food in children with autism spectrum disorder and typically developing children. *Journal of the Academy of Nutrition and Dietetics, 114*(12), 1981–1987. https://doi.org/10.1016/j.jand.2014.04.017

Hyman, S. L., Levy, S. E., & Myers, S. M. (2020). Identification, evaluation and management of children with autism spectrum disorder. *Pediatrics, 145*(1), e20193447. https://doi.org/10.1542/peds.2019-3447

Inoue, T., Otani, R., Iguchi, T., Ishii, R., Uchida, S., Okada, A., Kitayama, S., Koyanagi, K., Suzuki, Y., Suzuki, Y., Sumi, Y., Takamiya, S., Tsurumaru, Y., Nagamitsu, S., Fukai, Y., Fujii, C., Matsuoka, M., Iwanami, J., Wakabayashi, A., Sakuta, R., et al. (2021). Prevalence of autism spectrum disorder and autistic traits in children with anorexia nervosa and avoidant/restrictive food intake disorder. *BioPsychoSocial Med, 15*(9), 1–11. https://doi.org/10.1186/s13030-021-00212-3

Jack, A., Sullivan, C. A. W., Aylward, E., Bookheimer, S. Y., Dapretto, M., Gaab, N., Horn, J. D. V., Eilbott, J., Jacokes, Z., Torgerson, C. M., Bernier, R. A., Geschwind, D. H., McPartland, J. C., Nelson, C. A., Webb, S. J., Pelphrey, K. A., Gupta, A. R., Consortium, the G., Van Horn, J. D., & GENDAAR Consortium. (2021). A neurogenetic analysis of female autism. *Brain: A Journal of Neurology, 144*(6), 1911–1926. https://doi.org/10.1093/brain/awab064

Johns, M. (2021). *The Epworth Sleepiness Scale and the Epworth Sleepiness Scale for Children and Adolescents.* https://epworthsleepinessscale.com/

Katz, T., Shui, A. M., Johnson, C. R., Richdale, A. L., Reynolds, A. M., Scahill, L., et al. (2018). Modification of the Children's Sleep Habits Questionnaire for children with autism spectrum disorder. *Journal of Autism and Developmental Disorders, 48,* 2629–2641. https://doi.org/10.1007/s10803-018-3520-2

Kliem, S., Schmidt, R., Vogel, M., Hiemisch, A., Kiess, W., & Hilbert, A. (2017). An 8-item short form of the Eating Disorder Examination-Questionnaire adapted for children (ChEDE-Q8). *The International Journal of Eating Disorders, 50*(6), 679–686. https://doi.org/10.1002/eat.22658

Kopp, S., & Gillberg, C. (1992). Girls with social deficits and learning problems: Autism, atypical Asperger syndrome or a variant of these conditions. *European Child & Adolescent Psychiatry, 1*(2), 89–99. https://doi.org/10.1007/BF02091791

Kuschner, E. S., Morton, H. E., Maddox, B. B., de Marchena, A., Anthony, L. G., & Reaven, J. (2007). The BUFFET program: Development of a cognitive behavioral treatment for selective eating in youth with autism spectrum disorder. *Clinical Child and Family Psychology Review, 20*(4), 403–421. https://doi.org/10.1007/s10567-017-0236-3

Lai, M.-C., Kassee, C., Besney, R., Bonato, S., Hull, L., Mandy, W., Szatmari, P., & Ameis, S. H. (2019). Prevalence of co-occurring mental health diagnoses in the autism population: A systematic review and meta-analysis. *The Lancet Psychiatry, 6*(10), 819–829. https://doi.org/10.1016/S2215-0366(19)30289-5

Lai, M.-C., Lombardo, M. V., Pasco, G., Ruigrok, A. N. V., Wheelwright, S. J., Sadek, S. A., Chakrabarti, B., & Baron-Cohen, S. (2011). A behavioral comparison of male and female adults with high functioning autism spectrum conditions. *PLoS One, 6*(6). https://doi.org/10.1371/journal.pone.0020835

Lord, C., Charman, T., Havdahl, A., Carbone, P., Anagnostou, E., Boyd, B., Carr, T., de Vries, P. J., Dissanayake, C., Divan, G., Freitag, C. M., Gotelli, M. M., Kasari, C., Knapp, M., Mundy, P., Plank, A., Scahill, L., Servili, C., Shattuck, P., . . . McCauley, J. B. (2022). The Lancet Commission on the future of care and clinical research in autism. *Lancet, 399*(10321), 271–334. https://doi.org/10.1016/S0140-6736(21)01541-5

Lord, C., Luyster, R. J., Gotham, K., & Guthrie, W. (2012a) *Autism Diagnostic Observation Schedule, 2nd Edition,* Toddler Module. Western Psychological Services.

Lord, C., Rutter, M., Di Lavore, P. C., Risi, S., Gotham, K., & Bishop, S. L. (2012b). *Autism Diagnostic Observation Schedule, 2nd Edition,* Modules. Western Psychological Services.

Mallory, C., & Keehn, B. (2021). Implications of sensory processing and attentional differences associated with autism in academic settings: An integrative review. *Frontiers in Psychiatry, 12,* 695825. https://doi.org/10.3389/fpsyt.2021.695825

Mandy, W., Chilvers, R., Chowdhury, U., Salter, G., Seigal, A., & Skuse, D. (2012). Sex differences in autism spectrum disorder: Evidence from a large sample of children and adolescents. *Journal of Autism and Developmental Disorders, 42*(7), 1304–1313. https://doi.org/10.1007/s10803-011-1356-0

Matheis, M., Matson, J. L., Hong, E., & Cervantes, P. E. (2019). Gender differences and similarities: Autism symptomatology and developmental functioning in young children. *Journal of Autism and Developmental Disorders, 49*(3), 1219–1231. https://doi.org/10.1007/s10803-018-3819-z

Mayes, S. D., & Zickgraf, H. (2019). Atypical eating behaviors in children and adolescents with autism, ADHD, other disorders, and typical development. *Research in Autism Spectrum Disorders, 64,* 76–83. https://doi.org/10.1016/j.rasd.2019.04.002

McConachie, H., Livingstone, N., Morris, C., Beresford, G., & Le Couteur, A., Gringras, P. Garland, D. Jones, D., Macdonald, G., Williams, K., & Parr, J. R. (2018). Parents suggest which indicators of progress and outcomes should be measured in young children with autism spectrum disorder. *Journal of Autism and Developmental Disorders, 48,* 1041–1051. https://doi.org/10.1007/s10803-017-3282-2

McLean, K. J., Eack, S. M., & Bishop, L. (2021). The impact of sleep quality on quality of life for autistic adults. *Research in Autism Spectrum Disorders, 88,* 1–9. https://doi.org/10.1016/j.rasd.2021.101849

Miller., J.K. (ed.) 2015. *Women from another planet? Our lives in the universe of autism.* AuthorHouse.

Miller, D., Rees, J., & Pearson, A. (2021). "Masking is life": Experiences of masking in autistic and nonautistic adults. *Autism in Adulthood, 3*(4), 330–338. https://doi.org/10.1089/aut.2020.0083

Milner, V., McIntosh, H., Colvert, E., & Happé, F. (2019). A qualitative exploration of the female experience of autism spectrum disorder (ASD). *Journal of Autism & Developmental Disorders, 49*(6), 2389–2402. https://doi.org/10.1007/s10803-019-03906-4

Moseley, R. L., Druce, T., & Turner-Cobb, J. M. (2020). 'When my autism broke': A qualitative study spotlighting autistic voices on menopause. *Autism: The International Journal of Research and Practice, 24*(6), 1423–1437. https://doi.org/10.1177/1362361319901184

Mullen, E. M. (1995). *Mullen Scales of Early Learning*. Pearson.

Nadon, G., Feldman, D. E., Dunn, W., & Gisel, E. (2011). Association of sensory processing and eating problems in children with autism spectrum disorders. *Autism Research and Treatment, 541926*. https://doi.org/10.1155/2011/541926

Narzisi, A., Masi, G., & Grossi, E. (2021). Nutrition and autism spectrum disorder: Between false myths and real research-based opportunities. *Nutrients, 13*(6), 2068. https://doi.org/10.3390/nu13062068

Nicolaidis, C., Kripke, C. C., & Raymaker, D. (2014). Primary care for adults on the autism spectrum. *Medical Clinics, 98*(5), 1169–1191. https://doi.org/10.1016/j.mcna.2014.06.011

Nisticò, V., Faggioli, R., Tedesco, R., Giordano, B., Priori, A., Gambini, O., & Demartini, B. (2022). Brief report: Sensory sensitivity is associated with disturbed eating in adults with autism spectrum disorders without intellectual disabilities. *Journal of Autism and Developmental Disorders*. https://doi.org/10.1007/s10803-022-05439-9

Øien, R. A., Schjølberg, S., Volkmar, F. R., Shic, F., Cicchetti, D. V., Nordahl-Hansen, A., Stenberg, N., Hornig, M., Havdahl, A., Øyen, A.-S., Ventola, P., Susser, E. S., Eisemann, M. R., & Chawarska, K. (2018a). Clinical features of children with autism who passed 18-month screening. *Pediatrics, 141*(6), 1–10. https://doi.org/10.1542/peds.2017-3596

Øien, R. A., Vambheim, S. M., Hart, L., Nordahl-Hansen, A., Erickson, C., Wink, L., Eisemann, M. R., Shic, F., Volkmar, F. R., & Grodberg, D. (2018b). Sex-differences in children referred for assessment: An exploratory analysis of the Autism Mental Status Exam (AMSE). *Journal of Autism & Developmental Disorders, 48*(7), 2286–2292. https://doi.org/10.1007/s10803-018-3488-y

Osorio, J. M. A., Rodríguez-Herreros, B., Richetin, S., Junod, V., Romascano, D., Pittet, V., Chabane, N., Jequier, Gygax, M., & Maillard, A. M. (2021). Sex differences in sensory processing in children with autism spectrum disorder. *Autism Research*, 1–12. https://doi.org/10.1002/aur.2580

Owens, J. A., Spirito, A., & McGuinn, M. (2000). The Children's Sleep Habits Questionnaire (CSHQ): Psychometric properties of a survey instrument for school-aged children. *Sleep, 23*(8), 1043–1051. https://doi.org/10.1007/s10803-020-04752-5

Packard, A., Bautista, R., Smotherman, C., & Gautham, S. (2021). Gender differences in Epworth Sleepiness Scale revealed by paired patient-spouse scoring. *Epilepsy & Behavior, 114*(Pt A), 107272. https://doi.org/10.1016/j.yebeh.2020.107272

Page, S. D., Souders, M. C., Kral, T. V. E., Chao, A. M., & Pinto-Martin, J. (2021). Correlates of feeding difficulties among children with autism spectrum disorder: A systematic review. *Journal of Autism and Developmental Disorders, 5*, 1–20. https://doi.org/10.1007/s10803-021-04947-4

Peverill, S., Smith, I. M., Duku, E., Szatmari, P., Mirenda, P., Vaillancourt, T., Volden, J., Zwaigenbaum, L., Bennett, T., Elsabbagh, M., Georgiades, S., & Ungar, W. J. (2019). Developmental trajectories of feeding problems in children with autism spectrum disorder. *Journal of Pediatric Psychology, 44*, 988–998. https://doi.org/10.1093/jpepsy/jsz033

Phung, J. N., & Goldberg, W. A. (2019). Promoting executive functioning in children with autism Spectrum disorder through mixed martial arts training. *Journal of Autism and Developmental Disorders, 49*, 3669–3684. https://doi.org/10.1007/s10803-019-04072-3

Postorino, V., Sanges, V., Giovagnoli, G., Fatta, L. M., De Peppo, L., Armando, M., et al. (2015). Clinical differences in children with autism spectrum disorder with and without food selectivity. *Appetite, 92*, 126–132. https://doi.org/10.1016/j.appet.2015.05.016

Rynkiewicz, A., Schuller, B., Marchi, E., Piana, S., Camurri, A., Lassalle, A., & Baron-Cohen, S. (2016). An investigation of the 'female camouflage effect' in autism using a computerized ADOS-2 and a test of sex/gender differences. *Molecular Autism, 7*(1), 10. https://doi.org/10.1186/s13229-016-0073-0

Romeo, D. M., Cordaro, G., Macchione, E., Venezia, I., Brogna, C., Mercuri, E., & Bruni, O. (2021). Application of the Sleep Disturbance Scale for Children (SDSC) in infants and toddlers (6-36 months). *Sleep Medicine, 81*, 62–68. https://doi.org/10.1016/j.sleep.2021.02.001

Saré, R. M., & Smith, C. B. (2020). Association between sleep deficiencies with behavioral problems in autism spectrum disorder: Subtle sex differences. *Autism Research: Official Journal of the International Society for Autism Research.* Advance online publication. https://doi.org/10.1002/aur.2396

Schröder, A., van Wingen, G., Eijsker, N., San Giorgi, R., Vulink, N. S., Turbyne, C., & Denys, D. (2019). Misophonia is associated with altered brain activity in the auditory cortex and salience network. *Scientific Reports, 9*, 7542. https://doi.org/10.1038/s41598-019-44084-8

Semple, R. J. (2018). Review: Yoga and mindfulness for youth with autism spectrum disorder: Review of the current evidence. *Child and Adolescent Mental Health, 24*(1), https://doi.org/10.1111/camh.12295

Sharp, W., Berry, R., McCracken, C., Nuhu, N., Marvel, E., Saulnier, C., Klin, A., Jones, W., & Jaquess, D. (2013). Feeding problems and nutrient intake in children with autism spectrum disorders: A meta-analysis and comprehensive review of the literature. *Journal of Autism & Developmental Disorders, 43*(9), 2159–2173. https://doi.org/10.1007/s10803-013-1771-5

Shmaya, Y., Eilat-Adar, S., Leitner, Y., Reif, S., & Gabis, L. (2015). Nutritional deficiencies and overweight prevalence among children with autism spectrum disorder. *Research in Developmental Disabilities, 38*, 1–6. https://doi.org/10.1016/j.ridd.2014.11.020

Simone, R. (2010). *Aspergirls: Empowering females with Asperger syndrome.* Jessica Kingsley.

Sparrow, S. S., Cicchetti, D. V., & Saulnier, C. A. (2016). *Vineland Adaptive Behavior Scales: Third Edition* (Vineland-3). NCS Pearson.

Sproston, K., Sedgewick, F., & Crane, L. (2017). Autistic girls and school exclusion: Perspectives of students and their parents. *Autism and Developmental Language Impairments, 2*. https://doi.org/10.1177/2396941517706172

Supekar, K., & Menon, V. (2015). Sex differences in structural organization of motor systems and their dissociable links with repetitive/restricted behaviors in children with autism. *Molecular Autism, 6*(1), 1–13. https://doi.org/10.1186/s13229-015-0042-z

Tang, J. W., Li, J. W., Baulderstone, D., & Jeyaseelan, D. (2021). Presenting age and features of females diagnosed with autism spectrum disorder. *Journal of Paediatrics & Child Health, 57*(8), 1182–1189. https://doi.org/10.1111/jpc.15417

Taylor, E., Holt, R., Tavassoli, T., Ashwin, C., & Baron-Cohen, S. (2020). Revised scored Sensory Perception Quotient reveals sensory hypersensitivity in women with autism. *Molecular Autism, 11*(18). https://doi.org/10.1186/s13229-019-0289-x

Tse, C. Y. A., Lee, H. P., Chan, K. S. K., Edgar, V. B., Wilkinson-Smith, A., & Lai, W. H. E. (2019). Examining the impact of physical activity on sleep quality and executive functions in children with autism spectrum disorder: A randomized controlled trial. *Autism, 23*(7), 1699–1710. https://doi.org/10.1177/1362361318823910

Tsuji, Y., Matsumoto, S., Saito, A., Imaiszumi, S., Yamazaki, Y., Kobayashi, T., Fujiwara, Y., Omori, M., & Sugawara, M. (2022). Mediating role of sensory differences in the relationship between autistic traits and internalizing problems. *BMC Psychol, 10*, 148. https://doi.org/10.1186/s40359-022-00854-0

Tye, C., Runicles, A. K., Whitehouse, A. J., & Alvares, G. A. (2019). Characterizing the interplay between autism spectrum disorder and comorbid medical conditions: An integrative review. *Frontiers in Psychiatry, 9*, 751. https://doi.org/10.3389/fpsyt.2018.00751

van't Hof, M., Ester, W. A., Serdarevic, F., van Berckelaer-Onnes, I., Hillegers, M. H. J., Tiemeier, H., Hoek, H. W., & Jansen, P. W. (2020). The sex-specific association between autistic traits and eating behavior in childhood: An exploratory study in the general population. *Appetite, 147*, 104519. https://doi.org/10.1016/j.appet.2019.104519

Wallace, G. L., Richard, E., Wolff, A., Nadeau, M., & Zucker, N. (2021). Increased emotional eating behaviors in children with autism: Sex differences and links with dietary variety. *Autism: The International Journal of Research and Practice, 25*(3), 603–612. https://doi. org/10.1177/1362361320942087

Wardle, J., Guthrie, C. A., Sanderson, S., & Rapoport, L. (2001). Development of the Children's Eating Behavior Questionnaire. *Journal of Child Psychology and Psychiatry, 42*(7), 963–970. https://doi.org/10.1111/1469-7610.00792

Weir, E., Allison, C., Ong, K. K., & Baron-Cohen, S. (2021). An investigation of the diet, exercise, sleep, BMI, and health outcomes of autistic adults. *Molecular Autism, 12*(1), 31. https://doi. org/10.1186/s13229-021-00441-x

Chapter 5
Autism Assessment of Female Social Skills, Play, Imitation, Camouflaging, Intense Interests, Stimming Behaviors, and Safety

Introduction

One of the impacts of the male bias in autism research (see Chap. 1) is that the context in which a child, adolescent or adult is evaluated is treated as if it is universal across genders. This is not likely to be true. Gender bias is discussed in Chapter 1, but the different social worlds inhabited by different genders is an important consideration in the diagnostic or identification process. Male clinicians are certainly capable of accurate diagnoses of females with autism, but their expertise must be well-informed by female input regarding the context in which a girl is growing up.

> *"Autistic girls may be able to mimic certain aspects of play and social skills, but the learning curve in the girl world is steep. "* -*Karen Lean* (Ballou et al., 2021, p. 52)

Case Study—Kyra: Outgoing, Active Imagination, and Special Interest in Observing and Analyzing Peers

When Kyra was 5 years old, her parents described her as having been very social. They noted that she would frequently walk up to children on the playground and try to engage with them, and she was "always in the group." Parents felt Kyra had a "rich inner life," and she was described as very imaginative. They didn't recall any unusual or intense interests or behaviors when she was younger. When Kyra, who was now 12 years old, was asked about her experiences with friendships, she described feeling like she knew how to "make the first move" in meeting peers, but she wasn't sure what to do after that. She identified several peers she considered friends whom she had known since elementary school, but she didn't see them outside the school setting. Kyra further described a lot of time spent watching her peers interacting with one another. She said she was like a "scientist" who was studying

T. P. Gabrielsen et al., *Assessment of Autism in Females and Nuanced Presentations*, https://doi.org/10.1007/978-3-031-33969-1_5

"kids in the wild." She explained that she started doing this close study of peers in fourth grade because she began to see that sometimes children would purposefully be mean to other children. She was on the receiving end of this behavior more than once, and she wanted to understand why. Kyra decided it was "safer" to be an observer, and she credited her observations with helping her "avoid trouble at school." Although Kyra still enjoys spending time with her friends during school hours, she prefers to spend time alone in her imagination outside of school.

Social Skills

First Person Narratives

> *Autism makes me very unique, and in principle I don't mind being different. I know I am very capable and very intelligent in a unique way. I just wish I had the social skills to be able to do something good with that set of skills. Woman with autism* (Hendrickx, 2015, p. 122)

> *Like many females on the spectrum, I am very sensitive to the untouchable feelings of others. I can walk into a room of strangers and within moments, be drawn to the person in the most psychological pain.* (Willey, 2012, p. 65)

> *Emily: It feels like in my classroom that I'm surrounded by lions… I feel like a mouse and everyone else is like a giant cat or something.* (Tierney et al. 2016)

> *My days were filled with: exhaustion, insomnia, depression, anger, obsessive-compulsive disorder, chronic panic attacks (meltdowns), migraines, stress, anxiety, self-inflicted psychological abuse, low self-esteem, paranoia, unhealthy relationships, distrust of most people because I didn't fully understand social interaction or social cues, emotional confusion, constant frustration due to misunderstanding social situations. -Anonymous* (Ballou et al., 2021, p. 154)

Very early social communication skills may differ between genders, even in infancy. Early eye-tracking studies document differences in siblings with a high likelihood of autism. Male high-likelihood infants looked more at mouths than other males or high-likelihood females did, but high-likelihood females looked *less* at mouths than female controls did (Kleberg et al., 2019). Harrop et al. (2019) found similar results for faces in general, with autistic females paying more attention to faces in a parallel play scenario than autistic males, and comparable to neurotypical males overall. Other studies suggest that toddler/preschool-age females showed less-developed social communication than their male counterparts at the same ages. This may not necessarily be true of all very young females with autism, however, as only parents with existing concerns about their daughters were included in the study (Ros-Demarize et al., 2020). The opposite has also been found—there are far fewer differences in social skills across genders at very young ages, specifically for children participating in autism evaluations, i.e., during the Autism Diagnostic Observation Schedule, 2nd Ed. (ADOS-2; Lord et al., 2012). No differences were found across genders *in a clinically referred sample* at ages 14–30 months with 28% of participants who were female (Ronkin et al., 2021).

A commonality in these studies of very young children is that the females may not be as well-represented in the samples as males and that they are clinical samples in which concerns have already been noticed and evaluation has already been sought. Females with advanced skills in this age range, or less noticeable social differences for whatever reason, may not be represented by these findings. On the other hand, perhaps if we had been able to evaluate girls or effectively screen a wider range of girls, their social differences might have been more evident earlier than at later ages after camouflaging behaviors have begun to develop. This is included in the DSM-5-TR discussion of autism, which explains that core diagnostic features are evident in early development, but compensation, intervention, and supports may mask the magnitude of difficulties in some, but not all, contexts (APA, 2022).

By school age, teachers may have a harder time picking up on autistic traits in females, reporting fewer concerns about social skills and externalizing behaviors (Hiller et al., 2014). Teachers are less likely to associate autism with observed or reported traits when the student is female vs. male and are dramatically less likely to bring concerns to the school psychologist for females, even with the same traits and behaviors as males (Whitlock et al., 2020). Teacher reports and school observations may also not indicate some behaviors at school because of strong gender expectations for following rules (Simcoe et al., 2022). Compared to males with autism spectrum disorder, females may have stronger reciprocal conversation and be more likely to share interests, integrate verbal and nonverbal behavior, and modify their behavior by situation, despite having similar social understanding difficulties as males (Lai et al., 2015).

Evidence of empathy may also affect the consideration of an autism diagnosis for females. Standard autism assessment measures often rate the lack of empathy or identification of emotions in others as an autistic trait (Lord et al., 2012, LeCouteur et al., 2003). Pre-adolescent autistic females were shown to provide empathetic support and emotional comfort when presented with someone who was hurt—more than their autistic male peers but less than allistic females. This is consistent with overall patterns of more emotionally empathetic responses from females than males regardless of autism status (Rieffe et al., 2021). Empathy is mentioned as a positive aspect of autism by adult women (Milner et al., 2019), which may be a barrier to diagnosis if clinicians assume that the presence of empathy means the person is not autistic (Belcher et al., 2022; Rieffe et al., 2021).

In older autistic girls, or females identified at older ages, Head et al. (2014) documented significantly higher scores on the Friendship Questionnaire in autistic females vs. autistic males and further found autistic female social skills to be roughly equivalent to typically developing boys. Some have suggested that more than one observation of social skills will be necessary to get a true picture of skills and inclusion or exclusion (Barnes et al., 2018). It is also possible that camouflaging behavior or imitating abilities may increase positive perceptions of social skills such as conversation. Sasson et al. (2017) concluded that if only the content of a conversation (i.e., transcript) was rated by peers, there were no differences between autistic and allistic transcripts. When conversations were viewed, however, neurotypical raters were more likely to rate autistic conversations negatively, presumably because of audio/visual (e.g., behaviors or prosody) rather than content cues.

There may be underlying differences in brain function that can explain why autistic females have stronger conventional social skills than autistic males. More cognitive flexibility in attention to social-emotional stimuli might allow for better social skills and also social camouflaging (Lacroix et al., 2021). Females and children assigned female at birth may also receive more direct instruction and pressure to use conventional social skills. Flexibility in applying the skills can continue to be a problem for females, however. See Chap. 7 for a more extensive discussion of executive function.

Finally, it is also common for autistic females to be socially isolated because although they can imitate, they may lack understanding of underlying social dos and don'ts, including when to tell the absolute truth or not based on the social context. They may be inaccurately viewed or mislabeled—as rude, condescending, intolerant, oppositional, selfish, aloof, self-involved, manipulative, attention-seeking, anxious, and withdrawn—before they are perceived as possibly autistic (Eckerd, 2020).

In assessment, it is critical that clinicians are aware that the presence of some expected social skills may still be consistent with autism. The spectrum of core social skills may range from complete disinterest in others to strong social motivation for acceptance, with successful interactions only with adults, other high-masking adults or younger children, or only brief, non-sustained social interactions or socialization around special interests in between these two extremes. This variability in presentations of autism can lead to delayed detection, misdiagnosis, and delayed or lack of evidence-based treatments (Duvall et al., 2021).

To better assess social skills, observations beyond clinical settings are required. Parent or teacher reports are helpful, but if this is the only method of data collection (e.g., no direct observations of play are possible), consider the following: parent or other report may not be available (e.g., for an adult); environment has strong effects on social behaviors, which may result in different perceptions of social interactions by family members vs. others; sometimes ongoing adaptations in some environments create perceptions of social flexibility that may not generalize to other settings; and parents may not be able to provide accurate or detailed observations of their child's social abilities with peers (Duvall et al., 2021).

Play and Imagination

First Person Narratives

It is often said that those with Asperger's have little imagination and do not engage in imaginative play as children. I think this is erroneous and may be a hindrance to identifying those with Asperger's who do possess a vivid imagination… But the stories I made up in my head were far more interesting than the ones I could enact with my dolls—rigid, unconvincing bits of plastic....we all seem to start out by copying what we admire and some will stop there, at being great emulators. (Simone, 2010, p. 22)

Playtime was very difficult. I didn't know how other kids just sort of knew what to do and who to play with. So, I just hung out by myself, wandered around the playground, sometimes standing weirdly in a group of kids, not saying much, thinking that was enough to be included and considered a part of whatever game they were playing. Mostly I just watched. Woman with autism (Hendrickx, 2015, p. 77)

My classmates in third grade played a game I didn't understand. It involved the girls running away from the boys. I could see that, but I didn't understand why, nor could I figure out the rules. When I tried to join in by imitating, it didn't work. I didn't know how to shriek properly, nor did I want to (it hurt my ears), but I considered myself pretty good at running. The trouble was that nobody chased me. Jane Meyerding (Miller, 2015, p. 184)

Even for girls who loved having soft, cuddly toys and dolls, the play was more in organising, collecting and sorting rather than interactive and imaginative play with these items. (Hendrickx, 2015, p. 63)

When a child would like more friends but clearly has little success in this area, one option is to create imaginary friends.... Girls with Asperger's Syndrome can create imaginary friends and elaborate doll play that superficially resembles the play of other girls, but there can be several qualitative differences. They often lack reciprocity in their natural social play and can be too controlling when playing with their peers. This is illustrated in Liane Holliday-Willey's autobiography. 'The fun came from setting up and arranging things. Maybe this desire to organize things rather than play with things, is the reason I never had a great interest in my peers. They always wanted to use the things I had so carefully arranged. They would want to rearrange and redo. They did not let me control the environment.' (Attwood et al., 2006, p. 5)

As long as things followed a set of rules, I could play along. Rules were – and are – great friends of mine. I like rules. They set the record straight and keep it that way. You know where you stand with rules and you know how to act with rules. Trouble is, rules change and if they do not, people break them. I get terribly annoyed when either happens. (Willey, 2014, p. 46)

To me dolls seemed like the stiff corpses of small people....I would comply: dress on, dress off. "Mom, I took the dress off and put it on five times. Is that enough? Can I go outside and play in the woods now?" -Diana Krumins (Miller, 2015, p. 103)

School-age children are most likely to play with same-gender friends, but when autistic girls seek out friends to play with, they are often overlooked but not necessarily rejected. One possible reason girls are not identified sooner might be that they appear to be less isolated than the more obviously rejected autistic boys in elementary school. This puts additional stress on females, as they are less likely to have adult assistance or guidance. It is harder to observe that a child is being left out or not included than it is to see a child who is overtly rejected (Dean et al., 2014).

Although female play skills may look typical at first glance, extended observation may show a stronger tendency toward rigidity in play that may explain why non-inclusion is overlooked after what may appear to be some initial success (Barnes et al., 2018). One phenomenon reported in the literature is "flitting," or moving from group to group without ever truly being accepted into the play group.

This has the outward appearance of playing with many friends. On closer inspection, autistic girls are often not included or do not know how to integrate themselves into group play very well, so they "flit" from the outer edges of one group to another throughout recess or at a social event. Autistic girls used compensatory behaviors that may have masked their social difficulties. They were described as weaving in and out of activities and staying in close proximity to peers before eventually seeking out solitary play (Dean et al., 2017). This is in contrast to typical male play, often centered around group activities or team sports, making a boy who is not included more obvious to onlookers.

Pretend play consistent with gender expectations in particular is observed more often in autistic girls than boys (Knickmeyer et al., 2008), which can interfere with the identification of autism traits. In a very early study (likely to be somewhat biased, as females in the study were found to have consistently lower IQ than males), autistic females were still found to have less unusual visual stimming behaviors and more conventional, less stereotypic play than males (Lord et al., 1982). There are some differences, however, surrounding playing games. Rigid expectations in setting up or organizing a game as opposed to flexible play during a game and a strong tendency to control or dominate games have been reported (Hiller et al., 2014).

More recently, although girls showed less typical play than their peers, autistic girls showed more typical play than autistic boys (Tang et al., 2021). Perhaps the best conclusion regarding play is aligned with Hull et al. (2017), suggesting that core autism traits are fundamentally similar across genders, but that sex/gender variations that are found in neurotypical children are also present in autistic children. Thus, the dimensional nature of autism is one example of the human condition where sex and gender differences are as important as they are in neurotypical development. Including the overarching differences across sex and gender roles when assessing for autism may temper the possibly exclusionary effects of rigid scoring criteria and mental checklists.

In our clinical experiences, imagination in autistic girls can sometimes be extreme, as in almost living within imaginary worlds through play or intense interests in reading. This may interfere with autism identification if clinicians fail to notice that input from playmates or others is often ignored, that the strong "vision" for pretend play is not picked up by peers, and that representational pretend play (using objects to represent other things) might be more delayed than that of peers. Extended and repeated observations of play are recommended during assessment. More in-depth observations of play, particularly interactive play, is also advised, as young autistic girls may appear to have doll collections similar to their peers for example, but play may be more isolated, repetitive, or non-imaginative (Lord et al., 2022), which merits interactive play assessment and/or extended parent interview on this topic. As they move into adolescence, preferences for imaginative and fantasy play are less likely to be shared by their peers.

Imitation and Camouflaging

First Person Narratives

> *It's as though the challenge of quickly creating a new persona to deal with them is very interesting to me: Can I do it or not? I could now say to them that actually, far from being understood, they have never been imitated so well. Sometimes the imitation becomes almost a parody...I very rarely meet an NT that I have trouble understanding if I study them long enough. By understanding I mean predicting or anticipating their most likely response, though why they do what they do is often still a mystery. April Masilamani* (Miller, 2015, p. 127)

> *When I did agree to play it was more out of curiosity about what they were doing. Since I didn't understand what they were doing, I would simply wait until someone told me what to do. Later, I learned to ask for certain roles. I realized that if I asked to be the servant or child in pretend play, that someone would always direct me. That way I didn't need to figure out what the game was all about. It was the first of many ways I learned to hide my social confusion. I never did catch on, but I was learning to be like them. -Susan Golubock* (Miller, 2015, p. 148)

> *Having Asperger's means relearning for every situation what I need to know. It means copying. It means acting sometimes. It means studying what people do so as to better fit (as much as I detest conformity) because sometimes it is necessary to be in social situations where I am required to play a role I do not feel cut out for. - Kimberly Tucker* (Miller, 2015, p. 257)

> *I found that I needed to put myself in situations that helped and supported me as a person, rather than try to mask and pretend all the time to fit into an unmanageable role that wasn't designed for my neurology. -Barb Cook* (Cook & Garnett, 2018 p. 87)

Imitation

In autism assessments, lack of imitation skills is one of the behaviors observed for differences in young children (Lord, Rutter et al., 2012; Lord, Luyster et al., 2012). Imitation skills and related brain functions have been studied to provide some clues as to why autistic girls may have stronger imitation abilities than their male counterparts to the extent that autism might be dismissed in an evaluation process. Eye-tracking investigations found that autistic females paid more attention to faces in socially "lean" (i.e., limited social engagement) videos (such as parallel play) than autistic males and attention to faces in socially "rich" or complex interactive play was different for autistic females only compared to typically developing females. This study (Harrop et al., 2019) agreed with Lei et al. (2019), Jack et al. (2021), etc. that differences are consistently found between autistic females and neurotypical females, indicating that **the most appropriate comparison group when evaluating females for differences is a same-sex peer group—not autistic males.**

Imitation skills may also highlight differences in understanding and preferences related to gender. One study found that girls were more likely to imitate TV characters of the opposite sex during childhood compared to boys, suggesting at least the possibility that identification with assigned gender roles is lower in autistic females in their early years (Brunissen et al., 2021).

Camouflaging

In autism research, camouflaging is defined as using behavioral and/or cognitive strategies to adapt to or cope within the predominantly non-autistic social world (Cook et al., 2021), but it is not a specifically autistic trait (Fombonne, 2020). Camouflaging is probably one of the biggest barriers to autism identification and possibly a trait with significant adverse effects in terms of co-occurring mental health issues (Cook et al., 2021). Higher levels of self-reported autistic traits and sex and gender differences are also associated with camouflaging in scientific literature (Cook et al., 2021).

Autistic women who are verbally fluent, with average or higher cognitive abilities, and who appear to be doing well might *not* be functioning well emotionally (Beck et al., 2020). The conflict and stress described by many autistic females are tied to desire for acceptance (Tierney et al., 2016), lack of autism identity, and the intense effort to maintain a facade that does not match the "true" person or personality. Camouflaging is described as one way to avoid bullying (Cage & Troxell-Whitman, 2020) and/or as a social coping mechanism (Lai et al., 2017). It is also possible that some individuals are "switchers," who camouflage more in some settings than others (Tubío-Fungueiriño et al., 2020). There is no single motivation for camouflaging, but loneliness often predicts it (Millner et al., 2023). Other terms used to describe these behaviors have included compensation, masking, and adaptive morphing (Cook et al., 2021), with a call for consulting within the autistic community for preferred terminology (Lai et al., 2020). Libsack et al. (2021) outlined the difficulties in not just labeling these behaviors but interpreting them as well. They used the term passing as non-autistic (PAN) to succinctly attempt to capture both the behavior and interpretation.

Camouflaging is often associated with suicidality (Cassidy et al., 2018), but camouflaging with thwarted belonging has been found to mediate suicidal thoughts and behaviors more than camouflaging alone (Cassidy et al., 2020). Exhaustion, time to recover, and negative self-perceptions are all associated with camouflaging behaviors (Hull et al., 2017). Despite the personal cost, the motivation for camouflaging is to be accepted in society. The cumulative effects of camouflaging and extensive camouflaging in daily life were reported as the most damaging to mental health (Bradley et al., 2021).

Camouflaging does not always meet social acceptance goals, with many individuals experiencing the costs, but not enjoying the anticipated benefits of camouflaging (Halsall et al., 2021). Self-perceived stigma associated with autism is also associated with self-reports of camouflaging (Perry et al., 2022), but Han et al. (2022) found that camouflaging is not reliably protective against internalized or stigma-related stress. While neurotypical adolescents and autistic males do not report specific reasons for camouflaging, autistic females have detailed reasons and reported negative emotions and feeling drained following camouflaging (Bargiela et al., 2016; Bernardin et al., 2021).

Camouflaging is not a universal behavior, nor is it one-dimensional. Also referred to as "impression management" (Schneid & Raz, 2020), it has been conceptualized as having three manifestations: masking, compensation, and assimilation (Hull et al., 2019). Camouflaging rates are not different across genders in neurotypical populations, but it is more prevalent in autistic females than other groups, and not enough is known about camouflaging in non-binary individuals (Hull et al., 2020). Camouflaging can vary from refraining from autistic tendencies in social situations, developing rules for more successful social interactions, or complicated imitation of typical behaviors to more successfully navigate social situations (Mandy, 2019). Subjective experiences are important for differential diagnosis of autism, and camouflaging behaviors are not exclusive to females (Lai et al., 2020).

Camouflaging may be situational or contextual. In nuanced autism, females may demonstrate stronger conventional social and emotional skills (superficially) than autistic males, more closely resembling neurotypical male skills. This highlights the importance of selecting the right comparison group in assessment (Head et al., 2014). Choice of measures should also be carefully considered, as interview measures such as the ADI-R (LeCouteur et al., 2003) may miss females with higher cognitive abilities more often than direct observational measures. However, parent report measures were also found to report higher levels of impairment in adaptive and conventional social skills, illustrating possible inconsistencies in current assessment procedures (Ratto et al., 2018).

New aspects of camouflaging behaviors were discovered recently using qualitative methods by Cook et al. (2022). They asked autistic adults to describe their camouflaging strategies that may not have been obvious to the observer. Almost 40 behaviors were described by participants watching video of their own social interactions. Main themes among these behaviors included masking, "innocuous engagement," modeling neurotypical communication, and active self-presentation. They included behaviors such as passive encouragement (eye contact, smiling, laughing, etc.), centering social partners (focusing on social partners and allowing them to guide the interaction), deferential engagement (apologizing, seeking approval, and avoiding confrontation), and actions to reduce social risk (staying with small talk, avoiding controversy, jokes, and honest, direct communication) as part of innocuous engagement. The category of "active self-presentation" included a range of social behaviors from reciprocal (asking questions, balancing participation, finding common ground, and sharing facts) to risky (jokes and disclosures) to comfortable/familiar social behaviors (comfortable topics and/or scripts).

Awareness of small differences may also aid in assessment. Linguistic camouflage has been examined for differences, with females using the filler word "um" more often than "uh," which is considered more typical and socially sophisticated, whereas males used "uh" (Parrish-Morris et al., 2017). Also look for scores on social awareness to be in the more typical range despite other social scores showing as more impaired (Jorgenson et al., 2020). Reciprocity is also more present in autistic females than males, closer to rates for neurotypical females (Wood-Downie et al., 2021).

Camouflaging behaviors for social acceptance in school are also a possible reason for discrepancies between parent and teacher report measure results, which can sometimes be a barrier in accurate identification (Tsirgiotis et al., 2021). Assessment processes also need to consider that camouflaging may be disguising underlying learning disabilities (Halsall et al., 2021). Another key to accurate assessment is awareness that females may imitate or reflect their female assessors, including their emotional states, and that they may be more in tune with emotional states of others (Rieffe et al., 2021).

When autistic identity self-ratings are high and autism is disclosed, camouflaging behaviors decrease, with accompanying decrease in conflict and stress. If autism is not disclosed, however, and autistic identity is high, camouflaging may still be significant (Cage & Troxell-Whitman, 2020). The message behind these findings is that safe non-discriminatory environments that foster disclosure are likely to reduce camouflaging behaviors.

Restricted (Special) Interests and Repetitive (Stimming) Behaviors

First Person Narratives

> *The stereotype of autistic men collecting train timetables, model cars, or sports statistics contributes to the male bias in ASD diagnosis and research, and in recent studies has been linked to the skewed gender ratio in autism rates. This impedes timely female identification--the women I've known are multifaceted and have several co-existing interests. —Christine Jenkins* (Cook & Garnett, 2018, p. 271)

> *Our girls [with ASD] really do seem different than autistic boys we know. For instance, the boys seem to hyperfocus on certain interests like trains, weather, etc. Our girls don't do that at all. In fact, our 18-year-old can't stand to be with her [male] Aspie counterparts because they only talk about science and sports or whatever their thing is. She wants to talk about relationships, art, music, and feelings. I think it all goes back to the typical differences between boys and girls. Since the girls are less likely to have these keen interests I think some doctors don't catch their autism. Mother of four daughters, oldest 18 with Asperger's syndrome and youngest 9 with classic autism* (Nichols, 2009, pp. 20–21)

> *Animals. They are what I consider my true friends. I do indeed feel like I have a natural affinity to them, since a very tender age. I feel like I'm better able to read them than humans [...] Sometimes I do wish I were an animal, or at the very least someone who was 'as one with the wild', such as in some tribal communities, and lived a simpler yet inevitably more physically taxing life - Woman with autism* (Hendrickx, 2015, p. 150)

> *In the future, clinicians should be encouraged to consider all behaviors/characteristics of females as a whole and look for repetitive behaviors of any kind, even seemingly benign ones.* (Halladay et al., 2015)

Restricted Interests

Of all findings in the scientific literature, the most consistent seems to be that special interests and stimming behaviors (also referred to as RRBIs) are definitely different and not observed or detected as often in females as they are in males (Corbett et al., 2021; Duvekot et al., 2017; Kaat et al., 2021; Lai & Szatmari, 2020; McFayden et al., 2019; Rubenstein et al., 2015; Tang et al., 2021; Tillman et al., 2018; Wilson et al., 2016). Across studies, intense or special interests may indeed be present, but interests are more likely to be mainstream in terms of the subject. This may lead to RRBIs being less recognized, despite the intensity of the interest or mismatched age appropriateness (APA, 2022; Sutherland et al., 2017). Reported interests include animals, unicorns, video games, YouTube, and dolls (Tang, et al., 2021) and celebrities and science (McFayden et al., 2019). Stimming behaviors may be more discreet, such as hair twirling, teeth clenching, lip biting, or subtle hand movements, all of which are easily missed (Suckle, 2021).

Development of RRBIs is also notably different across genders. Fewer *differences* related to RRBIs are noticed in early years (Ros-Demarize et al., 2020), but this reverses in adolescence, where RRBIs are more noticeable in females (Jamison et al. 2017; Kaat et al., 2021). Developmental trajectories relative to RRBIs begin to diverge by gender during primary school age (6–11 years; Bourson & Prevost, 2022). These data and the preponderance of findings of different RRBIs in females led to a comparison of imaging data. This study found robust evidence for reduced levels of identified RRBIs in autistic girls compared to autistic boys and gray matter differences in the brain associated with RRBIs and social communication by gender (differences that were not present across genders in neurotypical individuals), specifically in motor regions and in areas thought of as social (Supekar & Menon, 2015):

RRBIs can be socially isolating in some settings, but can also be a way to connect with people in others. They may also serve a function to reduce anxiety. Withdrawing into a special interest can decrease external data streams that are difficult to sort through and process. There is also a sense of pleasure engaging in RRBIs that can create opportunities to refuel and recover (Bourson & Prevost, 2022).

Assessment is Key

Assessment of RRBIs in females and nuanced autism is more involved than standard questionnaires or observations. Interviews are critical. Asking questions to get examples for quality and intensity of the interest, interference with social or academic experiences, and what happens if you prevent the RRBI can provide the context needed to identify a seemingly typical interest or behavior as RRBIs (Young et al., 2018). Ask about camouflaging behaviors around intense or special interests to see if they are limiting their talk about their interest or inhibiting stimming behaviors because they know they will not be accepted. Kavanaugh et al. (2021) studied two very large datasets ($n > 20{,}000$; 20% female) and found low levels of recognized RRBIs interacted with sex to result in later (delayed) diagnoses. The DSM-5-TR acknowledges that even if RRBIs are not observed or reported in the present, that does not preclude a diagnosis of autism if there have been reports of RRBIs in the past (APA, 2022).

Safety (Bullying and Victimization)

First Person Narratives

> *Physical signs [of bullying]: torn clothing or backpacks, ruined homework or employment projects, bruises, cuts, bloody noses, bumps, black eyes, etc., gum, mud or other nasty things squished in your hair, clothing, personal property, etc., chunks of hair cut off, name-calling on the internet, in person or behind your back, scratches on your car or damage done to your personal property, suggestions from others that you should do your make-up, hair-dos, and personal style in ways you don't see anyone else doing. … Physiological and psychological signs [of bullying]: developing gastrointestinal problems, stomachaches, shaking, headaches, etc., showing personality changes, creating frightening or violent drawings and art, expressing a heightened interest in violence, weapons, violent films, etc., beginning to act like a bully, showing signs of poor self-esteem, exhibiting a feeling of disempowerment, becoming insecure, becoming more agitated and anxious than usual, developing depression, developing eating disorders?* (Willey, 2012, pp. 44–45)

> *I have endured numerous insults, particularly in school not so much away from school … but numerous insults about being lazy, not trying, not paying attention. People just thought you were awkward or selfish or just kind of … just some sort of prima donna who couldn't behave reasonably.* (Punshon et al., 2009, p. 276)

Bullying

Bullying and victimization in childhood, including sexual victimization, were reported by 90% of autistic adults (Weiss et & Fardella, 2018). Autistic and gender non-conforming individuals are at even higher risk of bullying and victimization (Strang et al., 2018). Bullying has been reported to be experienced more often in autistic females than males, perhaps because of increased social interaction and less obvious differences (Sanchez et al., 2022). Bullying is cited as a reason for camouflaging to avoid negative experiences, but bullying is also reported as a result of attempts at camouflaging (Bernardin et al., 2021).

> *"When I was being bullied, I was told not to antagonise these girls, and actually I was only antagonizing them by being myself. -P03"* (Bargiela et al., 2016, p. 3286)

From an assessment standpoint, school refusal should be considered one possible sign of bullying, which is more common among children with autism (Ochi et al., 2020). Relational victimization is reported to increase in adolescence, as social norms and inter-group expectations exceed their social navigation skills, and is associated with more impairment of social functioning, RRBIs, and anxiety (Greenlee et al., 2020). Suicidality is also documented as an outcome related to peer victimization (Segers & Rawana, 2014). Unfortunately, some bullying may also come from parents, teachers, and other adults:

> *"In secondary school I just got the shit kicked out of me mentally, physically, emotionally, the works, and the teachers joined in." - Gemma* (Kanfiszer et al., 2017, p. 666)

Victimization

Sexual victimization is not just an adult issue (Beteta, 2009; Cazalis et al., 2022) and not particular to autism (Benedet & Grant, 2014; Gotby et al., 2018). Neurodiversity and low understanding of social cues, combined with high social motivation and imitation or camouflaging in females with autism, create heightened risk for sexual victimization at all ages. Careful consideration of sexual victimization can be part of the assessment process. Be careful about bias. It is not only possible that an autistic child or adolescent has experienced some type of sexual contact; it is more likely that they may have been victimized. Equally important is consideration of recommendations for sex education, sexual health, and teaching about consent in recommendations. For more about sexuality and victimization in adults, see Chap. 12.

> *When the bullying turned sexual, I assumed it was more of the same: my fault....So, I kept it secret and tried my best to avoid everyone--an impossinle goal when you're locked up together inside a school building....So, again, the problem was all my fault, and I was left to suffer at the hands of others with the conviction that it was only what I deserved. Those were nightmare years for me. Maxfield Sparrow* (Ballou et al., 2021, p.140)

Supports and Recommendations

Social Skills

There is a distinct lack of social skills interventions specifically designed for females. One that has shown considerable success and longevity is the Girls Night Out model from the University of Kansas (Jamison & Schuttler, 2017), a program providing girls with social skills specific to the lives of adolescent and young adult females with additional focus on health, wellness, and self-esteem. Another female-specific model is Felicity House in Manhattan, New York (USA): "It is a free social community space just for women with autism. We come here to meet, to socialize, to pursue interests, to learn, to create, to connect to other resources, to find supportive people, to laugh" https://felicity-house.org/. Most social skills interventions will serve females as well as males, but care must be taken to not isolate one female in a group otherwise composed of all males.

Play and Imagination

There are infinite ways to play. Solitary play may be preferred and very fulfilling for some, but if observations show that a child is seeking opportunities to play with peers but is not consistently included, consider including some peer-mediated interventions for inclusion at recess (see Kretzman et al., 2018). Sometimes intense imaginative or fantasy play is helpful to recover from social stress, but also watch for signs or comments that social frustrations are occurring and brainstorm ways to support the type of success the child is seeking.

Imitation

Imitation can be beneficial in learning new skills and fitting in, but frequent check-ins with teachers and parents are helpful to ensure safety and the appropriateness of models being imitated. Supports such as the Circles® curriculum (https://stanfield. com) can help children with less life experience to learn to make judgments about safe people for imitation and people to ask a trusted adult about.

Camouflaging

Most women report relief from camouflaging upon diagnosis, as they feel more free to be themselves with an explanation for how and why they are different. This can often relieve many of the costs and burdens of camouflaging outlined above. In ongoing counseling or targeted lessons, consider the topic of when camouflaging might be helpful and when there is no longer a need to adopt a non-authentic persona in order to be accepted. It may also be necessary to help her identify activities or groups in which her authentic self is the norm instead of a difference (e.g., social skills groups, shared interest groups).

Intense or Special Interests and Repetitive or Stimming Behaviors

Consider that a noticeable escalation or increased visibility of RRBIs in adolescence might be a possible coping strategy to deal with anxiety. Addressing the anxiety is the primary goal. Explore ways in which intense interests and stimming behaviors are helping, and ask if they are interfering with any goals that they are also trying to achieve. If there is any interference, you can work on ways to increase the repertoire of strategies available for dealing with anxiety. Many intense interests can lead to career choices as well.

Safety (Bullying and Victimization)

Start early and often with sex education, using concrete terminology and activities to help her develop abilities to protect herself from victimization. Terminology and frequent reminders are ways to increase likelihood of reporting victimization for earlier action. Reporting or even recognizing bullying or victimization may be difficult to communicate, however, so look for other signs of distress, and talk with teachers and others to look for possible victimization. The Circles® curriculum mentioned earlier is a good resource for teaching how to discern safety in social circles. Sexual health considerations and education about consent need to begin no later than puberty, which is likely to be earlier for autistic females than others (Corbett et al., 2020). Menarche has also been found to be delayed (Knickmeyer et al., 2006), which does not mean sex education should be postponed, as victimization can still occur.

Return to the Case Study

Through her targeted observations, Kyra has already discovered several effective strategies to help her better contextualize the actions of her peers. However, these observations haven't been as helpful in maintaining longer-term friendships. While Kyra enjoys solitary play, and this is a big positive in her day, she also expressed a desire to connect with peers she considered friends at a deeper level. Her parents were thrilled to discover a local social group for girls with similar interests to Kyra (e.g., animals, anime). She also joined an afterschool club focused on environmental issues, where they did things like organize campus clean-up days, create posters to encourage good environmental habits, and write letters to companies. Having specific topics on which to focus during each group or club meeting was helpful in finding common ground to develop friendships based on interest. Participation in these activities also helped Kyra develop stronger skills in negotiating and resolving conflict, with the support of Kyra's parents and her counselor. Having someone to reach out to and ask about why things went a certain way during a conversation and how to move forward was a helpful support for Kyra in learning how to manage the nuances of a more mature friendship. See Table 5.1 for a summary of assessment strategies.

Table 5.1 At-a-glance summary—social skills, play, imitation, camouflaging, intense interests, stimming behaviors, and safety

Domain	Focus	Assessment planning and age ranges
Play	Flexibility in play, ability to initiate and follow, taking turns	**Interview and observation (see Chap. 2 for more play measures)**
Play	Adapting the other person's ideas in play	*Autism Diagnostic Observation Schedule*, **ADOS-2, Modules T, 1, 2, and 3** (Lord et al., 2012): 12 mos. to adult; see Rea et al. 2022—autistic girls 8–17 likely to score lower than autistic males on the ADOS-2 on social communication, total, and subscale scores
Play	Pretend play, approaching other children, playing in a group of more than one other child	*Autism Diagnostic Interview-Revised* (**ADI-R**): 2 and older (LeCouteur et al., 2003) (with published algorithms for children younger than 4—see Kim & Lord, 2012, and Kim et al., 2013). Autistic females with high cognitive abilities may have lower scores on the ADI-R, however
Camouflaging and imitation	Degree of camouflaging present (not as a diagnostic feature, but to provide context for other results)	*Camouflaging Autistic Traits-Questionnaire* (**CAT-Q**) (**self-report**): 16 and older (Hull et al., 2019)
Social impairment	Social impairment (could also indicate anxiety, however)	*Social Responsiveness Scales, 2nd Ed.* (**SRS-2**)—gender norms available for school age only: 30 mos. to adult (Constantino & Gruber, 2012)
RRBIs	Ritualistic/sameness behavior, stereotypic behavior, self-injurious behavior, compulsive behavior, and special interests	*Repetitive Behavior Scales Revised* (**RBS-R**) all ages (Lam & Aman, 2007)
RRBIs	Repetitive motor, special interests and behavior, ritual and routine, and self-directed behavior	*Repetitive Behavior Scale for Early Childhood*: ages 17 to 25 months (Wolff et al., 2016)
RRBIs	Repetitive behaviors noted	*Toddler Autism Symptom Inventory* (**TASI**): ages 12–36 months (Coulter et al., 2021)
RRBIs/special interests and stimming behaviors	Unusual sensory interests, repetitive motor movements, rigidity/adherence to routine, and preoccupations with special interest	*Repetitive Behaviors Questionnaire-2*: ages 15–35 months (Leekam et al., 2007)

(continued)

Table 5.1 (continued)

Domain	Focus	Assessment planning and age ranges
RRBIs	Repetitive sensory and motor behaviors and insistence on sameness	*The Repetitive Behaviors Questionnaire-2 for Adults*: ages 16 to 66 (Barrett et al., 2015, 2018)
Bullying	Direct questions on bullying and teasing	**ADOS-2, Modules 3 and 4**: ages 4 to adult (Lord et al., 2012)
Bullying	Look deeper into school refusal behavior for evidence of bullying	**Interview and observation**
Victimization	Look for changes in behavior such as declines in academic performance and other signs of unusual anxiety	**Interview and observation**

Please see the References section in this chapter for additional information on measures.
Not all measures and processes listed are available in all settings or appropriate for all cases. Qualification levels apply. Multiple measures in a single domain are not necessary. Some measures can provide data in multiple domains. This is meant to provide a relatively quick reference for assessment planning and implementation, not an endorsement of any particular measure as "best." Emphasis here is on readily available, commonly used measures, but similar measures may also be useful.

References

American Psychiatric Association. (2022). *Diagnostic and statistical manual of mental disorders, Fifth Ed., Text Revision*. Author.

Attwood, T., Grandin, T., Bolic, T., Faherty, C., Iland, L., Myers, J. M., Snyder, R., Wagner, S., & Wrobel, M. (2006). *Asperger's and girls*. Future Horizons.

Ballou, E. P., da Vanport, S., & Onaiwu, M. G. (Eds.). (2021). *Sincerely, your autistic child*. Beacon Press.

Bargiela, S., Steward, R., & Mandy, W. (2016). The experiences of late-diagnosed women with autism spectrum conditions: An investigation of the female autism phenotype. *Journal of Autism and Developmental Disorders, 46*(10), 3281–3294. https://doi.org/10.1007/s10803-016-2872-8

Barnes, K., Petersen, J., & Harrington, N.L. (2018). *Autism 208: Hiding in plain sight: Girls with autism spectrum disorder, Seattle Children's Hospital*. https://www.youtube.com/watch?v=XJ0weHzBagU

Barrett, S. L., Uljarevic, M., Baker, E. K., Richdale, A. L., Jones, C. R. G., & Leekam, S. R. (2015). The adult repetitive behaviours questionnaire-2 (RBQ-2A): a self-report measure of restricted and repetitive behaviours. *Journal of Autism and Developmental Disorders, 45*(11), 3680–3692. https://doi.org/10.1007/s10803-015-2514-6

Barrett, S. L., Uljarevic, M., Jones, C. R. G., & Leekam, S. R. (2018). Assessing subtypes of restricted and repetitive behaviour using the Adult Repetitive Behaviour Questionnaire-2 in autistic adults. *Molecular Autism, 9*, 58. https://doi.org/10.1186/s13229-018-0242-4

Beck, J. S., Lundwall, R. A., Gabrielsen, T., Cox, J. C., & South, M. (2020). Looking good but feeling bad: "Camouflaging" behaviors and mental health in women with autistic traits. *Autism: The International Journal of Research & Practice, 24*(4), 809–821. https://doi.org/10.1177/1362361320912147

Belcher, H. L., Morein-Zamir, S., Stagg, S. D., & Ford, R. M. (2022). Shining a light on a hidden population: Social functioning and mental health in women reporting autistic traits but lacking diagnosis. *Journal of Autism and Developmental Disorders, 1-15.* https://doi.org/10.1007/s10803-022-05583-2

Benedet, J., & Grant, I. (2014). Sexual assault and the meaning of power and authority for women with mental disabilities. *Feminist Legal Studies, 22*(2), 131–154. https://doi.org/10.1007/s10691-014-9263-3

Bernardin, C. J., Mason, E., Lewis, T., & Kanne, S. (2021). "You must become a chameleon to survive": Adolescent experiences of camouflaging. *Journal of Autism and Developmental Disorders, 51*(12), 4422–4435. https://doi.org/10.1007/s10803-021-04912-1

Beteta, L. M. (2009). A phenomenological study of the lived experiences of adolescent females with Asperger Syndrome [ProQuest Information & Learning]. In *Dissertation Abstracts International Section A: Humanities and Social Sciences, 70,* (1–A), p. 138. https://scholarworks.waldenu.edu/dissertations/649/

Bourson, L., & Prevost, C. (2022). Characteristics of restricted interests in girls with ASD compared to boys: A systematic review of the literature. *European Child & Adolescent Psychiatry,* 1–18. https://doi.org/10.1007/s00787-022-01998-5

Bradley, L., Shaw, R., Baron-Cohen, S., & Cassidy, S. (2021). Autistic adults' experiences of camouflaging and its perceived impact on mental health. *Autism in Adulthood, 3*(4), 320–329. https://doi.org/10.1089/aut.2020.0071

Brunissen, L., Rapoport, E., Chawarska, K., & Adesman, A. (2021). Sex differences in gender-diverse expressions and identities among youth with autism spectrum disorder. *Autism Research: Official Journal of the International Society for Autism Research, 14*(1), 143–155. https://doi.org/10.1002/aur.2441

Cage, E., & Troxell-Whitman, Z. (2020). Understanding the relationships between autistic identity, disclosure, and camouflaging. *Autism in Adulthood, 2*(4), 334–338. https://doi.org/10.1089/aut.2020.0016

Cassidy, S., Bradley, L., Shaw, R., & Baron-Cohen, S. (2018). Risk markers for suicidality in autistic adults. *Molecular Autism, 9*(42), 1–14. https://doi.org/10.1186/s13229-018-0226-4

Cassidy, S. A., Gould, K., Townsend, E., Pelton, M., Robertson, A. E., & Rodgers, J. (2020). Is camouflaging autistic traits associated with suicidal thoughts and behaviours? Expanding the interpersonal psychological theory of suicide in an undergraduate student sample. *Journal of Autism & Developmental Disorders, 50*(10), 3638–3648. https://doi.org/10.1007/s10803-019-04323-3

Cazalis, F., Reyes, E., Leduc, S., & Gourion, D. (2022). Evidence that nine autistic women out of ten have been victims of sexual violence. *Frontiers in Behavioral Neuroscience, 16.* https://doi.org/10.3389/fnbeh.2022.852203

Constantino, J., & Gruber, C. P. (2012). *Social Responsiveness Scale, Second Edition.* Western Psychological Services.

Cook, J., Crane, L., Hull, L., Bourne, L., & Mandy, W. (2022). Self-reported camouflaging behaviours used by autistic adults during everyday social interactions. *Autism, 26*(2), 406–421. https://doi.org/10.1177/13623613211026754

Cook, B., & Garnett, M. (Eds.). (2018). *Spectrum women: Walking to the beat of autism.* Jessica Kingsley.

Cook, J., Hull, L., Crane, L., & Mandy, W. (2021). Camouflaging in autism: A systematic review. *Clinical Psychology Review, 89.* https://doi.org/10.1016/j.cpr.2021.102080

Corbett, B. A., Schwartzman, J. M., Libsack, E. J., Muscatello, R. A., Lerner, M. D., Simmons, G. L., & White, S. W. (2021). Camouflaging in autism: Examining sex-based and compensatory models in social cognition and communication. *Autism Research: Official Journal of the International Society for Autism Research, 14*(1), 127–142. https://doi.org/10.1002/aur.2440

Corbett, B. A., Vandekar, S., Muscatello, R. A., & Tanguturi, Y. (2020). Pubertal timing during early adolescence: Advanced pubertal onset in females with autism spectrum disorder. *Autism Research: Official Journal of the International Society for Autism Research, 13*(12), 2202–2215. https://doi.org/10.1002/aur.2406

Coulter, K. L., Barton, M. L., Boorstein, H., Cordeaux, C., Dumont-Mathieu, T., Haisley, L., Herlihy, L., Jashar, D. T., Robins, D. L., Stone, W. L., & Fein, D. A. (2021). The Toddler Autism Symptom Inventory: Use in diagnostic evaluations of toddlers. *Autism, 25*(8), 2386–2399. https://doi.org/10.1177/13623613211021699

Dean, M., Harwood, R., & Kasari, C. (2017). The art of camouflage: Gender differences in the social behaviors of girls and boys with autism spectrum disorder. *Autism, 21*(6), 678–689. https://doi.org/10.1177/1362361316671845

Dean, M., Kasari, C., Shih, W., Frankel, F., Whitney, R., Landa, R., Lord, C., Orlich, F., King, B., & Harwood, R. (2014). The peer relationships of girls with ASD at school: Comparison to boys and girls with and without ASD. *Journal of Child Psychology & Psychiatry, 55*(11), 1218–1225. https://doi.org/10.1111/jcpp.12242

Duvall, S., Armstrong, K., Shahabuddin, A., Grantz, C., Fein, D., & Lord, C. (2021). A road map for identifying autism spectrum disorder: Recognizing and evaluating characteristics that should raise red or "pink" flags to guide accurate differential diagnosis. *The Clinical Neuropsychologist,* 1–36. Advance online publication. https://doi.org/10.1080/13854046.2021.1921276.

Duvekot, J., van der Ende, J., Verhulst, F. C., Slappendel, G., van Daalen, E., Maras, A., & Greaves-Lord, K. (2017). Factors influencing the probability of a diagnosis of autism spectrum disorder in girls versus boys. *Autism: The International Journal of Research and Practice, 21*(6), 646–658. https://doi.org/10.1177/1362361316672178

Eckerd, M. (2020). Detection and diagnosis of ASD in females. *Journal of Health Service Psychology, 46*(1), 37–47. https://doi.org/10.1007/s42843-020-00006-1

Fombonne, E. (2020). Camouflage and autism. *Journal of Child Psychology and Psychiatry, 61*(7), 735–738. https://doi.org/10.1111/jcpp.13296

Greenlee, J. L., Winter, M. A., & Marcovici, I. A. (2020). Brief report: Gender differences in experiences of peer victimization among adolescents with autism spectrum disorder. *Journal of Autism and Developmental Disorders, 50*(10), 3790–3799. https://doi.org/10.1007/s10803-020-04437-z

Gotby, V. O., Lichtenstein, P., Långström, N., & Pettersson, E. (2018). Childhood neurodevelopmental disorders and risk of coercive sexual victimization in childhood and adolescence – a population-based prospective twin study. *Journal of Child Psychology & Psychiatry, 59*(9), 957–965. https://doi.org/10.1111/jcpp.12884

Han, E., Scior, K., Avramides, K., & Crane, L. (2022). A systematic review on autistic people's experiences of stigma and coping strategies. *Autism Research, 15*(1), 12–26. https://doi.org/10.1002/aur.2652

Halladay, A. K., Bishop, S., Constantino, J. N., Daniels, A. M., Koenig, K., Palmer, K., Messinger, D., Pelphrey, K., Sanders, S. J., Singer, A. T., Taylor, J. L., & Szatmari, P. (2015). Sex and gender differences in autism spectrum disorder: Summarizing evidence gaps and identifying emerging areas of priority. *Molecular Autism, 6*(1), 1–5. https://doi.org/10.1186/s13229-015-0019-y

Halsall, J., Clarke, C., & Crane, L. (2021). "Camouflaging" by adolescent autistic girls who attend both mainstream and specialist resource classes: Perspectives of girls, their mothers and their educators. *Autism: The International Journal of Research and Practice, 25*(7), 2074–2086. https://doi.org/10.1177/13623613211012819

Harrop, C., Jones, D., Zheng, S., Nowell, S., Schultz, R., & Parish-Morris, J. (2019). Visual attention to faces in children with autism spectrum disorder: Are there sex differences? *Molecular Autism, 10,* 1–10. https://doi.org/10.1186/s13229-019-0276-2

Head, A. M., McGillivray, J. A., & Stokes, M. A. (2014). Gender differences in emotionality and sociability in children with autism spectrum disorder. *Molecular Autism, 5*(1), 1–9. https://doi.org/10.1186/2040-2392-5-19

Hendrickx, S. (2015). *Women and girls with autism spectrum disorder: Understanding life experiences from early childhood to old age.* Jessica Kingsley.

Hiller, R. M., Young, R. L., & Weber, N. (2014). Sex differences in autism spectrum disorder based on DSM-5 criteria: Evidence from clinician and teacher reporting. *Journal of Abnormal Child Psychology, 42*(8), 1381–1393. https://doi.org/10.1007/s10802-014-9881-x

Hull, L., Lai, M.-C., Baron-Cohen, S., Allison, C., Smith, P., Petrides, K. V., & Mandy, W. (2020). Gender differences in self-reported camouflaging in autistic and non-autistic adults. *Autism, 24*(2), 352–363. https://doi.org/10.1177/1362361319864804

Hull, L., Mandy, W., Lai, M.-C., Baron-Cohen, S., Allison, C., Smith, P., & Petrides, K. V. (2019). Development and validation of the Camouflaging Autistic Traits Questionnaire (CAT-Q). *Journal of Autism and Developmental Disorders, 49*(3), 819–833. https://doi.org/10.1007/s10803-018-3792-6

Hull, L., Mandy, W., & Petrides, K. V. (2017). Behavioural and cognitive sex/gender differences in autism spectrum condition and typically developing males and females. *Autism, 21*(6), 706–727. https://doi.org/10.1177/1362361316669087

Jack, A., Sullivan, C. A. W., Aylward, E., Bookheimer, S. Y., Dapretto, M., Gaab, N., Horn, J. D. V., Eilbott, J., Jacokes, Z., Torgerson, C. M., Bernier, R. A., Geschwind, D. H., McPartland, J. C., Nelson, C. A., Webb, S. J., Pelphrey, K. A., Gupta, A. R., Consortium, the G., Van Horn, J. D., & GENDAAR Consortium. (2021). A neurogenetic analysis of female autism. *Brain: A Journal of Neurology, 144*(6), 1911–1926. https://doi.org/10.1093/brain/awab064

Jamison, R., Bishop, S. L., Huerta, M., & Halladay, A. K. (2017). The clinician perspective on sex differences in autism spectrum disorders. *Autism, 21*(6), 772–784. https://doi.org/10.1177/1362361316681481

Jamison, T., & Schuttler, J. (2017). Overview and preliminary evidence for a social skills and self-care curriculum for adolescent females with autism: The girls night out model. *Journal of Autism & Developmental Disorders, 47*(1), 110–125. https://doi.org/10.1007/s10803-016-2939-6

Jorgenson, C., Lewis, T., Rose, C., & Kanne, S. (2020). Social camouflaging in autistic and neurotypical adolescents: A pilot study of differences by sex and diagnosis. *Journal of Autism and Developmental Disorders, 50*(12), 4344–4355. https://doi.org/10.1007/s10803-020-04491-7

Kaat, A. J., Shui, A. M., Ghods, S. S., Farmer, C. A., Esler, A. N., Thurm, A., Georgiades, S., Kanne, S. M., Lord, C., Kim, Y. S., & Bishop, S. L. (2021). Sex differences in scores on standardized measures of autism symptoms: A multisite integrative data analysis. *Journal of Child Psychology & Psychiatry, 62*(1), 97–106. https://doi.org/10.1111/jcpp.13242

Kanfiszer, L., Davies, F., & Collins, S. (2017). "I was just so different": The experiences of women diagnosed with an autism spectrum disorder in adulthood in relation to gender and social relationships. *Autism: The International Journal of Research and Practice, 21*(6), 661–669. https://doi.org/10.1177/1362361316687987

Kavanaugh, B. C., Schremp, C. A., Jones, R. N., Best, C. R., Sheinkopf, S. J., & Morrow, E. M. (2021). Moderators of age of diagnosis in >20,000 females with autism in two large US studies. *Journal of Autism and Developmental Disorders, 1-6*. https://doi.org/10.1007/s10803-021-05026-4

Kim, S. H., & Lord, C. (2012). New Autism Diagnostic Interview-Revised Algorithms for Toddlers and Young Preschoolers from 12 to 47 Months of Age. *Journal of Autism and Developmental Disorders, 42*, 82–93. https://doi.org/10.1007/s10803-011-1213-1

Kim, S. H., Thurm, A., Shumway, S., & Lord, C. (2013 July). Multisite study of new autism diagnostic interview-revised (ADI-R) algorithms for toddlers and young preschoolers. *Journal of Autism and Developmental Disorders, 43*(7), 1527–1538. https://doi.org/10.1007/s10803-012-1696-4

Kleberg, J. L., Nyström, P., Bölte, S., & Falck-Ytter, T. (2019). Sex differences in social attention in infants at risk for autism. *Journal of Autism and Developmental Disorders, 49*(4), 1342–1351. https://doi.org/10.1007/s10803-018-3799-z

Knickmeyer, R. C., Wheelwright, S., & Baron-Cohen, S. B. (2008). Sex-typical play: Masculinization/defeminization in girls with an autism spectrum condition. *Journal of Autism and Developmental Disorders, 38*(6), 1028–1035. https://doi.org/10.1007/s10803-007-0475-0

Knickmeyer, R. C., Wheelwright, S., Hoekstra, R., & Baron-Cohen, S. (2006). Age of menarche in females with autism spectrum conditions. *Developmental Medicine & Child Neurology, 48*(12), 1007–1008. https://doi.org/10.1017/S0012162206222229

Kretzmann, M., Shih, W., & Kasari, C. (2018). Improving peer engagement of children with autism on the school playground: a randomized controlled trial. *Behavior Therapy, 46*(1), 20–28. https://doi.org/10.1016/j.beth.2014.03.006

Lacroix, A., Dutheil, F., Logemann, A., Cserjesi, R., Peyrin, C., Biro, B., Gomot, M., & Mermillod, M. (2021). Flexibility in autism during unpredictable shifts of socio-emotional stimuli: Investigation of group and sex differences. *Autism: The International Journal of Research and Practice*. https://doi.org/10.1177/13623613211062776

Lai, M., Hull, L., Mandy, W., Chakrabarti, B., Nordahl, C. W., Lombardo, M. V., Ameis, S. H., Szatmari, P., Baron, C. S., Happé, F., & Livingston, L. A. (2020). Commentary: 'Camouflaging' in autistic people—Reflection on Fombonne (2020). *Journal of Child Psychology and Psychiatry, 62*(8), 1037–1041. Advance online publication https://doi.org/10.1111/jcpp.13344.

Lai, M. C., Lombardo, M. V., Auyeung, B., Chakrabarti, B., & Baron-Cohen, S. (2015). Sex/gender differences and autism: setting the scene for future research. *Journal of the American Academy of Child and Adolescent Psychiatry, 54*(1), 11–24. https://doi.org/10.1016/j.jaac.2014.10.003

Lai, M.-C., Lombardo, M. V., Ruigrok, A. N. V., Chakrabarti, B., Auyeung, B., Szatmari, P., Happé, F., & Baron-Cohen, S. (2017). Quantifying and exploring camouflaging in men and women with autism. *Autism, 21*(6), 690–702. https://doi.org/10.1177/1362361316671012

Lai, M. C., & Szatmari, P. (2020). Sex and gender impacts on the behavioural presentation and recognition of autism. *Current Opinion in Psychiatry, 33*(2), 117–123. https://doi.org/10.1097/YCO.0000000000000575

Lam, K. S. L., & Aman, M. G. (2007). The Repetitive Behavior Scale-Revised: Independent validation in individuals with autism spectrum disorders. *Journal of Autism and Developmental Disorders, 37*(5), 855–866. https://doi.org/10.1007/s10803-006-0213-z

Le Couteur, A., Lord, C., & Rutter, M. (2003). *Autism diagnostic interview-revised*. Western Psychological Services.

Leekam, S., Tandos, J., McConachie, H., Meins, E., Parkinson, K., Wright, C., Turner, M., Arnott, B., Vittorini, L., & Le Couteur, A. (2007). Repetitive behaviours in typically developing 2-year-olds. *Journal of Child Psychology and Psychiatry, 48*(11), 1131–1138. https://doi.org/10.1111/j.1469-7610.2007.01778.x

Lei, J., Lecarie, E., Jurayj, J., Boland, S., Sukhodolsky, D. G., Ventola, P., Pelphrey, K. A., & Jou, R. J. (2019). Altered neural connectivity in females, but not males with autism: Preliminary evidence for the female protective effect from a quality-controlled diffusion tensor imaging study. *Autism Research, 12*(10), 1472–1483. https://doi.org/10.1002/aur.2180

Libsack, E. J., Keenan, E. G., Freden, C. E., Mirmina, J., Iskhakov, N., Krishnathasan, D., & Lerner, M. D. (2021). A *systematic review of passing as non-autistic in autism spectrum disorder*. *Clinical Child and Family Psychology Review, 24*(4), 783–812. https://doi.org/10.1007/s10567-021-00365-1

Lord, C., Charman, T., Havdahl, A., Carbone, P., Anagnostou, E., Boyd, B., Carr, T., de Vries, P. J., Dissanayake, C., Divan, G., Freitag, C. M., Gotelli, M. M., Kasari, C., Knapp, M., Mundy, P., Plank, A., Scahill, L., Servili, C., Shattuck, P., ... McCauley, J. B. (2022). The Lancet commission on the future of care and clinical research in autism. *Lancet, 399*(10321), 271–334. https://doi.org/10.1016/S0140-6736(21)01541-5

Lord, C., Luyster, R. J., Gotham, K., & Guthrie, W. (2012). *Autism diagnostic observation schedule* (Toddler module) (2nd ed.).

Lord, C., Rutter, M., DiLavore, P. C., Risi, S., Gotham, K., & Bishop, S. L. (2012). *Autism Diagnostic Observation Schedule, 2nd edition, modules 1–4*. Western Psychological Services.

Lord, C., Schopler, E., & Revicki, D. (1982). Sex differences in autism. *Journal of Autism and Developmental Disorders, 12*(4), 317–330. https://doi.org/10.1007/BF01538320

McFayden, T. C., Albright, J., Muskett, A. E., & Scarpa, A. (2019). Brief report: Sex differences in ASD diagnosis—A brief report on restricted interests and repetitive behaviors. *Journal of Autism and Developmental Disorders, 49*(4), 1693–1699. https://doi.org/10.1007/s10803-018-3838-9

Mandy, W. (2019). Social camouflaging in autism: Is it time to lose the mask? *Autism, 23*(8), 1879–1881. https://doi.org/10.1177/1362361319878559

Miller, J. K. (Ed.). (2015). *Women from another planet? Our lives in the universe of autism.* AuthorHouse.

Milner, V., Mandy, W., Happé, F., & Colvert, E. (2023) Sex differences in predictors and outcomes of camouflaging: Comparing diagnosed autistic, high autistic trait and low autistic trait young adults *Autism,27*(2) 402–414 1–13. https://doi.org/10.1177/13623613221098240.

Milner, V., McIntosh, H., Colvert, E., & Happé, F. (2019). A qualitative exploration of the female experience of autism spectrum disorder (ASD). *Journal of Autism and Developmental Disorders, 49*(6), 2389–2402. https://doi.org/10.1007/s10803-019-03906-4

Nichols, S. (2009). *Girls growing up on the autism spectrum: What parents and professionals should know about the pre-teen and teenage Years.* Jessica Kingsley.

Ochi, M., Kawabe, K., Ochi, S., Miyama, T., Horiuchi, F., & Ueno, S. I. (2020). School refusal and bullying in children with autism spectrum disorder. *Child and Adolescent Psychiatry and Mental Health, 14,* 17. https://doi.org/10.1186/s13034-020-00325-7

Parish-Morris, J., Liberman, M. Y., Cieri, C., Herrington, J. D., Yerys, B. E., Bateman, L., Donaher, J., Ferguson, E., Pandey, J., & Schultz, R. T. (2017). Linguistic camouflage in girls with autism spectrum disorder. *Molecular Autism, 8,* 1–12. https://doi.org/10.1186/s13229-017-0164-6

Perry, E., Mandy, W., Hull, L., & Cage, E. (2022). Understanding camouflaging as a response to autism-related stigma: A social identity theory approach. *Journal of Autism and Developmental Disorders, 52*(2), 800–810. https://doi.org/10.1007/s10803-021-04987-w

Punshon, C., Skirrow, P., & Murphy, G. (2009). The not guilty verdict: Psychological reactions to a diagnosis of Asperger syndrome in adulthood. *Autism The International Journal of Research and Practice, 13*(3), 265–283. https://doi.org/10.1177/1362361309103795

Ratto, A. B., Kenworthy, L., Yerys, B. E., Bascom, J., Wieckowski, A. T., White, S. W., Wallace, G. L., Pugliese, C., Schultz, R. T., Ollendick, T. H., Scarpa, A., Seese, S., Register-Brown, K., Martin, A., & Anthony, L. G. (2018). What about the girls? Sex-based differences in autistic traits and adaptive skills. *Journal of Autism and Developmental Disorders, 48*(5), 1698–1711. https://doi.org/10.1007/s10803-017-3413-9

Rea, H. M., Øien, R. A., Shic, F., Webb, S. J., & Ratto, A. B. (2022). Sex differences on the ADOS-2. *Journal of Autism and Developmental Disorders,* 1–13. https://doi.org/10.1007/s10803-022-05566-3

Rieffe, C., O'Connor, R., Bülow, A., Willems, D., Hull, L., Sedgewick, F., Stockmann, L., & Blijd-Hoogewys, E. (2021). Quantity and quality of empathic responding by autistic and non-autistic adolescent girls and boys. *Autism: The International Journal of Research and Practice, 25*(1), 199–209. https://doi.org/10.1177/1362361320956422

Ronkin, E., Tully, E. C., Branum-Martin, L., Cohen, L. L., Hall, C., Dilly, L., & Tone, E. B. (2021). Sex differences in social communication behaviors in toddlers with suspected autism spectrum disorder as assessed by the ADOS-2 toddler module. *Autism: The International Journal of Research and Practice, 26*(5), 1282–1295. https://doi.org/10.1177/13623613211047070

Ros-Demarize, R., Bradley, C., Kanne, S. M., Warren, Z., Boan, A., Lajonchere, C., Park, J., & Carpenter, L. A. (2020). ASD symptoms in toddlers and preschoolers: An examination of sex differences. *Autism Research, 13*(1), 157–166. https://doi.org/10.1002/aur.2241

Rubenstein, E., Wiggins, L. D., & Lee, L. C. (2015). A review of the differences in developmental, psychiatric, and medical endophenotypes between males and females with autism spectrum disorder. *Journal of Developmental and Physical Disabilities, 27*(1), 119–139. https://doi.org/10.1007/s10882-014-9397-x

Sanchez, M., Bullen, J. C., Zajic, M. C., McIntyre, N., & Mundy, P. (2022). Behavioral gender differences in school-age children with autism. *European Child & Adolescent Psychiatry,* 10.1007/s00787-022-02036-0. Advance online publication. https://doi.org/10.1007/s00787-022-02036-0.

Sasson, N. J., Faso, D. J., Nugent, J., Lovell, S., Kennedy, D. P., & Grossman, R. B. (2017). Neurotypical peers are less willing to interact with those with autism based on thin slice judgments. *Scientific Reports, 7,* 40700. https://doi.org/10.1038/srep40700

Schneid, I., & Raz, A. E. (2020). The mask of autism: Social camouflaging and impression management as coping/normalization from the perspectives of autistic adults. *Social Science & Medicine, 248*. https://doi.org/10.1016/j.socscimed.2020.112826

Segers, M., & Rawana, J. (2014). What do we know about suicidality in autism spectrum disorders? A systematic review. *Autism Research : Official Journal of the International Society for Autism Research, 7*(4), 507–521. https://doi.org/10.1002/aur.1375

Simcoe, S. M., Gilmour, J., Garnett, M. S., Attwood, T., Donovan, C., & Kelly, A. B. (2022). Are there gender-based variations in the presentation of Autism amongst female and male children? *Journal of autism and developmental disorders*. Advance online publication. https://doi.org/10.1007/s10803-022-05552-9

Simone, R. (2010). *Aspergirls: Empowering females with Asperger syndrome*. Jessica Kingsley.

Strang, J. F., Meagher, H., Kenworthy, L., de Vries, A. L. C., Menvielle, E., Leibowitz, S., Janssen, A., Cohen-Kettenis, P., Shumer, D. E., Edwards-Leeper, L., Pleak, R. R., Spack, N., Karasic, D. H., Schreier, H., Balleur, A., Tishelman, A., Ehrensaft, D., Rodnan, L., Kuschner, E. S., … Anthony, L. G. (2018). Initial clinical guidelines for co-occurring autism spectrum disorder and gender dysphoria or incongruence in adolescents. *Journal of Clinical Child and Adolescent Psychology, 47*(1), 105–115. https://doi.org/10.1080/15374416.2016.1228462

Suckle, E. K. (2021). DSM-5 and challenges to female autism identification. *Journal of Autism and Developmental Disorders, 51*(2), 754–759. https://doi.org/10.1007/s10803-020-04574-5

Supekar, K., & Menon, V. (2015). Sex differences in structural organization of motor systems and their dissociable links with repetitive/restricted behaviors in children with autism. *Molecular Autism, 6*(1), 1–13. https://doi.org/10.1186/s13229-015-0042-z

Sutherland, R., Hodge, A., Bruck, S., Costley, D., & Klieve, H. (2017). Parent-reported differences between school-aged girls and boys on the autism spectrum. *Autism, 21*(6), 785–794. https://doi.org/10.1177/1362361316668653

Tang, J. W., Li, J. W., Baulderstone, D., & Jeyaseelan, D. (2021). Presenting age and features of females diagnosed with autism spectrum disorder. *Journal of Paediatrics & Child Health, 57*(8), 1182–1189. https://doi.org/10.1111/jpc.15417

Tierney, S., Burns, J., & Kilbey, E. (2016). Looking behind the mask: Social coping strategies of girls on the autistic spectrum. *Research in Autism Spectrum Disorders, 23*, 73–83. https://doi.org/10.1016/j.rasd.2015.11.013

Tillmann, J., Ashwood, K., Absoud, M., Bölte, S., Bonnet-Brilhault, F., Buitelaar, J. K., Calderoni, S., Calvo, R., Canal-Bedia, R., Canitano, R., De Bildt, A., Gomot, M., Hoekstra, P. J., Kaale, A., McConachie, H., Murphy, D. G., Narzisi, A., Oosterling, I., Pejovic-Milovancevic, M., … Charman, T. (2018). Evaluating sex and age differences in ADI-R and ADOS scores in a large European multi-site sample of individuals with autism spectrum disorder. *Journal of Autism and Developmental Disorders, 48*(7), 2490–2505. https://doi.org/10.1007/s10803-018-3510-4

Tsirgiotis, J. M., Young, R. L., & Weber, N. (2021). A mixed-methods investigation of diagnostician sex/gender-bias and challenges in assessing females for autism spectrum disorder. *Journal of Autism and Developmental Disorders, 52*, 4474–4489. https://doi.org/10.1007/s10803-021-05300-5

Tubío-Fungueiriño, M., Cruz, S., Sampaio, A., Carracedo, A., & Fernández-Prieto, M. (2020). Social camouflaging in females with autism spectrum disorder: A systematic review. *Journal of Autism and Developmental Disorders., 51*(7), 2190–2199. https://doi.org/10.1007/s10803-020-04695-x

Young, H., Oreve, M. J., & Speranza, M. (2018). Clinical characteristics and problems diagnosing autism spectrum disorder in girls. *Archives de Pédiatrie, 25*(6), 399–403. https://doi.org/10.1016/j.arcped.2018.06.008

Weiss, J. A., & Fardella, M. A. (2018). Victimization and perpetration experiences of adults with autism. *Frontiers in Psychiatry, 9*. https://doi.org/10.3389/fpsyt.2018.00203

Whitlock, A., Fulton, K., Lai, M.-C., Pellicano, E., & Mandy, W. (2020). *Recognition of girls on the autism spectrum by primary school educators: An experimental study*. Autism Research: Official Journal of the International Society for Autism Research, 13(8), 1358–1372. https://doi.org/10.1002/aur.2316

Willey, L. H. (2012). *Safety skills for Asperger women: How to save a perfectly good female life.* Jessica Kingsley Publishers.

Willey, L. H. (2014). *Pretending to be normal: Living with Asperger's syndrome (autism spectrum disorder) expanded edition.* Jessica Kingsley.

Wilson, C. E., Murphy, C. M., McAlonan, G., Robertson, D. M., Spain, D., Hayward, H., Woodhouse, E., Deeley, P. Q., Gillan, N., Ohlsen, J. C., Zinkstok, J., Stoencheva, V., Faulkner, J., Yildiran, H., Bell, V., Hammond, N., Craig, M. C., & Murphy, D. G. M. (2016). Does sex influence the diagnostic evaluation of autism spectrum disorder in adults? *Autism, 20*(7), 808–819. https://doi.org/10.1177/1362361315611381

Wolff, J. J., Boyd, B. A., & Elison, J. T. (2016). A quantitative measure of restricted and repetitive behaviors for early childhood. *Journal of Neurodevelopmental Disorders, 8*(27). https://doi.org/10.1186/s11689-016-9161-x

Wood-Downie, H., Wong, B., Kovshoff, H., Mandy, W., Hull, L., & Hadwin, J. A. (2021). Sex/gender differences in camouflaging in children and adolescents with autism. *Journal of Autism & Developmental Disorders, 51*(4), 1353–1364. https://doi.org/10.1007/s10803-020-04615-z

Chapter 6
Interpreting Female Social Relationships: Autism Friendships and Pragmatic Language

Introduction

In our clinical experience, we have heard statements indicating that a girl or woman could not possibly have autism because she had at least one friend. Having one good friend is fairly common in the first person literature, however. These friendships are described as very important, but also difficult to navigate for multiple reasons.

> *There is so much that autistic women and girls can give to each other, including love, laughter, joy, kind smiles, critical thought, understanding, and true safety. Instead of striving to conform to a neurotypical norm, these friendships can let our young women be who they are on their own terms. Navigating the complicated social rules of girls and women is so very difficult. Doing it with a friend or two who truly understand and like you for who you are makes it, if not easier, at least less painful. -Jean Winegardner,* (Ballou et al., 2021, p. 175)

Case Study—Aaliyah: Online Friendships, Imaginative Ideas, and Scripted Socializing

Aaliyah is 17 years old. Her parents felt she was very social as a younger child, but they wonder why she no longer seeks out interactions with peers and prefers to chat with "strangers" online. Her teachers report that she seems to get along with peers in the classroom, but she doesn't seem particularly close to anyone. Aaliyah reported that she sometimes talks to peers she has known since elementary school, but she didn't feel like she had a lot in common with them anymore. Specifically, they didn't share her specific interests in anime and manga, and Aaliyah was not interested in clothes, boys, and the types of books her friends were reading. Spending just a few minutes with them at school each day felt like plenty of time for Aaliyah.

T. P. Gabrielsen et al., *Assessment of Autism in Females and Nuanced Presentations*, https://doi.org/10.1007/978-3-031-33969-1_6

Aaliyah described engaging in a detailed imaginative world that included several anime characters from her two favorite shows. She found a few Discord servers devoted to these interests and happily spends most of her free time each day engaging with peers from around the world. While Aaliyah sees this as an active social life, her parents would prefer she engage with peers in person. Aaliyah's previous interest in studying her peers and their interactions has helped her develop several appropriate responses in common social situations (e.g., when peers were excited or upset about a romantic partner, when a peer would say they were "depressed" or would say negative things about a class or a teacher, etc.). This has been very helpful, as she otherwise struggles to respond to comments peers make in the moment. Aaliyah feels any sort of small talk is unnecessary, and she would much rather not "waste time" so she can get right to the interesting parts of conversation—talking about her interests. Aaliyah's ready-made list of things to say and ways to respond to common situations has also helped her to, as she put it, "avoid detection as an alien" by her peers. Aaliyah often uses the imagery of feeling like an "alien" among classmates, and she now knows that the differences that make her "alien" also make her a target for bullying.

Gender Differences

The term *biopsychosocial* was first introduced in 1977 as a medical model for understanding the key to the assessment and treatment of medical issues (biological) that also involved both psychological and social dimensions (Engel, 1977). This concept and terminology are still commonly used in medical settings, but can just as easily apply to better understanding of nuanced autism that we are beginning to acknowledge. The underpinnings for the behaviors described in this chapter begin with differences in the neurobiological processing (biology) of social information in autistic females that is more like their neurotypical counterparts than their autistic male peers (Kirkovski et al., 2016). This finding may also explain the psychological findings of gender differences in social motivation and imitation abilities (compared to autistic males). The social dimensions of gendered expectations may be the more difficult barrier to overcome in terms of assessment, however. Beginning in 2020, Lai and Szatmari called for a holistic (biopsychosocial) approach to understanding individuals within sex and gender contexts as an essential key to accurate and timely diagnosis and support.

To adult clinicians, the skills evaluated in autism assessment may seem to be gender neutral, but that is likely to be a crucial mistake (Tierney et al., 2016). Autistic females have less-developed friendship skills than their neurotypical (NT) female peers, but perhaps because their social skills are relatively close to NT boys, their differences are not as noticeable to adults (Head et al., 2014). For example, the different ways in which autistic girls engage in special interests and stimming behaviors, their higher level of social and conversation skills, and their ability to initiate friendships can all lead to lack of concern from teachers (Hiller et al., 2014). An experimental study among teachers found bias against girls when asked about autism. As they reviewed vignettes of different phenotypes of autism, ADHD, and separation anxiety with gendered names, primary school educators (even those with autism training) were less sensitive to autism in girls and more sensitive to autism in males (Whitlock et al., 2020). Further complicating identification in school settings are findings that while noncompliance is often reported in autistic girls by their parents, it is often not seen at school, perhaps because of gender expectations for following rules (Simcoe et al., 2022). The energy needed to regulate emotions and reactions at school may result in lower resilience at the end of the day at home. Other school research has found that social pressures and challenges are different by gender, with girls being overlooked more than overtly excluded (Dean et al., 2014). Differences in social pressures can include more subtle nuances in interaction, more intimate interactions, and the stronger need to conform with group interests (Dean, et al., 2013). In contrast to structured play with relatively clear hierarchies seen in boys' play, girls play in smaller, fluid, intimate groups with conversation and less structured play, based on reciprocal friendships (Blatchford et al., 2003).

Internalized gender expectations (of themselves) may also affect self-reporting of social functioning and empathy that can lead clinicians away from autism identification. Belcher et al. (2022) concluded that results of their study showing higher levels of self-reported empathy and social motivation among autistic women (diagnosed or probably autistic) could have been affected by internalized gender norms. In this case, the internalization of gender norms refers to an autistic person, but clinicians across genders may also be vulnerable to their own internalized gender expectations.

The subtle nuances of female friendships (e.g., protecting secrets, relational aggression, exclusivity, and interdependence) that are difficult for autistic females to navigate are not easily identifiable in assessment processes, as they may not always be noticed by adults. Dean et al. (2017) concluded that for most adults observing children on the playground, male social groups (because of the activities typical for each gender) were just as conducive to exposing the social challenges of autistic boys as the female group activities were likely to obscure social challenges of autistic girls. These subtleties are magnified in importance in adolescence, when autistic girls have much more difficulty understanding and meeting inter-group expectations. Neurotypical adolescent female groups require sophisticated skills of navigation that often exceed the social communication skill sets and experiences of autistic girls, who are ultimately excluded (Greenlee et al., 2020). Some may argue that many adolescents have difficulty navigating social norms in adolescence, but autistic girls are likely to have more difficulty. If these patterns continue into adulthood, Oswald et al. (2016) concluded that the interaction of autism traits with societal expectations for women leads to difficulties in maintaining jobs and educational placements.

Social Motivation

First Person Narratives

But, day in and day out, rejection began to lay heavy on my shoulders most likely because I did not understand why I was being excluded. To choose to be left out is one thing, but to be locked out, is quite another. A smile and a few minutes of conversation used to be enough to make a friend, and for the life of me, I could not figure out when or why this had stopped being the rule. -(Willey, 2014, p. 56)

While it is true that some Aspergirls just don't want friends and are happy being alone, the thing I have found in my research is not so much an innate lack of desire for friends, but an acceptance of the fact they will never have them. (Simone, 2010, p. 100).

I deeply wanted to engage my peers and make connections as others did, but the map to them was beyond cryptic, if not altogether missing. The words I needed were buried in some language that I had not mastered at all. After I failed repeatedly and sometimes watched helplessly, I withdrew into my own private prison. I desperately studied humans and I later developed an "appropriate" monologue of responses and conversation starters. I found ways to look "normal" while inside I felt very far away from everyone. Through pattern seeking, I learned that people loved to talk about themselves and that I could be the grand listener. It served me and fooled many people into thinking I was doing well socially and had a lot of friends. But the truth was that as a teenager and young adult, I simply had a lot of pretend therapy clients. - Jennifer St. Jude (Ballou et al., 2021, p. 58)

Although many consider lack of social motivation to be an important consideration in autism assessment, current diagnostic criteria acknowledge this as possibly a myth or misunderstanding:

There may be an apparent preference for solitary activities or for interacting with much younger or older people. Frequently, there is a desire to establish friendships without a complete or realistic idea of what friendship entails (e.g., one-sided friendships or friendships based solely on shared special interests). Relationships with siblings, coworkers, and caregivers are also important to consider (in terms of reciprocity). (APA, 2022)

This update to the description of autism in general regarding social motivation is noted extensively in the scientific literature about autistic females. In most studies, social motivation, awareness, and friendships of autistic girls are more similar to neurotypical (NT) females than autistic boys (Jorgenson et al., 2020; Sedgewick et al., 2016; Sproston et al., 2017; Vine Foggo & Webster, 2017). These findings reinforce the importance of choosing appropriate comparison groups and to not compare girls with autistic boys in the assessment process.

Researchers and first-person narratives emphasize the importance of friendships and social connectedness for the sense of confidence, companionships, and happiness that can come with friendship (Botha et al., 2022). Accounts of successful and long-lasting friendships are reported in people across the spectrum of autistic traits, including friendships around sharing common interests or similar social preferences (Duvall et al., 2021). Social motivation is not always followed by social success, however, as difficulty maintaining friendships is also noted throughout the literature

(Bottema-Beutel et al., 2016; Mademtzi et al., 2018). Unfortunately, despite social motivation and awareness, autistic children across genders face more peer rejection than their peers (Dean et al., 2014):

> *"I had many friends [...] until adolescence. All at once, my idiosyncrasies became very uncool, almost overnight. My social deficits became glaring holes in my persona."* (Simone, 2010, p. 28)

Given that there are likely to be reports of friendship in the data collection for autism assessment, it is important to explore the quality, reciprocity, and duration of these relationships. For example, initiating and maintaining play with unfamiliar children on the playground may seem like good evidence of social success, but look for more evidence of successfully maintaining relationships over time (Duvall et al., 2021).

Imitation Skills and Social Relationships

First Person Narratives

> *I was very conscious of the rules my friends set for themselves and the group, particularly as they applied to behaviors and other social skills. As if I had a Rolodex in my mind, I would categorize the actions of people, noting their differences and subtleties with a mix of abstract appreciation and real curiosity about why they acted as they did. I became very aware of the smallest and most subtle aspects of my peers' movements.* (Willey, 2014, p. 45)

> *Being so focused on fitting in, I had pretty much stopped caring about academics and grades. I wanted to fit in with the kids I hung out with. I also began to obsess awkwardly about looking and acting as much like my peers as I could and about boys. Meltdowns mainly transpired at home, but I recall having a really intense one at school over a misunderstanding where friends ignored me after I said something wrong. I wanted to know what I had said wrong and fix it, but when no one would talk to me, I ended up extremely distraught. I started attending counseling. I wanted to know why I kept struggling but was not prepared for the answer.* - Jen Elcheson (Cook & Garnett, 2018, p. 37)

In assessment, it is important to consider the difference between a person's intuitive ability to connect in a developmentally typical way with their peers and applied skills in using learned social scripts and rules in social interactions to increase success (Duvall et al., 2021). Imitation skills that are often thought of as deficient or missing in autism are actually quite variable across the spectrum. These imitation skills, which help autistic girls assimilate into social groups, may be more evident particularly when higher cognitive abilities are present (Vanvuchelen et al., 2011). Imitating others and adhering to self-generated complex rules for social interaction may result in a social veneer that is not obviously different upon casual inspection (Duvall et al., 2021). The ability to imitate as a developed "survival" skill may also explain why many with nuanced autism find cultural and performing arts groups to be very welcoming and tolerant of autistic differences (Willey, 2014).

Possible Differences in Autistic Friendships

First Person Narratives

> If we have a best friend who is not on the spectrum, this friend can become both caretaker and cruise director, and without them we can be totally lost in social situations....We think of ourselves as loyal, but they may find us clingy and stifling if we insist on having only them as our friend. Artemesia (Cook & Garnett, 2018, p. 48)

> I realized if I could start faking a persona, I could gain more normal friends and after trying to act more normal in front of people my motive for making friends began to work and I gained a best friend. I was so happy to have a best friend that I became too attached to her and very clingy towards her and very protective as well. I wouldn't let anyone else be with her because I was so excited to have a best friend. I didn't know how to have a healthy friendship... I continued to create exhausting personas towards people in my grade so they would not talk down to me or treat me like a baby or a five year old....but as I matured I became more aware of my autistic behaviors and one of them is to become over emotional in public. So if one of them said something critical towards me I would fake a smile and end up saving my tears and crying at home. Madeline Martin (TEDx, 2019)

> When I finally decided that I couldn't take the pain of being emotionally hypersensitive in an environment that didn't support it (of course I didn't know I was any different from anyone else at the time), I decided to stop feeling. - Sue (Miller, 2015)

> I did have friends but the relationships were through shared interests. Carol and I were good friends because we both loved horses and riding. Other friendships were formed through interests in model rockets and electronics. . . . In high school it was horses and later in life it was friends in the construction industry. We had a good time because we built things together. - Temple Grandin (Attwood et al., 2019, p. 206)

> What was wonderful, though, about developing friends through this internet support group was that it was in writing! I could see and re-read their words. I could respond or not respond as I was ready. Things didn't move at the rapid pace that overwhelmed me in real-time. Most importantly, these people understood me. They experienced life in much the same way I did. I was valued for the inner me that I shared with them. - Susan Golubock. (Miller, 2015, p. 88)

One Friend is Typical

As early as 2000, Bauminger and Kasari documented the typicality of at least one friendship in the lives of autistic children (described at the time as high functioning), but also that the quality of friendships was different from neurotypical peers in terms of companionship, security, and help.

> "As a child, I interacted with one friend at a time, distressed when that person wanted to socialize with others," (Cohen, 2017, p. 65)

The ability to focus on more than one friend in a social situation may be affected by sensory and/or language differences that prohibit the "multitasking" that is often required to participate in friend groups:

"Girls with ASD may appear to have friends or, more accurately, often just one friend...in other cases, women with ASD say that large groups were the best places for them," (Hendrickx, 2015, p. 81)

It is also possible that the multitude of emotions present in any group may be overwhelming to try to deal with or interpret. In both scientific and first-person literature, there are also mentions of friendships with boys as being easier than same-sex friendships (Cridland et al., 2014; Fowler & O'Connor, 2021; Hendrickx, 2015).

"Generally, I had one friend in each class throughout my school years. Whichever other girl in the class was not accepted by the others would end up sitting with me during lunch--Jane Meyerding," (Miller, 2015, p. 185)

Imaginary friends are also reported frequently (Hendrickx, 2015). Relationships with friends who share common interests are often the easiest to initiate and maintain (Attwood et al., 2019):

I often hated getting out of bed because that was a great place to think about my imaginary friends undisturbed, and having to drag myself away from that and return to reality was horrible and depressing. (Hendrickx, 2015, p. 67)

Although there are risks associated with online friendships (Gillespie-Smith et al., 2021), having the luxury of being able to focus on the interaction without the burden of trying to read body language, a wider group to choose from, and the ability to seek out a group with existing common interests may outweigh the risks of victimization and talking to strangers. Relationships and connections made through videogames or similar digital platforms are also variations of friendships that may be either the only type of friendships or additional friendships for any gender (Duvall et al., 2021).

Tierney et al. (2016) conducted a qualitative study, interviewing adolescent autistic girls. Regarding friendship, they reported there was abundant motivation for emotionally intimate same-gender friendship. The complication was that the autistic girls did not understand the covert rules of such friendships, making it impossible to abide by those rules. Because they inevitably break the rules that neurotypical peers have already internalized, they are often rejected as different. The most successful and long-lasting friendships described in the first-person and scientific literature are friends who share interests and/or are similarly left out of the more mainstream social groups (Attwood et al., 2019).

I felt at secondary school that they were kind of the left-over girls [...] I did feel that they were girls that kind of drifted together because they weren't in any other group. FP03 (parent) (Milner et al., 2019, pg. 2392).

Conflicts and Sensitivity

First Person Narratives

> It is tiring [interacting with neurotypicals], I have only realized this since I got autistic friends. It is so much easier … it is effortless. Participant 10 (Crompton et al., 2020, pg. 1443)

> I wish people could understand that I can soak up all I need from most friends in just a few minutes, then walk away happy and content, knowing I have just spent time with a friend. I am not trying to be at all evasive or unfriendly, I just fill up fast. - (Willey, 2014, p. 78)

> I vividly remember hating to see her with anyone other than me. I don't believe I was jealous. I know it wasn't simple insecurities. I didn't give other children enough thought to warrant those emotions. I simply could not see the point in having more than one friend and I could never imagine Maureen might feel any differently. To me, the logic was simple. I had my friend. She had me. End of story. (Willey, 2014, p. 21)

> Opinions on social relationships, particularly with other girls, are a clear indicator that these young women thought and felt differently to their peers. They had different agendas, different interests and different requirements from a friendship. Some were bullied, some were excluded and some were permitted to exist on the fringes. (Hendrickx, 2015, p. 89)

> I didn't understand that this was a natural thing people did, moving on, shifting directions. I didn't understand that it didn't mean they weren't my friends anymore.…just when I thought things were starting to make sense, confusion and frustration took over once again. - Susan Golubock (Miller, 2015, p. 87)

> It was easy for me to give my opinions on things, virtually all the time. I was by far the most blunt and outspoken of our group, even when my friends suggested I had gone too far. I never knew how far was too far. Even now, I cannot find one reliable reason for keeping my thoughts to myself. (Willey, 2014, p. 34)

Autistic girls may be more socially motivated and have more intimate friendships than autistic boys, but they are still not as skilled as girls without autism at recognizing conflict in those friendships (Sedgewick et al., 2019). Multiple studies of first-person accounts note that conflict is particularly difficult for autistic females to identify, understand, and manage within social relationships (Sedgewick et al., 2016).

> "All my life is like I didn't fit in, like I had friends and they weren't like my proper friends and I'd fall out with them. -FF17" (Milner et al., 2019, p. 2392)

Difficulties understanding how other girls perceive them, expectation of peers, and expectations of socializing within groups are all listed as factors that impact success in maintaining relationships (Vine Foggo & Webster, 2017). Another obstacle to social success may also be the need to de-stress after social interactions and pursue solitary interests for a while, disrupting participation with the rest of the group on a somewhat regular basis (Vine Foggo & Webster, 2017).

Gender expectations are also a factor in difficulties understanding social cues and expected behaviors (Cridland et al., 2014; Kirkovski et al., 2013). In studies of autistic adolescents, gender is suggested to play a more critical role than autism traits or diagnoses in perceptions and experiences with social relationships (Sedgewick et al., 2019). Rigidity as an autistic trait was also implicated in lack of insight into the reciprocal nature of friendship and what that entails (Trubanova et al., 2014).

Lai and Szatmari (2020) summarized scientific findings regarding equity of access to the identification of autism for girls and women as related to deficiencies in standard measures that fail to take into account the higher social attention, linguistic ability, and motivation for friendship in autistic females. Increases in problems with adaptive functioning and social challenges as the gap between NT and autistic females widens in adolescence were also noted.

Clinicians should pay attention to the many comments in the first-person literature about not understanding the natural ebb and flow of friendships. Not understanding that a friendship is changing or cooling and the sense of confusion about these changes could be evidence for not understanding social relationships well, even if someone has had friends or does have a current friend. Some are devastated when friendships end (Fowler & O'Conner, 2021).

Pragmatic Language (Social Communication)

First Person Narratives

I also really struggle to make friends because social chitchat doesn't come naturally to me. I don't know what's expected and I don't know what other people want me to say. I learned to hide it at a young age and I learned to mimic the behavior of other people. Carrie Beckwith-Fellows (TED-X speaker, 2017)

I can listen or look, talk or do, but not both at the same time. To compensate for my decreased auditory processing as I visually focused on people's faces, I learned to nod, smile or frown to make it appear I was listening....Later, I learned from watching a friend how asking questions kept conversations going....I often wondered, though, why no one ever asked me to talk. Didn't matter. It was too hard to shift gears from listening to talking anyway. Susan Golubock (Miller, 2015, p. 173)

Maybe I was experiencing sensory overload. Maybe I was frazzled because I did not have any way of predicting what would come next. Or, maybe I simply felt uncomfortable sharing close space with people so foreign to me. All I know for certain is that these moments were terrible. Faces began to merge together, voices sounded out of sync and my perception fooled me. Things ran on slow speed then, letting an eternity slip by until I could find a quiet corner or an empty room to gather myself up again. It was hard to make me right at that point, but given time, I always did. (Willey, 2014, p. 41–42)

The other girls had become friends with one another. Alone there, with no adult present to direct us, they chatted and whispered and laughed and interacted with seamless ease. How did they know what to say? They weren't talking about anything, and yet they talked constantly. Jane Myerding (Miller, 2015, p. 183)

People would share information about themselves with me, yet I didn't know what I was supposed to do with it. People would call themselves my friends, but I couldn't figure out what I was supposed to do with a friend. Without this sharing of thoughts and feelings between myself and others, I had no clue just how much I thought or felt differently from others. It was quite a shock when I finally did discover how much of myself I had hidden even from myself all those years. -Susan Golubock (Miller, 2015, p. 86)

Recent trends toward more acceptance of qualitative research in the scientific literature have allowed us to learn more about relationships between language abilities (particularly conversation) and social relationships throughout life. Even young children report that language and communication difficulties, along with their own emotional responses, have an effect on their social relationship. Listening difficulties and subsequent confusion, stress, and annoyance were also identified as interfering with social success (Sturrock et al., 2022).

It may be that the uses of language beyond pragmatic needs have not yet been discovered or internalized by some autistic children, adolescents, or adults (Willey, 2014). The diagnostic criteria for autism includes struggling to understand behaviors considered appropriate in one situation but not another (e.g., casual behavior at home vs. professional behavior during a job interview) or nuances in the ways that language may be used to communicate (e.g., irony, white lies) (APA, 2022).

Differences in the language of girls and women as they talk about their social lives have also been investigated as an indicator of autism in females. Song et al. (2021) found autistic females used "they" to describe social groups in their settings vs. the use of the word "we" among neurotypical females. Their hypothesis was that diminished membership in social groups (and heightened discussion of social groups) in pre-teen and adolescent years was manifest in the choice of words:

"All my friendships died a quick death because I couldn't keep up my end of a conversation. The subject matter had to be something I found interesting, otherwise my brain would freeze. End of friendship. -Gail Pennington" (Miller, 2015, p. 216)

Bullying and Abuse

First Person Narratives

I had no idea I was a regular victim of abuse until my counselor made it abundantly clear some of my so-called friends, mentors, and trusted bosses were nothing more than abusers who must have picked up on the fact I was an easy mark because of the very things that make me autistic. Liane Holliday Willey (Cook & Garnett, 2018, p. 95)

At first glance, this seems like an obvious abuse to detect. But the shrewd predator will know how to hurt you without leaving a visible mark and they will know how to convince you either that they aren't abusing you or that you deserve the abuse they are giving, or that they are sorry and are so thankful they have you to understand they aren't bad people even though they beat you to pieces. So many of us on the spectrum will fall into these traps for all sorts of fine and not so fine reasons. Maybe we have an admirably strong sense of loyalty or a deep sense of empathy and concern. Or maybe we have no self-worth, or a desperate need to keep a friend no matter how horrible the friend is. Liane Holliday Willey (Cook & Garnett, 2018, p. 100)

All at once, my idiosyncrasies became very uncool, almost overnight. My social deficits, which prior to that point had just been differences, became glaring holes in my persona. At first I was merely ostracized, losing friends one by one, but then, the threats began....I developed ulcers first, by age 12....After a year or more of baiting me with hints of future physical pain, she finally made good her threat and I was badly beaten in front of a very large crowd of cheering kids, mostly older teenagers. I went from obsessive reading to obsessive push-ups to strengthen my weak limbs. Singing and laughing–my two favorite things--were supplanted by mutism and crying. I developed very low self-esteem and PTSD....How does a girl who was once a gifted and popular student fall so far? Home was dysfunctional, and I'd already become mute and withdrawn there, long before I did at school. (Simone, 2010, p. 28)

Growing up, I wish my parents had known that teaching me to fight for my rights was more important than forcing me to fit in. I was conditioned early to know that my saying "no" was not an option, certain "atypical" behaviors needed to be eliminated, and being compliant made me "good." I spent a lot of time learning to deny my natural impulses and feelings in order to conform to what was expected of a "good girl." In doing so, I opened myself up to become a victim of both emotional and sexual abuse from adults and intense bullying from my peers. The way I experienced the world around me was supposedly wrong, and there was no argument. So, I remained silent. Always. -Lei Wiley-Mydske (Ballou et al., 2021, p. 31)

It was probably the culmination of everything, but the bullying was I think was the catalyst for the breakdown. The trigger that sent her into freefall. -P12 - Mother. (Fowler & O'Connor, 2021)

Vulnerability and Bullying

Temple Grandin describes her friendships with individuals with mutual interests as "refuge" from bullying and teasing (Attwood et al., 2019). For individuals with social communication difficulties, lack of understanding of social expectations, and limited reciprocal friendship behaviors and skills, the likelihood of bullying, teasing, and rejection can be high, even within social or friend groups. Autistic females have been described as naive and easily deceived, perhaps because of intense motivation to be accepted by peers (M. Wrobel, in Attwood et al., 2019).

While bullying and abuse can happen at any time, there are multiple studies showing that autistic traits and isolation increase from childhood to adolescence, when anxiety, depression, and other mental health issues can begin to dominate (Greenlee et al., 2017; Lai & Szatmari, 2020).

Greenlee et al. (2020) studied relational aggression across genders. It can be more complicated in autistic girls compared to autistic boys, however, as in boys, the primary difficulty may be just social cognition, or understanding social contexts for social decision-making. For autistic girls, social cognition with increased motivation, awareness, and communication skills and rigid or special interests and stimming behaviors were factors in relational aggression incidents. Additionally, depression and anxiety were predicted by victimization only in the girls in the study. Misunderstanding conflict as noted above was mentioned by Sproston et al. (2017) as possibly associated with more relational victimization of autistic girls. The compensatory skills that were sufficient for younger friendships were not sophisticated enough to navigate adolescent friendships, resulting in higher rates of exclusion (Greenlee et al., 2020).

Assessment Planning

Interpreting Standardized Measures for Females

Scientific and first-person literature agree that autism assessment requires more details on friendships than are currently collected using standardized measures. Although specific items from the Autism Diagnostic Interview-Revised (ADI-R; Lecouteur et al., 2003) are listed below, Ratto et al. (2018) found the ADI-R to be less likely to identify autistic females with higher cognitive levels. Interviews and observations are likely to provide this additional information, while new and more detailed measures are under development, including some with gendered distinctions.

Clark et al. (2021) piloted an additional coding scheme based on information provided through Autism Diagnostic Observation Schedule, Second Edition (ADOS-2; Lord et al., 2012) administrations to explore additional autistic features characterizing nuanced autism. They are developing a Gendered Autism Behavior Scale to specifically gather data regarding the known autistic traits that are sometimes missed. Although this measure is still in development and validation phases, the concepts of focus include social adaptations, managing emotions, social relationships, and interests. Within these categories, consideration of characteristics such as camouflaging, self-reflection on social behavior, self-reporting about friends, understanding of friendships, and quality of friendships (including age of friends) is evaluated in addition to the items scored on the ADOS-2. Other categories are also explored in this preliminary work, including social interest and responding to conversational cues and internalizing and externalizing behaviors. Emotions are also explored with focus on discomfort talking about emotions, social acceptance/rejection and emotions, and emotions related to rigid expectations and requirements. Assessment of interests in terms of frequency and intensity and the quality and nature of the interests are also captured in this proposed additional assessment.

Additional Measures to Inform the Assessment Process

Because more information is needed to fully understand the nature of friendships in assessment, consider additional sources of information from adaptive measures (social activity and independence, leadership, and functional communication). Social-emotional measures (atypicality, withdrawal) are also helpful. We also find value in the comprehensive evaluation of receptive and expressive language abilities that may seem to be typical within highly structured, short interactions, but may be more limited when investigated in depth (interdisciplinary teaming or collaboration between psychology and speech and language).

Interviews and Observations

Interviews with the individual are likely to provide considerably more relevant data regarding friendships than standardized measures alone. Questions about the history of a friendship (particularly the end of friendships), quality of friendship (reciprocity), and shared interests in friendship can help determine the nature of friendship skills and relationships. Observations in classrooms, cafeterias, and playgrounds can provide information on the inclusion and balance of participation with friends. For adults, this is obviously more difficult, but observations of social interactions in waiting rooms, at meals, and in group sessions can provide some detailed information.

Supports and Recommendations

Managing Conflict

With consistent reports of difficulties understanding and navigating conflict, this can be a primary topic of therapy to preserve existing social relationships. Teaching specific social repair strategies, even if the source of the conflict is not understood immediately, can be beneficial. Social stories and video modeling for targeted situations can be used to accomplish this goal.

Recognizing and Avoiding Abuse

Developing a sense of self and self-esteem independent of the acceptance of others is also a worthy target for support and therapy. Some of us use Brené Brown's books as resources.

Expanding Friendships Beyond One Friend

Developing a sense of curiosity and opening up social circles is dependent on trust and security within existing friendships that may have been hard won. Possessiveness, rigidity, and anxiety about losing a friend can be addressed through diversification of existing friendship activities, including gradual exposure to others with similar interests. With purposeful and planned exploration, anxiety about losing a friend in a larger group may be reduced as success and confidence are gained.

Compensatory Language Processing Behaviors

Teach compensatory behaviors for when language processing speed is not keeping up with conversational speed. Behaviors designed to give additional time for processing can include "Wait, what did you just say?", "I am not sure how to react to that," "I'm going to need a minute to think about that," etc. can slow down the speed of interaction enough to allow for additional processing time, clarification, or a graceful "out" if unsure about how to continue.

Gaining Confidence in Casual Social Relationships

The Girls Night Out program at the University of Kansas provides a model for increasing social confidence and skills in social relationships by way of gaining experience in self-care and typical adolescent activities in a group setting. Felicity House in Manhattan, NY, provides a model for working within groups to seek new experiences, creativity, and knowledge to build social relationships in adult women. Many universities offer social groups for autistic women as well. Because of the relatively lower number of identified autistic girls and women, it may be harder to find female-only groups for younger children, but asking school psychologists, speech and language pathologists, and social workers in schools is the first step to creating these experiences for students with nuanced autism.

Resources Created by Autistic Authors

There are a variety of resources created for autistic children and adults by the autistic community. We are listing a broad range here as representative of what is available.

- Cook, J. (2022) *The Asperkid's (Secret) Book of Social Rules, Tenth Anniversary Edition.* Jessica Kingsley [book].
- Natasha, (n.d.) The Cool Calming Corner (https://supernovamomma.com/the-coolcalmingcorner/) [posters].
- Whelton, E. (2018) Konfident Kidz (https://konfidentkidz.ie), run by autistic speech and drama teacher Evaleen Whelton, offers neurodiversity-affirming classes and resources.
- Gill, V.C. (2023) Ava: SEL game for neurodivergent youth ages 10–15. https://www.socialciphergame.com.
- Outschool.com offers autistic-led social/learning opportunities by autistic teachers such as Gabrielle Hughes and Heather Cook.

Return to the Case Study

Aaliyah reports being very happy with the level of engagement she has with peers online. Helping her parents understand the validity of these relationships can ease some of the tension Aaliyah feels when parents ask why she isn't more social. Since Aaliyah doesn't feel she can connect to classmates she used to be close with, it might be helpful to seek out (or even create) social clubs outside school hours that focus on Aaliyah's interests. Finding classmates with whom she has common interests through a semi-structured club experience may prove easier than seeking out such relationships from the large pool of high schoolers. Aaliyah is successfully using some scripted language to respond to common situations. Increasing her repertoire of situations and preparing ahead of time for situations that will likely occur in the near future (e.g., asking for support from counselors for college/career planning, inquiring about jobs) will help Aaliyah to feel more prepared for upcoming changes as she prepares to transition away from high school. While Aaliyah strongly dislikes small talk, having a few key phrases and nonverbal/minimally verbal responses (e.g., nodding, utterances that convey possible agreement or attention) prepared for when those situations become more necessary (e.g., with a potential employer) would be helpful. See Table 6.1 for an at-a-glance summary of assessment strategies related to friendships and pragmatic language.

Table 6.1 At-a-glance summary of social relationships, autism friendships, and pragmatic language

Domain	Focus	Assessment planning (age ranges)
Social-emotional reciprocity	"Have you ever tried to change anything about yourself to fit in with other people?" (Clark et al., 2021) Listen for examples of understanding definitions of social relationships, but lack of reciprocity or sense of own role in maintaining relationships	**Interview**—Individual **ADOS-2, Module 3 or 4** *(generally age 4+ language levels with fluent speech including ability to talk about abstract concepts;* Lord et al., 2012*)*
Turn taking and reciprocity	Imbalanced participation—Too much direction of others with frustration with disagreements Not keeping up with rapid changes in social dynamics or conversation	**Playground observation** *Autism diagnostic interview-revised* **(ADI-R)** *social development and play section* (2 and older; Le Couteur et al., 2003) *(For published algorithms for children younger than 4—see* Kim and Lord, 2012, *and* Kim et al. 2013) **Classroom observations**
Nonverbal communication	Watch for more-than-expected check-ins for clarification of expectations	
Developing, maintaining, and understanding relationships	When describing friendships: "Would you say that you have a best friend or friends? Is there anyone you are friendly with, but not that close to?" (Clark et al., 2021) Listen for mystification about relationships that have ended.	

(continued)

Table 6.1 (continued)

Domain	Focus	Assessment planning (age ranges)
Developing, maintaining, and understanding relationships	Early friendships, behavior on the playground when other children are present, how friendships are made Who are friends? Is there a range of friends? What ages? (above or below chronological age) Nature of friendships? Intense? Distant? Online? How do friendships end?	**Interviews—Individual, parents, and teachers**
Conversation	Imbalanced participation—More than expected or not enough (not keeping up with rapidly changing conversation or dominating)	**Cafeteria, playground, and classroom observations**
Language	Difficulty with subtext and pragmatic language, reliance on scripts	**Receptive and expressive language evaluation** *SLPs have a variety of measures to choose from according to the individual*
Nonverbal communication	Not reading or using nonverbal cues or slow to understand and respond to nonverbal cues	**ADOS-2, Module 3 or 4** *(generally age 4+ language levels with fluent speech including ability to talk about abstract concepts;* Lord et al., 2012)
Bullying and abuse	If reports being bullied or teased: "How did you feel when that happened?" (Clark et al., 2021) Ask about understanding in the moment and later when enough time to process has passed	**ADOS-2, Module 3 or 4** *(generally age 4+ language levels with fluent speech including ability to talk about abstract concepts;* Lord et al., 2012) Also, interview and observation
Restricted, special, or intense interests	In addition to "happiness" question: "Do you have any hobbies or interests that make you feel happy?" (Clark et al., 2021)	**ADOS-2, Module 3 or 4** *(generally age 4+ language levels with fluent speech including ability to talk about abstract concepts;* Lord et al., 2012) Also, interview and observation
Emotional regulation	In addition to "frightened or anxious" question: "How often do you feel that way?" (Clark et al., 2021)	**ADOS-2, Module 3 or 4** *(generally age 4+ language levels with fluent speech including ability to talk about abstract concepts;* Lord et al., 2012) Also, interview and observation

(continued)

Table 6.1 (continued)

Domain	Focus	Assessment planning (age ranges)
Emotional regulation	In addition to "sad" question: "How often do you feel that way?" or "Do you ever feel hopeless or that good things don't ever happen to you?" (Clark et al., 2021)	**ADOS-2, Module 3 or 4** (*generally age 4+ language levels with fluent speech including ability to talk about abstract concepts;* Lord et al., 2012) Also, interview and observation

Please see the "References" section in this chapter for additional information on measures.

Not all measures and processes listed are available in all settings or appropriate for all cases. Qualification levels apply. Multiple measures in a single domain are not necessary. Some measures can provide data in multiple domains. This is meant to provide a relatively quick reference for assessment planning and implementation, not an endorsement of any particular measure as "best." Emphasis here is on readily available, commonly used measures, but similar measures may also be useful

References

American Psychiatric Association. (2022). *Diagnostic and statistical manual of mental disorders* (Text revision) (15th ed.). American Psychiatric Association.

Attwood, T., Garnett, M., Grandin, T., Faherty, C., McIlwee Meyers, J., Snyder, R., Wagner, S., Wrobel, M., Iland, L., & Bolick, T. (2019). *Autism and girls*. Future Horizons.

Ballou, E. P., da Vanport, S., & Onaiwu, M. G. (Eds.). (2021). *Sincerely, your autistic child*. Beacon Press.

Bauminger, N., & Kasari, C. (2000). Loneliness and friendship in high-functioning children with autism. *Child Development, 71*(2), 447–456. https://doi.org/10.1111/1467-8624.00156

Belcher, H. L., Morein-Zamir, S., Stagg, S. D., & Ford, R. M. (2022). Shining a light on a hidden population: Social functioning and mental health in women reporting autistic traits but lacking diagnosis. *Journal of Autism and Developmental Disorders, 1-15*. https://doi.org/10.1007/s10803-022-05583-2

Blatchford, P., Baines, E., & Pellegrini, A. (2003). The social context of school playground games: Sex and ethnic differences, and changes over time after entry to junior school. *British Journal of Developmental Psychology, 21*, 481–505. https://doi.org/10.1348/026151003322535183

Botha, M., Dibb, B., & Frost, D. M. (2022). 'It's being a part of a grand tradition, a grand counter-culture which involves communities': A qualitative investigation of autistic community connectedness. *Autism: The International Journal of Research & Practice.* https://doi.org/10.1177/13623613221080248

Clark, E., Hull, L., Loomes, R., McCormick, C. E. B., Sheinkopf, S. J., & Mandy, W. (2021). Assessing autism spectrum disorder using the Gendered Autism Behavioral Scale (GABS): An exploratory study. *Research in Autism Spectrum Disorders, 88*, 101844. https://doi.org/10.1016/j.rasd.2021.101844

Cohen, T. (2017). *Six-word lessons on female Asperger syndrome: 100 lessons to understand and support girls and women with Asperger's*. Pacelli Publishing.

Cook, B., & Garnett, M. (Eds.). (2018). *Spectrum women: Walking to the beat of autism*. Jessica Kingsley.

Cook, J. (2022). *The Asperkid's (secret) book of social rules:.Tenth anniversary edition*. Jessica Kingsley.

Cridland, E. K., Jones, S. C., Caputi, P., & Magee, C. A. (2014). Being a girl in a boys' world: Investigating the experiences of girls with autism spectrum disorders during adolescence. *Journal of Autism and Developmental Disorders, 44*(6), 1261–1274. https://doi.org/10.1007/s10803-013-1985-6

Crompton, C. J., Hallett, S., Ropar, D., Flynn, E., & Fletcher-Watson, S. (2020). I never realised everybody felt as happy as I do when I am around autistic people: A thematic analysis of autistic adults' relationships with autistic and neurotypical friends and family. *Autism: The International Journal of Research and Practice, 24*(6), 1438–1448. https://doi.org/10.1177/1362361320908976

Dean, M., Adams, G. F., & Kasari, C. (2013). How narrative difficulties build peer rejection: A discourse analysis of a girl with autism and her female peers. *Discourse Studies, 15*(2), 147–166. https://doi.org/10.1177/1461445612471472

Dean, M., Kasari, C., Shih, W., Frankel, F., Whitney, R., Landa, R., Lord, C., Orlich, F., King, B., & Harwood, R. (2014). The peer relationships of girls with ASD at school: Comparison to boys and girls with and without ASD. *Journal of Child Psychology & Psychiatry, 55*(11), 1218–1225. https://doi.org/10.1111/jcpp.12242

Dean, M., Harwood, R., & Kasari, C. (2017). The art of camouflage: Gender differences in the social behaviors of girls and boys with autism spectrum disorder. *Autism, 21*(6), 678–689. https://doi.org/10.1177/1362361316671845

Duvall, S., Armstrong, K., Shahabuddin, A., Grantz, C., Fein, D., & Lord, C. (2021). A road map for identifying autism spectrum disorder: Recognizing and evaluating characteristics that should raise red or "pink" flags to guide accurate differential diagnosis. *The Clinical Neuropsychologist, 36*(5), 1172–1207. https://doi.org/10.1080/13854046.2021.1921276

Engel, G. L. (1977). The need for a new medical model: A challenge for biomedicine. *Science, 196*(4286), 129–136. https://doi.org/10.1126/science.847460

Fowler, K., & O'Connor, C. (2021). "I just rolled up my sleeves": Mothers' perspectives on raising girls on the autism spectrum. *Autism: The International Journal of Research and Practice, 25*(1), 275–287. https://doi.org/10.1177/1362361320956876

Gillespie-Smith, K., Hendry, G., Anduuru, N., Laird, T., & Ballantyne, C. (2021). Using social media to be 'social': Perceptions of social media benefits and risk by autistic young people, and parents. *Research in Developmental Disabilities, 118*, 104081. https://doi.org/10.1016/j.ridd.2021.104081

Greenlee, J. L., Winter, M. A., & Marcovici, I. A. (2020). Brief report: Gender differences in experiences of peer victimization among adolescents with autism spectrum disorder. *Journal of Autism and Developmental Disorders, 50*(10), 3790–3799. https://doi.org/10.1007/s10803-020-04437-z

Head, A. M., McGillivray, J. A., & Stokes, M. A. (2014). Gender differences in emotionality and sociability in children with autism spectrum disorder. *Molecular Autism, 5*(1), 1–9. https://doi.org/10.1186/2040-2392-5-19

Hendrickx, S. (2015). *Women and girls with autism spectrum disorder: Understanding life experiences from early childhood to old age*. Jessica Kingsley.

Hiller, R. M., Young, R. L., & Weber, N. (2014). Sex differences in autism spectrum disorder based on DSM-5 criteria: Evidence from clinician and teacher reporting. *Journal of Abnormal Child Psychology, 42*(8), 1381–1393. https://doi.org/10.1007/s10802-014-9881-x

Jorgenson, C., Lewis, T., Rose, C., & Kanne, S. (2020). Social camouflaging in autistic and neurotypical adolescents: A pilot study of differences by sex and diagnosis. *Journal of Autism and Developmental Disorders, 50*(12), 4344–4355. https://doi.org/10.1007/s10803-020-04491-7

Kim, S. H., & Lord, C. (2012). New autism diagnostic interview-revised algorithms for toddlers and young preschoolers from 12 to 47 months of age. *Journal of Autism and Developmental Disorders, 42*, 82–93. https://doi.org/10.1007/s10803-011-1213-1

Kim S. H., Thurm A, Shumway S, Lord C. (2013). multisite study of new *Autism Diagnostic Interview-Revised* (ADI-R) algorithms for toddlers and young preschoolers. *Journal of Autism and Developmental Disorders 43*(7):1527–1538. https://doi.org/10.1007/s10803-012-1696-4.

Kirkovski, M., Enticott, P., & Fitzgerald, P. (2013). A review of the role of female gender in autism spectrum disorders. *Journal of Autism & Developmental Disorders, 43*(11), 2584–2603. https://doi.org/10.1007/s10803-013-1811-1

Kirkovski, M., Enticott, P., Hughes, M., Rossell, S., & Fitzgerald, P. (2016). Atypical neural activity in males but not females with autism spectrum disorder. *Journal of Autism & Developmental Disorders, 46*(3), 954–963. https://doi.org/10.1007/s10803-015-2639-7

Lai, M. C., & Szatmari, P. (2020). Sex and gender impacts on the behavioural presentation and recognition of autism. *Current Opinion in Psychiatry, 33*(2), 117–123. https://doi.org/10.1097/YCO.0000000000000575

Le Couteur, A., Lord, C., & Rutter, M. (2003). *Autism Diagnostic Interview-Revised*. Western Psychological.

Lord, C., Rutter, M., DiLavore, P. C., Risi, S., Gotham, K., & Bishop, S. L. (2012). *Autism Diagnostic Observation Schedule* (2nd ed., pp. 1–4). Western Psychological Services.

Mademtzi, M., Singh, P., Shic, F., & Koenig, K. (2018). Challenges of females with autism: A parental perspective. *Journal of Autism & Developmental Disorders, 48*(4), 1301–1310. https://doi.org/10.1007/s10803-017-3341-8

Miller, J. K. (Ed.). (2015). *Women from another planet? Our lives in the universe of autism.* AuthorHouse.

Milner, V., McIntosh, H., Colvert, E., & Happé, F. (2019). A qualitative exploration of the female experience of autism spectrum disorder (ASD). *Journal of Autism & Developmental Disorders, 49*(6), 2389–2402. https://doi.org/10.1007/s10803-019-03906-4

Oswald, T. M., Winter-Messiers, M. A., Gibson, B., Schmidt, A. M., Herr, C. M., & Solomon, M. (2016). Sex differences in internalizing problems during adolescence in autism spectrum disorder. *Journal of Autism and Developmental Disorders, 46*(2), 624–636. https://doi.org/10.1007/s10803-015-2608-1

Ratto, A. B., Kenworthy, L., Yerys, B. E., Bascom, J., Wieckowski, A. T., White, S. W., Wallace, G. L., Pugliese, C., Schultz, R. T., Ollendick, T. H., Scarpa, A., Seese, S., Register-Brown, K., Martin, A., & Anthony, L. G. (2018). What about the girls? Sex-based differences in autistic traits and adaptive skills. *Journal of Autism and Developmental Disorders, 48*(5), 1698–1711. https://doi.org/10.1007/s10803-017-3413-9

Sedgewick, F., Hill, V., & Pellicano, E. (2019). "It's different for girls": Gender differences in the friendships and conflict of autistic and neurotypical adolescents. *Autism: The International Journal of Research and Practice, 23*(5), 1119–1132. https://doi.org/10.1177/1362361318794930

Sedgewick, F., Hill, V., Yates, R., Pickering, L., & Pellicano, E. (2016). Gender differences in the social motivation and friendship experiences of autistic and non-autistic adolescents. *Journal of Autism and Developmental Disorders, 46*(4), 1297–1306. https://doi.org/10.1007/s10803-015-2669-1

Simcoe, S. M., Gilmour, J., Garnett, M. S., Attwood, T., Donovan, C., & Kelly, A. B. (2022). Are there gender-based variations in the presentation of autism amongst female and male children? *Journal of Autism and Developmental Disorders.* Advance online publication. https://doi.org/10.1007/s10803-022-05552-9

Simone, R. (2010). *Aspergirls: Empowering females with Asperger syndrome.* Jessica Kingsley.

Song, A., Cola, M., Plate, S., Petrulla, V., Yankowitz, L., Pandey, J., Schultz, R. T., & Parish-Morris, J. (2021). Natural language markers of social phenotype in girls with autism. *Journal of Child Psychology and Psychiatry, and Allied Disciplines, 62*(8), 949–960. https://doi.org/10.1111/jcpp.13348

Sproston, K., Sedgewick, F., & Crane, L. (2017). Autistic girls and school exclusion: Perspectives of students and their parents. *Autism & Developmental Language Impairments, 2.* https://doi.org/10.1177/2396941517706172

Sturrock, A., Chilton, H., Foy, K., Freed, J., & Adams, C. (2022). In their own words: The impact of subtle language and communication difficulties as described by autistic girls and boys without intellectual disability. *Autism: The International Journal of Research and Practice, 26*(2), 332–345. https://doi.org/10.1177/13623613211002047

TEDx. (2017, July). *Beckwith-Fellows, C.: Invisible diversity: A story of undiagnosed autism* [video]. TEDxVilnius https://www.youtube.com/watch?v=cF2dhWWUyQ4

TEDx. (2019, May). *Madeline Martin: Blending In and innocence: the autistic teenage girl* TEDxUnionvilleHS youtube.com/watch?v=VQZnNKP8Tc

Tierney, S., Burns, J., & Killbey, E. (2016). Looking beyond the mask: Social coping strategies of girls on the spectrum. *Research in Autism Spectrum Disorders, 23*, 73–83. https://doi.org/10.1016/j.rasd.2015.11.013

Trubanova, A., Donlon, K., Kreiser, N. L., Ollendick, T. H., & White, S. W. (2014). Underidentification of autism spectrum disorder in females: A case series illustrating the unique presentation of this disorder in young women. *Scandinavian Journal of Child and Adolescent Psychiatry and Psychology, 2*(2), 66–76. https://doi.org/10.21307/sjcapp-2014-010

Vanvuchelen, M., Roeyers, H., & De Weerdt, W. (2011). Imitation assessment and its utility to the diagnosis of autism: Evidence from consecutive clinical preschool referrals for suspected autism. *Journal of Autism and Developmental Disorders, 41*(4), 484–496. https://doi.org/10.1007/s10803-010-1074-z

Vine Foggo, R. S., & Webster, A. A. (2017). Understanding the social experiences of adolescent females on the autism spectrum. *Research in Autism Spectrum Disorders, 35*, 74–85. https://doi.org/10.1016/j.rasd.2016.11.006

Whitlock, A., Fulton, K., Lai, M.-C., Pellicano, E., & Mandy, W. (2020). Recognition of girls on the autism Spectrum by primary school educators: An experimental study. *Autism Research: Official Journal of the International Society for Autism Research, 13*(8), 1358–1372. https://doi.org/10.1002/aur.2316

Willey, L. H. (2014). *Pretending to be normal: Living with Asperger's syndrome (autism spectrum disorder) expanded edition.* Jessica Kingsley.

Chapter 7
Autism Assessment Including Reading, Learning, and Executive Function in Females

Introduction

Connections between reading acquisition and comprehension and executive function may help to explain some of the reasons why reading is such a big part of nuanced autism, yet there may still be significant difficulties present. Working memory and processing speed explain some of these differences. Amongst our colleagues, we are beginning to wonder if the function and purpose of reading may actually be different in nuanced autism, and the many autistic females who are voracious readers, yet may have lower comprehension skills may need to read for a variety of reasons.

> For example, there were a few book series I loved and collected. Many kids didn't understand why I had such an intense interest in these books, but they encompassed important social themes. They were more than a pastime, rather a crash course in social skills I didn't innately have. One would think I was teaching myself a new language, a hidden curriculum. In many ways I was. -Jen Elcheson (Cook & Garnett, 2018, p. 35)

Case Study—Julia: Voracious Reader with Difficulty Comprehending, Slow Processing of New Information, and Challenges with Routine Tasks

Julia's parents reported that she quickly picked up reading skills. In fact, she was identifying letters and starting to "crack the code" by the time she was 3 years old. From that time on, she's been a voracious reader who rereads her favorite books over and over. Adults have observed that Julia gravitates toward her favorite books when she is in stressful situations (e.g., during non-preferred subjects at school, when she is overwhelmed with auditory stimuli). She fully engages with the

T. P. Gabrielsen et al., *Assessment of Autism in Females and Nuanced Presentations*, https://doi.org/10.1007/978-3-031-33969-1_7

characters in her favorite stories, often integrating their catchphrases into her speech and creating elaborate stories in her head that star her as a story character. When Julia is required to read specific books for school, her teacher has noted that she has difficulty with comprehension questions, including summarizing what she has read, identifying the main idea, and making inferences. Her teacher also finds that Julia processes new information very slowly. Once she understands something and has had time to think about it at her own pace, she can demonstrate mastery of many new concepts. Julia also struggles with managing aspects of day-to-day life. She has difficulty regulating sensory input and becomes overwhelmed very quickly. While she is amazing at focusing on certain tasks (especially reading), Julia struggles to attend to non-preferred activities and appears to miss adult directions. She needs frequent reminders for even basic daily tasks, such as brushing her teeth, bathing, keeping track of her belongings, following classroom routines, and taking care of her basic needs.

Differences in Autistic Reading Skills

First Person Narratives

> *I wish I could learn by synthesis, but I can't seem to synthesize at all. I had to drop classes I otherwise could have managed because I was expected to draw things together and synthesize concepts and new ideas from all the things I'd been reading. I can't do that. I can put all the readings into categories, I can pull them apart and put them back together. I can find every symbol, every figure of speech, and every component of the characters and plot, and analyze them to death, but to know what it was about? To get a feeling or concept about it, to make a whole from all the parts I can so easily distinguish? Completely and totally beyond me. After two dismal failures, I've decided I'm not cut out for studying English Literature after all. I can write in this language, but I can't understand it. Kalen* (Miller, 2015, p. 38)

With exceptionally few studies focused on autistic females or even reported results by gender, most of what we know about autism traits and reading comprehension difficulties is reported across genders. These data may be informative for support and assessment, however. One known study of autistic *girls* by Äsberg et al. (2010) did not find significant differences across autism, ADHD, and neurotypical groups in *average* measures of reading performance, but 40% of autistic girls had reading and/or writing disorders. This is consistent with the broader findings across genders that around half of autistic students have reading comprehension difficulties (Solari et al., 2017).

> *"While we may struggle with the main idea of a paragraph or the clear point of a line of reasoning, we are typically able to vividly describe just about anything we see."* (Willey, 2012, p. 66)

Grimm et al. (2017) compared a sample of autistic students (86% male, with verbal IQ average of 95) to NT students (66% male, with verbal IQ average of 110) and found that students in the autistic sample were able to gain reading skills on the same trajectory as their peers, but that they started out at a lower level (3 time points were measured), putting them at a disadvantage. By the third time point (age 14), advances in linguistic comprehension began to decline in the autism group.

Jones et al. (2009) identified lower levels of reading comprehension as the most significant gap between cognitive and academic scores (sample = 90% male). However, this does not necessarily imply that this gap exists or does not exist in females with autism or in those with more nuanced autism.

McIntyre et al. (2017) looked specifically at students with age-typical cognitive and language performance levels (described as high functioning in the study). The high prevalence (51% of the group) of lower comprehension skills compared to neurotypical and ADHD peers was consistent with other studies and tied to higher levels of autism traits, mediated by oral language skills. Implicit and inferential reading difficulties were noted as aligned with core autism traits. Explicit reading skills were not different from peers, which may obscure the comprehension difficulties in elementary (primary) grades. Estes et al. (2011) found 90% of autistic students (age 9) showed discrepancies between cognitive and academic performance measures, but differences were manifest in higher and lower academic achievement in reading compared to cognitive scores.

While many autistic students may read at or above grade level, they may nonetheless read differently than their NT peers in subtle, less evident ways, such as how they conceptualize narratives. Diehl et al. (2006) discovered that autistic children's narratives were much less cohesive than those of NT peers, despite the fact that the length and syntactic complexity of their narratives were comparable.

In addition to documenting disparities in comprehension outcomes, current research has focused on identifying predictors for students whom Davidson (2021) characterized as discrepant poor comprehenders. These students have distinct gaps in decoding and cognitive skills relative to comprehension skills. When these gaps are suspected, speech-language pathologists will likely play a crucial role in assessing and intervening (Davidson, 2021).

Reading fluency measures may also be helpful in predicting difficulties in comprehension even when decoding skills appear to be typical. In autistic students, Solari et al. (2017) found lower oral reading fluency for connected text (vs. individual words) and lower scores on rapid automatic naming measures to predict lower comprehension. One hypothesis mentioned was that deficits in structural language might interfere with fluent text reading. Ricketts et al. (2013) added word recognition, oral language, and social impairments to the list of factors affecting comprehension for autistic students.

In all but one of these studies, the gender balance in the autism groups were skewed more heavily toward males than in the comparison groups, which was not explored as a factor. Delays in the development of higher-order language skills and higher levels of autistic traits are implicated in the increased prevalence of reading comprehension difficulty.

In nuanced autism and many autistic females, autistic traits may interfere less, and language skills may appear to be better developed, but reading comprehension difficulties may still be present and undetected. As individuals get older, the gaps in comprehension may widen if not addressed. Consistently across studies, recommendations are to support and monitor reading comprehension skills early in development. Word decoding and oral vocabulary training were noted as not sufficient for intervention targets because they may already be at average levels.

To summarize, reading comprehension differences are relatively common in autistic children, but difficulties may be hidden behind typical cognitive, decoding, and vocabulary skills. Early intervention is key, but comprehensive screening and in-depth assessment by speech and language pathologists and reading specialists may be required to identify "hidden" comprehension difficulties in young children, particularly females or others with more nuanced traits and reading skills that may appear to be typical.

Can Reading Be a Special (Restricted) Interest?

First Person Narratives

> *Girls with ASD may exhibit great interest in reading, family, peers, and other things that seem like gender-typical interests. The distinguishing factor is the intensity of the interest- -it may be over-the-top, constant, and interfering with their schoolwork and socializing.* (OCALI, 2021)

> *A small number of activities came up time and time again as being favourites for repetition: watching the same TV/video/DVD programme... reading the same book... listening to the same song/tape... Collecting and sorting specific objects were also mentioned ... The common interest of reading fiction seen in girls with autism is also a valuable tool in learning about communication and relationships.* (Hendrickx, 2015, p. 59, 82)

> *One thing as problematic in its own way as having personas is my fantasy world, the imaginative realm I invented to inhabit, that helps shut out the outside world. It is on a par with reading and fulfills a similar role of keeping me mentally safe and happy while having to exist as a real person. April Masilamani* (Miller, 2015, p. 117)

> *We don't feel as if we have enough personality to put pen to paper, much less fill so many pages. We then set out to find our personality and fill our notebooks. Before we write our story, we have to write ourselves. We start by taking in as many other people's stories as we can. Whether we gravitate towards fiction (often of the sci-fi or fantasy variety) or nonfiction (astronomy, history, etc.), we will want to hear, see, or read until our brains are stuffed and spilling over. Reading the dictionary and the encyclopedia used to be standard procedure. Artemisia* (Cook & Garnett, 2018, p. 47)

Beyond Knowledge or Entertainment

Intensive interest in reading has been characterized for both genders as an example of a special interest that might go unnoticed because it is viewed as positive and beneficial (McFayden et al., 2019). According to our understanding, this concept is not yet documented in the scientific literature, yet first-person narrative evidence is readily available:

> *"But what might not be realized is that behind our bedroom door, we may be reading the same book 124 times, because we are obsessed with it. Some Aspergirls do border on trainspotting."* (Simone, 2010, p. 25)

The voracious reading often reported in autistic females may serve a different purpose than reading for pleasure or knowledge if it is a special interest. This may be an additional reason for the disparity between decoding and reading comprehension; reading may be a distinct activity with different goals for autistic females compared to their allistic peers:

> *"I have spent much of my teenage and adult years reading fiction, playing computer games and watching fiction on TV. Many times I've felt closer to fictional characters than real-life people. (Woman with autism)"* (Hendrickx, 2015, p. 93)

What About Math?

Studies addressing specific math disabilities are even less prevalent in the literature than studies examining reading comprehension difficulties. Math studies that do exist point to the assumption that autistic students are inherently good at math as the reason for the paucity of studies. Jones et al. (2009) indicated that mathematical abilities were either above or consistent with cognitive scores in 97% of students tested. Over time, Kim et al. (2018) saw math scores that were slightly higher than reading scores in students with IQ >85 continue to develop, with larger differences at age 18 than at age 9. However, Oswald et al. (2016) looked at autistic adolescents with average or higher cognitive abilities and found 22% indeed had significant math disabilities.

One study examined the perceptions of autistic students compared to measurements of math fluency and math competency to provide an additional clue for the lack of focus on math disability. There was a strong correlation between math self-perception and math performance, but this was not the case with reading. Neurotypical student self-reports were fairly consistent with performance across subjects. The authors explored the idea that feedback in arithmetic is rather concrete (e.g., correct or incorrect responses) and that it may be easier to define competency in math than in reading (McCauley et al., 2018). One recommendation was to provide more specific and concrete feedback in reading to help students clarify their self-concept relative to reading to perhaps increase reading comprehension.

Executive Function

First Person Narratives

> *The calling card of autistic brains–the single most omnipresent, most impactful distinction of our minds versus the neurotypical–is the discrepancy between our executive function and ... everything else. Which means what, exactly? How and where are we focusing our attention? Trains and fireflies. Though not literally.* (O'Toole, 2018, p. 93)

> *The dichotomy of being emotionally immature yet intellectually sound; of being logical and regimented yet having executive dysfunction, is something that is difficult for others (social workers and Family Court judges for example) to get their heads around.* (Simone, 2010, p. 143)

> *Tasks that require planning, working memory, organization, time management or flexible thinking can become mammoth challenges. . . . EF speaks to how well we manage the unexpected, the unfamiliar, and the unstructured.* (O'Toole, 2018, pp. 94–95)

> *Professionals call these executive function problems, but generally confine their attention to the cognitive and motor effects (difficulty with planning, organization, etc.), whereas we experience them as pervasive, impinging on most aspects of our lives. Typically, we process slowly, consciously, with difficulty managing more than one type of data or process at a time. Our systems are easily overloaded by sensory, social, emotional, cognitive or chemical stimuli, resulting in fatigue and shutdowns which may be transient or last for hours, weeks or even years. - Ava Ruth Baker & Sola Shelley* (Miller, 2015, p. 32)

> *But there are practicalities to attend to. When we are in the zone, we do have a hard time with taking breaks, going to the toilet, eating, drinking, grooming, getting fresh air, or exercise. It can also impinge upon getting a job, going to work, and other crucial activities. Is it really just executive dysfunction causing this behavior--not knowing when to stop? Or is there something more?* (Simone, 2010, p. 24)

Executive Function in Autistic Females

In general, autistic children and adults are known to have executive function differences compared to NT groups (Happé et al., 2006; Lai et al., 2017). Jennifer Cook O'Toole (2018) defines her own executive function (EF) as a continuum across which she functions. On the one hand, she describes it as being able to focus intensely without a feeling of time, requiring effort to slow down or refocus (like a train). On the other end, she describes it can also be like fireflies, focusing on everything everywhere at once, being driven by novelty and unable to focus on details, structure, or monotony. She explains that she is acutely aware of the disparity between her executive function and her cognitive function, and she acknowledges that this is likely frustrating to people around her.

Given that executive function is likely going to be very different from NT peers, the question then becomes, are there differences in EF by gender within autism? Scientific literature includes varying results regarding EF in autistic samples by gender or sex or other factors. Lehnhardt et al. (2016), for instance, demonstrated that autistic females may have superior EF than autistic males; however, the study's sample consisted solely of those identified later in life (average age approximately 35 years). Measurements were also direct observations of standardized tasks. Bölte et al. (2011) found autistic females to have better EF than autistic males (average age, 14 years; IQ average, 99) on one specific task by direct observation and scoring, but less ability on a different specific task for visual attention. In Lai et al. (2012), autistic female performance on executive function tasks was similar to NT females. They concluded that performance in the social-cognitive domain is similarly impaired in both autistic male and female adults. However, in specific non-social-cognitive domains of EF, performance varied by sex (autistic males and females, respectively: average age, 27 and 28; average IQ, 112 and 114).

According to Lemon (2011), autistic girls have more depressed response inhibition times than autistic boys (average age, 11; IQ averages: female, 97, and male, 92). Hull et al. (2017) found no differences between genders on EF tasks other than those evident in the general population (systematic review). A relationship between EF difficulties and more social and communication difficulties has been found in autistic females, but not necessarily their autistic male counterparts (Torske et al., 2022; average age, 10–12; average IQ, 94–96). Lacroix et al. (2022) found a similar, but positive, correlation with autistic females showing better performance on an emotional switching task than their male counterparts, who did better on a task switching task (average age = 32).

In contrast, parent and self-reports of autistic girls' EF provide a more consistent story of variations and delays in the development of EF. White et al. (2017) reported findings in school-age children (7–18 years old), with consistently higher levels of difficulty in EF for females reported across all subdomains in a well-matched sample of autistic children and adolescents (average IQ = 101). In this sample, females also had less-developed adaptive skills and a relatively higher proportion of inattentive ADHD symptoms. In samples including only adults, there were no gender differences other than those in the general population, however, with autistic females generally showing better skills than autistic males (Demetriou et al., 2021). Strang et al. (2021) provided further considerations with lower EF skills in autistic transgender youth (average age around 17; IQ proxy T-scores = 54–58) related to barriers to care and more suicidality and other internalizing symptoms.

These contradictory findings may be attributable to the age of the individuals (children versus adults), the type of measurement used, and the identification of gender. Executive function concerns in daily life are more consistently described in personal accounts.

Assessment Planning for Reading, Learning, and Executive Function

Interpreting Standardized Measures for Females

Fortunately, most executive function questionnaire measures have gendered norms and should accurately reflect perceptions of executive function in daily life. Teacher and parent reports of executive function may vary from each other and from the individual's report of their skills. If direct observation standardized tasks are used, be careful to include these questionnaire data and interviews to ensure that demands of daily life are not interfering with executive function beyond what is seen in standardized, controlled conditions. Self-report measures, if available in the person's age range, are critical for interpreting other executive function measures and abilities in real life.

Additional Measures to Inform the Assessment Process

Early identification of reading comprehension difficulties is important for reading skill and overall academic development. In addition to monitoring decoding and vocabulary skills in young readers, closely monitor comprehension and narrative skills for differences. Assessing comprehension of sentences may not be sufficiently comprehensive. Seek out comprehension from longer passages to assess for coherence and synthesis of ideas and themes. Attend to inferencing skill and whether inferencing is easier with narrative (fiction) or expository (nonfiction) passages.

Speech and language pathologists in addition to reading specialists are likely to have multiple measures for reading comprehension that should be added to typical assessments for learning disabilities. Gaps between cognitive skills and academic performance are likely to be found if comprehension is thoroughly assessed. Finally, curriculum-based measurement (CBM) strategies for assessing comprehension should be included in assessment data. For psychologists, interview data and careful attention to standardized results that seem to be discrepant (even if within the average range) could be a signal that more assessment should be considered.

Interviews and Observations

As autistic students reach adolescence, many are aware that their comprehension skills are different from their peers. This is likely to show up in social contexts as well as in reading comprehension in academic work. Listen for comments indicating difficulties, such as "I just don't understand ...." or "Everyone seems to get it, but I don't understand how they knew...." Inferencing and going "beyond the page" to make assumptions and conclusions about implicit messaging may be particularly difficult. Observations of nervousness, avoidance, or memorized answers are additional behavioral clues that comprehension skills may not match other academic performance.

Supports and Recommendations

Supports for reading and executive function are fairly well-known and available in schools *if it is known that they are needed.* However, Gray et al. (2021) surveyed educators about actions to be taken if autism was identified in a female student. Only 5% of educators indicated that they would consider female-specific supports, and only 37% indicated individual supports. Responses were not mutually exclusive, but 85% indicated their first step would be to provide generic autism supports. This could be interpreted in several ways. The generic autism approach might provide reading and executive function support because of overall expectations. The smaller response for individualized or female-specific supports may reflect lack of training or awareness. Parents in Gray's study reported: Inconsistent supports, key difficulties, and availability of resources and support were the most frequently mentioned themes in their experiences with their daughters' school experience. Those with earlier intervention (from early identification) reported gains in skills and function.

Early Identification of Reading Comprehension

Expanding on the prior information regarding the comprehensive assessment of reading comprehension, our experience has shown that thorough assessment by speech and language pathologists, especially in early assessment, can provide crucial information regarding receptive language, expressive language, theory of mind, and inference skills, all of which are essential to reading comprehension. The fact that a young student is a skilled reader and has good vocabulary should not exempt them from language evaluation. Early signs that comprehension may be limited (perhaps in informal or curriculum-based measures) should not be ignored. Examine lengthier passages of connected text in particular to determine reading fluency as a predictor of comprehension difficulties. Also consider using different genres of books.

Reading Supports

A simple technique to improve implicit and inferential reading comprehension during guided reading sessions is to implement a "look-back" strategy (McIntyre et al., 2017). All studies agreed that reading comprehension abilities can be improved with supports and targeted interventions if students are identified early as needing supports.

One theory posed in the literature (McCauley et al., 2018) was that specific feedback provided in math lessons may be absent in reading instruction, which may contribute to self-report disparities. With the knowledge that negatively phrased feedback can have an amplified effect on autistic females and those with nuanced autism, consider providing as much concrete, precise reading feedback as possible.

Executive Function Supports

Just as providing reading comprehension support to all or most students, regardless of reading levels, may improve skills even in students not yet identified with comprehension delays, supporting the executive function of all students in the classroom can improve the skills and performance of an autistic female or student with nuanced autism.

Many executive function resources are available for autistic students (school age through adulthood) in both clinical manuals for intervention and parent and self-help versions. Many evidence-based resources also exist for reading comprehension and are well-known to educators (e.g., Cartwright & Duke, (2023).

As we work to achieve our goal of earlier detection of females and those with more nuanced autism, school personnel will need more extensive training to better support autistic females. Sarah Hendrickx has compiled a list that should be adaptable for autistic individuals' needs. These guidelines do not necessitate technique-specific instruction; therefore, they should all be accessible to any student with autism who requires them.

From a first-person point of view (Hendrickx, 2015, pp. 114–116):

Although every girl and young woman with autism will need an individualized support plan to meet her needs, there are a number of general approaches teachers can adopt that will certainly aid the child's process of transition and settling into a new educational setting:

(1) *Put the support in place before she starts at your school.*
(2) *Meet her before she starts, show her around - let her know where she will be and what's required.*
(3) *Use visuals, schedules and other concrete information to help her settle in and make sense of what will happen and when.*
(4) *Girls with ASD generally want to do well, comply and stay out of trouble. If this is not happening, the chances are she has a gap in her understanding of what's required.*
(5) *Do not take what she says or does personally. She is not meaning to annoy you.*
(6) *Consider your rules. Are you and others adhering to them?*
(7) *Staff need training in ASD and specifically how it manifests in girls.*
(8) *Don't assume that because she's smart (or average) she will be fine.*

  (9) *Teach the non-academic skills.*

 (10) *Consider language processing limitations - just because she is highly articulate (her words) doesn't mean that she can comprehend what you require (your words).*

 (11) *Pre-teach the content of lessons. Give her the heads-up on the topic area in advance and let her go and research it on her own.*

 (12) *Ensure that she understands the requirements of assignments.*

 (13) *Keep an eye on her. She may not ask for help.*

 (14) *Bring her interests into the curriculum.*

 (15) *If teamwork is necessary, give her a role that she can succeed in.*

 (16) *Reduce homework assignments. She is exhausted.*

Return to the Case Study

Julia's love of reading is a wonderful thing. It serves many roles in Julia's life, including as an avenue of learning, a coping strategy, and a leisure activity. While her parents and teachers empower Julia to continue reading, they see a need for supporting Julia's comprehension. In the early primary grades, comprehension was as easy as identifying the "who" and the "what." As Julia has advanced in grades, however, she is expected to pick up on increasingly more subtle cues to make accurate inferences. When her frustration came to a head with her mother ("If the author wanted me to know her message, she would have said it in the book!"), adults began to realize that Julia needed more explicit support in comprehending implicit messages in reading. Although Julia's reading skills far surpass many of her peers, her connection with the material was on a more surface level. Teachers supported Julia by verbally modeling inferencing skills. By walking Julia through identifying cues that were relevant and then verbally stating what meaning might be inferred from each, Julia began to develop her own problem-solving skills for inferencing that she was able to apply to other reading material. To support Julia's independence in daily living, Julia's parents implemented some targeted visual supports. For example, Julia and her father wrote out a list of night-time routine activities (e.g., brushing teeth, setting out clothes, setting an alarm clock) in Julia's preferred order of action. They posted the list on Julia's bathroom mirror as a daily check and reminder of what needed to be done before she went to bed. Julia found these lists useful and extended them to include written reminders in her school binder of things she needed to do in her various classes (e.g., turn homework in, get materials out). By working with Julia to develop strategies (rather than telling Julia what she should do), Julia had a stronger sense of ownership and was better able to make growth toward more independence in daily routines. See (Table 7.1) for a summary of assessment strategies for reading, learning and executive function.

Table 7.1 At-a-glance summary—reading, learning, and executive function

Domain	Focus	Assessment planning (age ranges)
Reading comprehension	Multiple measures of comprehension	Use both narrative and multiple-choice measures and academic work samples (e.g., journal entries, responses to story prompts)

Reading comprehension	Choose from among these commonly available <u>and other options</u> for assessing fluency and comprehension. Subtests are typically identified with titles similar to the following:
	
	    Reading or Passage Comprehension
	    Oral Reading Fluency
	    Sentence Reading Fluency
	    Connected Text Fluency (longer passages)
	    Listening or Oral Comprehension
	    Reading Recall
	    Rapid Naming
	Also consider:
	    Essay Composition
	    Written Expression
		Wechsler Individual Achievement Test (**WIAT-4**): ages 4:0–50:11 (Wechsler, 2020)
		Kaufman Test of Educational Achievement (**KTEA-3**): ages 4:0–25:11 (Kaufman & Kaufman, 2014)
		Woodcock-Johnson-IV Achievement and Oral Language (**WJ-IV**): ages 2: 0–90+ (Schrank et al., 2014a, b)
		Feifer Assessment of Reading (**FAR**): grades PK to college (Feifer, 2015)
		Nelson Denny Reading Test Forms I and J (**NDRT**): ages 14–24 (Fischo, 2019)
		Grey Oral Reading Test, 5th Ed. (**GORT-5**): ages 6:0–23:11 (Wiederholt & Bryant, 2012)
		Clinical Evaluation of Language Fundamentals, 5th Ed. (**CELF-5**), including Supplemental Tests of Reading and Writing: ages 5:0–21:11 (Wiig et al., 2013)

(continued)

Table 7.1 (continued)

Domain	Focus	Assessment planning (age ranges)

Executive function	Although there are directly observable measures of executive function used in neuropsychological examinations, the focus in a comprehensive autism assessment is generally more relevant in reports of everyday life (questionnaires)	*Behavior Rating Inventory of Executive Function-Adult Version* **(BRIEF-A)**: 18+ (Roth et al., 2005)
		    Self-report
		    Other report
		        (English and Spanish)
		Behavior Rating Inventory of Executive Function, 2nd Ed. **(BRIEF-2)** (Gioia et al., 2015)
		        BRIEF-2—Teacher Report: ages 5–18
		            BRIEF-2—Parent Report: ages 5–18
		                BRIEF-2—Self-Report: ages 11–18
		Comprehensive Executive Function Inventory **(CEFI)** (Naglieri & Goldstein, 2017)
		        CEFI Teacher Form: ages 5–18
		            CEFI Parent Form: ages 5–18
		                CEFI Self-Report Form: ages 12–18

Please see the "References" section in this chapter for additional information on measures. Not all measures and processes listed are available in all settings or appropriate for all cases. Qualification levels apply. Multiple measures in a single domain are not necessary. Some measures can provide data in multiple domains. This is meant to provide a relatively quick reference for assessment planning and implementation, not an endorsement of any particular measure as "best." Emphasis here is on readily available, commonly used measures, but similar measures may also be useful

References

Äsberg, J., Kopp, S., Berg-Kelly, K., & Gillberg, C. (2010). Reading comprehension, word decoding and spelling in girls with autism spectrum disorders (ASD) or attention-deficit/hyperactivity disorder (AD/HD): Performance and predictors. *International Journal of Language & Communication Disorders, 45*(1), 61–71. https://doi.org/10.3109/13682820902745438

Bölte, S., Duketis, E., Poustka, F., & Holtmann, M. (2011). Sex differences in cognitive domains and their clinical correlates in higher-functioning autism spectrum disorders. *Autism, 15*(4), 497–511. https://doi.org/10.1177/1362361310391116

Cartwright, K. B., & Duke, N. K. (2023). *Executive skills and reading comprehension: A guide for educators. Second Edition.* Guilford Press.

Cook, B., & Garnett, M. (Eds.). (2018). *Spectrum women: Walking to the beat of Autism.* Jessica Kingsley Publishers.

Davidson, M. M. (2021). Reading comprehension in school-age children with autism spectrum disorder: Examining the many components that may contribute. *Language, Speech, and Hearing Services in Schools, 52*(1), 181–196. https://doi.org/10.1044/2020_LSHSS-20-00010

Demetriou, E. A., Pepper, K. L., Park, S. H., Pellicano, L., Song, Y., Naismith, S. L., Hickie, I. B., Thomas, E. E., & Guastella, A. J. (2021). Autism spectrum disorder: An examination of sex differences in neuropsychological and self-report measures of executive and non-executive cognitive function. *Autism: The International Journal of Research and Practice, 25*(8), 2223–2237. https://doi.org/10.1177/13623613211014991

Diehl, J. J., Bennetto, L., & Young, E. C. (2006). Story recall and narrative coherence of high functioning children with autism spectrum disorders. *Journal of Abnormal Child Psychology, 34*(1), 83–98. https://doi.org/10.1007/s10802-005-9003-x

Estes, A., Rivera, V., Bryan, M., Cali, P., & Dawson, G. (2011). Discrepancies between academic achievement and intellectual ability in higher-functioning school-aged children with autism spectrum disorder. *Journal of Autism and Developmental Disorders, 41*(8), 1044–1052. https://doi.org/10.1007/s10803-010-1127-3

Feifer, S. G. (2015). *Feifer Assessment of Reading (FAR)*. Psychological Assessment Resources (PAR Inc.).

Fischo, V. V. (2019). *Nelson-Denny reading test, forms I & J*. Pro-Ed.

Gioia, G. A., Isquith, P. K., Guy, S. C., & Kenworthy, L. (2015). *Behavior rating inventory of executive function®, Second edition (BRIEF®2)*. Psychological Assessment Resources (PAR Inc.).

Gray, L., Bownas, E., Hicks, L., Hutcheson-Galbraith, E., & Harrison, S. (2021). Towards a better understanding of girls on the autism spectrum: Educational support and parental perspectives. *Educational Psychology in Practice, 37*(1), 74–93. https://doi.org/10.1080/02667363.2020.1863188

Grimm, R. P., Solari, E. J., McIntyre, N. S., Zajic, M., & Mundy, P. C. (2017). Comparing growth in linguistic comprehension and reading comprehension in school-aged children with autism versus typically developing children. *Autism Research, 11*(4), 624–635. https://doi.org/10.1002/aur.1914

Happé, F., Booth, R., Charlton, R., et al. (2006). Executive function deficits in autism spectrum disorders and attention-deficit/hyperactivity disorder: Examining profiles across domains and ages. *Brain and Cognition, 61*(1), 25–39. https://doi.org/10.1016/j.bandc.2006.03.004

Hendrickx, S. (2015). *Women and girls with autism spectrum disorder: Understanding life experiences from early childhood to old age*. Jessica Kingsley Publishers.

Hull, L., Mandy, W., & Petrides, K. V. (2017). Behavioural and cognitive sex/gender differences in autism spectrum condition and typically developing males and females. *Autism, 21*(6), 706–727. https://doi.org/10.1177/1362361316669087

Jones, C. R. G., Happé, F., Golden, H., Marsden, A. J. S., Tregay, J., Simonoff, E., Pickles, A., Baird, G., & Charman, T. (2009). Reading and arithmetic in adolescents with autism spectrum disorders: Peaks and dips in attainment. *Neuropsychology, 23*(6), 718–728. https://doi.org/10.1037/a0016360

Kaufman, A. S., & Kaufman, N. L. (2014). *Kaufman test of educational achievement* (3rd ed.). Pearson.

Kim, S. H., Lord, C., & Bal, V. H. (2018). Longitudinal follow-up of academic achievement in children with autism from age 2 to 18. *Journal of Child Psychology & Psychiatry, 59*(3), 258–267. https://doi.org/10.1111/jcpp.12808

Lacroix, A., Dutheil, F., Logemann, A., Cserjesi, R., Peyrin, C., Biro, B., Gomot, M., & Mermillod, M. (2022). Flexibility in autism during unpredictable shifts of socio-emotional stimuli: Investigation of group and sex differences. *Autism: The International Journal of Research and Practice, 26*(7), 1681–1697. https://doi.org/10.1177/13623613211062776

Lai, M.-C., Lombardo, M. V., Ruigrok, A. N. V., Chakrabarti, B., Wheelwright, S. J., Auyeung, B., Allison, C., & Baron-Cohen, S. (2012). Cognition in males and females with autism: Similarities and differences. *PLoS ONE, 7*(10), 1–15. https://doi.org/10.1371/journal.pone.0047198

Lai, C., Lau, Z., Lui, S., Lok, E., Tam, V., Chan, Q., Cheng, K. M., Lam, S. M., & Cheung, E. (2017). Meta-analysis of neuropsychological measures of executive functioning in children and adolescents with high-functioning autism spectrum disorder. *Autism Research: Official Journal of the International Society for Autism Research, 10*(5), 911–939. https://doi.org/10.1002/aur.1723

Lehnhardt, F. G., Falter, C. M., Gawronski, A., Pfeiffer, K., Tepest, R., Franklin, J., & Vogeley, K. (2016). Sex-related cognitive profile in autism spectrum disorders diagnosed late in life: Implications for the female autistic phenotype. *Journal of Autism and Developmental Disorders, 46*(1), 139–154. https://doi.org/10.1007/s10803-015-2558-7

Lemon, J. M., Gargaro, B., Enticott, P. G., & Rinehart, N. J. (2011). Brief report: Executive functioning in autism spectrum disorders: A gender comparison of response inhibition. *Journal of Autism and Developmental Disorders, 41*(3), 352–356. https://doi.org/10.1007/s10803-010-1039-2

McCauley, J. B., Zajic, M. C., Oswald, T. M., Swain-Lerro, L. E., McIntyre, N. C., Harris, M. A., Trzesniewski, K., Mundy, P. C., & Solomon, M. (2018). Brief report: Investigating relations between self-concept and performance in reading and math for school-aged children and adolescents with autism spectrum disorder. *Journal of Autism and Developmental Disorders, 48*(5), 1825–1832. https://doi.org/10.1007/s10803-017-3403-y

McFayden, T. C., Albright, J., Muskett, A. E., & Scarpa, A. (2019). Brief report: Sex differences in ASD diagnosis—A brief report on restricted interests and repetitive behaviors. *Journal of Autism and Developmental Disorders, 49*(4), 1693–1699. https://doi.org/10.1007/s10803-018-3838-9

McIntyre, N., Solari, E., Gonzales, J., Solomon, M., Lerro, L., Novotny, S., Oswald, T., & Mundy, P. (2017). The scope and nature of reading comprehension impairments in school-aged children with higher-functioning autism spectrum disorder. *Journal of Autism & Developmental Disorders, 47*(9), 2838–2860. https://doi.org/10.1007/s10803-017-3209-y

Miller, J. K. (Ed.). (2015). *Women from another planet? Our lives in the universe of autism.* AuthorHouse.

Naglieri, J., & Goldstein, S. (2017). *Comprehensive executive function inventory.* Western Psychological Services (WPS).

OCALI–OhioCenterforAutismandLow-Incidence.(2021).*Autisminternetmodules:Girlsandwomen on the spectrum.* https://www.ocali.org/project/Girls-and-Women-on-the-Autism-Spectrum

Oswald, T. M., Beck, J. S., Iosif, A.-M., McCauley, J. B., Gilhooly, L. J., Matter, J. C., & Solomon, M. (2016). Clinical and cognitive characteristics associated with mathematics problem solving in adolescents with autism spectrum disorder. *Autism Research, 9*, 480–490. https://doi.org/10.1002/aur.1524

O'Toole, J. C. (2018). *Autism in heels: The untold story of a female life on the spectrum.* Skyhorse Publishing.

Ricketts, J., Jones, C. R. G., Happé, F., & Charman, T. (2013). Reading comprehension in autism spectrum disorders: The role of oral language and social functioning. *Journal of Autism and Developmental Disorders, 43*(4), 807–816. https://doi.org/10.1007/s10803-012-1619-4

Roth, R. M., Isquith, P. K., & Gioia, G. A. (2005). *Behavior rating inventory of executive function®–Adult version.* Psychological Assessment Resources (PAR Inc.).

Schrank, F. A., Mather, N., & McGrew, K. S. (2014a). *Woodcock-Johnson-IV: Tests of Achievement.* Riverside.

Schrank, F. A., Mather, N., & McGrew, K. S. (2014b). *Woodcock-Johnson-IV: Tests of Oral Language.* Riverside.

Simone, R. (2010). *Aspergirls: Empowering females with Asperger syndrome.* Jessica Kingsley Publishers.

Solari, E. J., Grimm, R., McIntyre, N. S., Swain-Lerro, L., Zajic, M., & Mundy, P. C. (2017). The relation between text reading fluency and reading comprehension for students with autism spectrum disorders. *Research in Autism Spectrum Disorders, 41–42*, 8–19. https://doi.org/10.1016/j.rasd.2017.07.002

Strang, J. F., Anthony, L. G., Song, A., Lai, M.-C., Knauss, M., Sadikova, E., Graham, E., Zaks, Z., Wimms, H., Willing, L., Call, D., Mancilla, M., Shakin, S., Vilain, E., Kim, D.-Y., Maisashvili, T., Khawaja, A., & Kenworthy, L. (2021). In addition to stigma: Cognitive and autism-related predictors of mental health in transgender adolescents. *Journal of Clinical Child & Adolescent Psychology, 52*(2), 212–229. https://doi.org/10.1080/15374416.2021.1916940

Torske, T., Nærland, T., Quintana, D. S., Hypher, R. E., Kaale, A., Høyland, A. L., Hope, S., Johannessen, J., Øie, M. G., & Andreassen, O. A. (2022). Sex as a moderator between parent ratings of executive dysfunction and social difficulties in children and adolescents with autism spectrum disorder. *Journal of Autism and Developmental Disorders.* https://doi.org/10.1007/s10803-022-05629-5

Wechsler, D. (2020). *Wechsler Individual Achievement Test (4th ed.).* Pearson.

White, E. I., Wallace, G. L., Bascom, J., Armour, A. C., Register, B. K., Popal, H. S., Ratto, A. B., Martin, A., & Kenworthy, L. (2017). Sex differences in parent-reported executive functioning and adaptive behavior in children and young adults with autism spectrum disorder. *Autism Research, 10*(10), 1653–1662. https://doi.org/10.1002/aur.1811

Wiederholt, J. L., & Bryant, B. R. (2012). *Grey Oral Reading Test (5th ed.).* Pro-Ed..

Wiig, E. H., Semel, E., & Secord, W. A. (2013). *Clinical Evaluation of Language Fundamentals (5th ed.).* Pearson.

Willey, L. H. (2012). *Safety skills for Asperger women: How to save a perfectly good female life.* Jessica Kingsley Publishers.

Chapter 8
Differential or Co-occurring? Other Common Diagnoses Prior to Autism Assessment

Introduction

One of the most frequent comments we hear in practice from females is, "Thank you for believing me." Whether she is coming to an evaluation knowing that she is autistic or not, the experience of being "blown off" or dismissed is almost universal. Professionals are trained to identify the most pressing or evident need, which is often characterized as disconnected traits that we would call co-occurring conditions. While these traits and symptoms are usually correctly identified, the pattern they create that indicates a common, underlying reason for the constellation of difficulties and experiences is frequently missed because of the pressing need for support and treatment. The downside to missing the autism, unfortunately, is that the treatment for the pressing issue may not be effective if the autism is not taken into consideration.

> "One meaning is that [undiagnosed women with ASD] have no way of explaining themselves to themselves, thus no access to the support and positive sense of self they need." (Miller, 2015).

> My third high hope is to help professionals learn to spot the signs of AS [autism] in women. To stop in its tracks, and preferably before it starts, the long, tedious, unproductive pattern of misdiagnosis. Misdiagnoses have wasted a lot of time and energy on both our parts and have resulted, at our end, in a lack of trust in the medical profession, particularly general practitioners and mental health professionals. (Simone, 2010, p. 17–18).

Case Study—Jade: Diagnosed with ADHD, Anxiety, and Depression

Jade is 19 years old and a recent high school graduate. Their parents reported that Jade "always" seemed anxious as a younger child. Jade complained of stomachaches and headaches before social events, such as peer birthday parties and family

T. P. Gabrielsen et al., *Assessment of Autism in Females and Nuanced Presentations*, https://doi.org/10.1007/978-3-031-33969-1_8

gatherings. This anxiety extended to the classroom, where Jade tended to avoid peers and exhibited "perfectionist tendencies." Jade's parents sought some support from their pediatrician when Jade was in second grade, and Jade was diagnosed as having generalized anxiety disorder. As Jade became older, their teachers noted challenges paying attention and following directions in class. They seemed to be "in their own world" during class, and teachers reported that Jade appeared easily distracted by "stories within their own head." This led to another evaluation with their pediatrician and a subsequent diagnosis of ADHD while in third grade. More recently, Jade was diagnosed with unspecified depressive disorder based on symptoms of withdrawal, sadness, and loss of interest in many activities. Jade began seeing a therapist for symptoms of anxiety and depression 18 months ago. The therapist has noted that her usual approach doesn't seem to be effective with Jade. This led her to question whether Jade's diagnoses were appropriate or if there might be something else going on with Jade.

Diagnostic Odyssey

First Person Narratives

My head had been spinning all my life with trying to make sense of why these things happened to me, why I was so odd, why I couldn't live like other people. The diagnosis stopped my head from spinning. I was able to breathe a sigh of relief and relax. Woman with autism (Hendrickx, 2015, p. 118)

When I was a teenager one of my special interests was reading university psychology texts. I took my social worker's psychology texts off her shelf and ran around reading them. I wanted to know what they thought was wrong with me. They had me at the psychological research section at the university hospital from ages 6 to 12. They identified my brother as having ADHD, but I was a difficult case. -April Griffin (Griffin, 2016)

I now realize that anxiety, a curse to so many autistics, often plays quite a terrible role in our existence. If I had known who I was when I was so much younger and understood why I was different, I think my path would have been vastly different to the one that I endured. I would have chosen to meet people in the library or a park surrounded by nature, not meet in a pub to drink in order to fit into a role for which I was never designed. I would have chosen work that complimented my way of thinking and downtime consisting of mindfulness and reflective contemplation. - Barb Cook (Cook & Garnett, 2018, pp. 87–88)

Females, from the littlest of girls to the eldest of ladies, continue to fly under the radar of proper diagnosis, eventually landing in worlds where they don't belong. Neuroses, schizophrenia, obsessive-compulsive disorder, personality disorder, oppositional defiant disorder, anxiety issues, social phobia–these are familiar diagnoses for women beyond a certain age who struggle to make sense of the environment, society, relationship rituals and the like. Not that these diagnoses are completely off base. The chances are very good that any mix of these comorbid factors also lay on a lady's genetic code. The problem is many counselors and doctors seem unable to see AS crouching in the middle of the huddle. - Liane Holliday Willey (Simone, 2010 p. 9–10)

We had years of difficulty finding out what was going on with [our daughter] and what to do about it. At that time (1998), not many people knew about Asperger's. We certainly had never heard of it. I think because she was very bright there was the feeling that nothing was wrong; she just needed to learn some relaxation techniques. When she was finally diagnosed, her psychologist felt that she needed to see a psychiatrist for medication. That psychiatrist didn't believe she had AS because she was so intelligent and expressed herself so well. I knew those were not reasons that disproved AS. (Mother of a bright 16-year-old girl with Asperger's syndrome and depression) (Nichols, 2009, p. 25)

I can't even find therapists who know very much about autism spectrum disorders. So I have to continually be trying to tell them that my needs are not the same and it is a real challenge to sometimes work with these folks [therapists]. Participant 49 (Maddox et al., 2020, p. 923)

I felt that I was either a failure as a person for not controlling myself better, or else insane. So I went to the health care place assigned to me under my workplace health insurance and told them the circumstances. I said I had lost it while vacuuming, felt that this was not normal, and was turning myself in. They interviewed me a couple times and announced that I was bipolar and had to take medicine for the rest of my life. So I took it for 13 years, terrified that I would end up institutionalized for insanity, having no idea what was going on, or that my behavior was actually normal for a person in my circumstances. - Patricia Clark (Miller, 2015, p. 96)

The "List" of Diagnoses Preceding an Autism Diagnosis

The diagnostic odyssey or journey for autistic females often includes stops in which oppositional defiant disorder, attention-deficit/hyperactivity disorder(ADHD), anxiety, depression, obsessive-compulsive disorder, social anxiety, and eating disorder are identified as "the reason" for the current difficulties. There may also be diagnoses of schizophrenia or another psychotic disorder (Nichols, 2009). The individual is presented with several dilemmas when faced with this "list." First, which of these is correct? Is it possible that all are correct? If all are accurate, what does that say about me? From a clinical point of view, there are additional considerations. Is this an individual with multiple disorders or do the features of a single disorder encompass the patterns of traits and symptoms that have previously been identified singly? Let's say that each of these conditions is legitimately present and I am trying to treat them, but evidence-based approaches that typically bring change and relief are not working very well. How do I meet the needs of this client or student?

Diagnostic Overshadowing

First Person Narratives

When some of us end up in a therapist's or doctor's office with anxiety, depression, or autoimmune health challenges, our options are limited to talk therapy or medication because only these outer layers of emotion and behavior are probed. (Nerenberg, 2021, p. 5)

Some [women] end up in the mental health system labeled as "mentally ill." Every time I was at the point of withdrawal and in need of complete solitude, those around me could not comprehend my need, so they could not support it. Instead, they made it worse. Services under the heading of any mental diagnosis made it worse. I would take their diagnosis and work with it, but it never made sense and it never made a difference. I recall happily announcing that I had depression to a few friends and they all just looked at me with total disbelief. I can understand why. I was always cheerful, happy, and what some called vivacious. Of course then when I tried to explain this to a psychiatrist I was told I must be bipolar. I was extremely frustrated but worked with that one for a while too. It did not fit. Of course being a "mental" patient I had no authority to make rational or logical decisions because of my own "illness." The system that was set up to help me was, in fact, making me worse. I am sure it was not their intent; they just did not know how and still do not. (Snyder, 2006, p. 129)

We see a huge amount of anxiety. People who are very sensory defensive, super sensitive to sensory information, are being bombarded their whole lives with sensory input that is hard to manage--so essentially they are being exposed to ongoing trauma. The disorder itself is actually just life--it's traumatizing them. So those individuals are likely to have higher rates of anxiety because they've learned to live in a world where everything is making them anxious. Teresa May-Benson (Nerenberg, 2021, p. 100–101)

Anecdotally, it is often reported that women with autism are more likely to internalize the anxiety and stress they feel around change, not wanting to draw attention to their inability to cope with the situation. This leads other people to believe that they are coping, when in fact they are not. (Hendrickx, 2015, p. 92)

For the child with Autism Spectrum Disorder (ASD) school constitutes a lack of control in all aspects of their world and hence can be a place of great trauma and anxiety. It is a constantly social environment. (Hendrickx, 2015, p. 96)

I'm beginning to think that is why the antidepressants I took made me have such trouble with anxiety and panic attacks. It was doing away with the depression, which must have been buffering against the acute attacks... Wendy (Miller, 2015, pp. 48–49)

I'm even called bubbly by some and few have any idea about the depression because all they see is this sudden surge of electricity that configures itself into a person in front of them. I'm also liable to find humor in wordplay or idea play, even when the topic is serious so I'm capable of appearing ridiculing or uncaring because I've just made fun with (not of) a name or concept. - Jean (Miller, 2015, p. 49)

My days were filled with: exhaustion, insomnia, depression, anger, obsessive-compulsive disorder, chronic panic attacks (meltdowns), migraines, stress, anxiety, self-inflicted psychological abuse, low self-esteem, paranoia, unhealthy relationships, distrust of most people because I didn't fully understand social interaction or social cues, emotional confusion, constant frustration due to misunderstanding social situations. - Anonymous (Ballou et al., 2021, p. 154)

I have saved the most complicated suspect for last. Maybe because it plagues me when I am most vulnerable and exhausted. Maybe because it is still the greatest mystery to me. Mutism--or, most accurately, selective mutism--is a common symptom of anxiety and overwhelm. And trust me, nothing halts communication faster than a good old episode of mutism. I'm not sure where the words go exactly. It usual feels like huge, foggy fatigue. On heavy social or sensory days it happens the most. First, I struggle to find the words and then I can no longer form them. It is incredibly frustrating and can often exacerbate an already messy situation. It is hard for others to understand that all of a sudden words are not an option. I'm sure many of you have experienced your own version of mutism. I wonder if it differs from mine? I have only just begun to explore this topic for myself and have only gotten as far as to understand the "when" of it. I have yet to understand the "why". Becca Lory (Cook & Garnett, 2018, pp. 168–169)

Those who described positive support appeared to have received input that was directive and supported the learning of social understanding, rather than a more psychoanalytical, emotional 'talking' approach. An understanding of autism is crucial when considering any therapeutic support. (Hendrickx, 2015, p. 211)

How Common are Co-occurring Conditions?

Croen et al. (2015) found co-occurring conditions in autistic adults to be significantly more prevalent than in the neurotypical population. Medical records for autistic adults included notations and diagnoses of depression, anxiety, bipolar disorder, obsessive-compulsive disorder, schizophrenia, and suicidal thoughts and behaviors. Medical conditions were also noted to be significantly more common, including immune conditions, gastrointestinal and sleep disorder, seizures, obesity, dyslipidemia, hypertension, and diabetes. Even rare conditions such as stroke and Parkinson's disease were more common in autistic adults. The sample was primarily individuals without intellectual developmental disorders (80%).

Studies have reported that up to 90% of autistic individuals also meet the criteria for at least one other diagnosis (Hossain et al., 2020). Co-occurring conditions are then likely to occur, but the issue with nuanced autism is how these conditions may actually overshadow and *prevent* consideration of autism. As the sheer number of diagnoses begins to "add up," missing the diagnosis of autism is likely to result in less-than-effective treatment options for co-occurring conditions because the origin of the condition and the neurological differences are not incorporated into treatment.

Mayes et al. (2011) emphasized the higher prevalence of depression in autistic children, which should be assessed to inform intervention. A majority of mothers (54%) endorsed characteristics of depressed mood in their autistic children, with more symptoms in children with age-level cognitive and language performance (54%) and slightly less in children who experience more impact on language and cognitive performance (42%). The study also reported endorsement of anxiety symptoms at 79% and 67%, respectively. The authors concluded that these remarkably high percentages justify routinely assessing all children with autism for depression, anxiety, and irritability:

> Because of the overlap in symptoms across diagnoses, it is not unusual for an individual with ASD to be misdiagnosed with multiple disorders *rather than* ASD. A concept that may be helpful in clarifying the assessment in these cases is the notion of *parsimony*. For example, if a clinician finds themselves diagnosing or evaluating a patient previously diagnosed with ADHD, Social Anxiety Disorder, Language Disorder, Developmental Coordination Disorder *and* sensory processing differences, it may be worth reassessing the constellations of symptoms and considering if ASD is a more overarching, accurate and parsimonious diagnosis. (Duvall et al., 2021, p. 1181)

One study of adult men and women referred for autism diagnosis found no difference in prevalence of co-occurring disorders between genders, yet more males than females were ultimately diagnosed with autism in the study. Better understanding of special interests and stimming behaviors and interests in females and a call for female-specific assessment were some conclusions from the study (Wilson et al., 2016). In another adult study (n = 290), almost half of those diagnosed with bipolar disorder and schizophrenia also showed significant autism traits, although patients with remitted major depressive disorder did not (Matsuo et al., 2015).

Several recent meta-analytic and systematic review studies have analyzed existing scientific literature regarding the prevalence of co-occurring conditions that are documented in autistic groups. Specific methods, inclusionary and exclusionary criteria, age groups, and methodology were incorporated. Results do not vary widely, with inclusion of some conditions across all studies and other conditions addressed by only one study. Table 8.1 illustrates the range in terms of findings and conditions that may be associated with autism. Most of the studies examined primarily adult samples, with the exception of the Lancet Commission, which focused primarily on

Table 8.1 Prevalence studies of co-occurring conditions in autism

Condition	Prevalence (Lai et al. 2019) meta-analysis (%)	Prevalence (Hossain et al. 2020) umbrella review (%)	Lancet commission report (Lord et al. 2022) (%)
Anxiety	20	1.47–54	15–20
Attention-deficit/ hyperactivity disorder	28	25.7–65	22–28
Depressive disorders	11	2.5–47.1	8–11
Bipolar disorder	5	6–21.4	3–5
Mood disorders		4.4–37	
Sleep-wake disorders	13		11–13
Schizophrenia disorder spectrum	4	4–67	2–4
Obsessive-compulsive disorders	9	9–22	4–9
Disruptive, impulse control, and conduct disorders	12	12–48	7–12
Suicidal ideation		10.9–66	11–50
Suicidal behavior		1–35	7–15
Eating disorders		1.4–7.9	2–7
Substance use disorders		0.7–36	
Personality disorder		12.6	
Tourette's disorder		2.6–36	
Post-traumatic stress disorder		1–5	
Oppositional defiant disorder			28
Non-suicidal self-injury			27–50

Note: Insufficient data are available regarding gender-specific prevalence for these conditions children and adolescents. None of the studies separated prevalence estimates by gender, however.

See Chap. 10 for more details on suicidality, eating disorders, and non-suicidal self-injury.

The authors urge clinicians to integrate and carefully assess mental healthcare for all autistic individuals. By the same token, given the relatively more common occurrence of these conditions, if co-occurring conditions are diagnosed first, and multiple conditions seem to be evident, carefully consider autism as a possibility for better-informed care (Lai et al., 2019). In the Lancet Commission, Lord et al. (2022) discussed the practical issues for clinicians—namely, they should avoid either attributing all maladaptive behaviors to autism or neglecting to take into account that aspects of autism can include treatable co-occurring conditions.

Assessment Planning for Differential Diagnosis

General Guidance

Given the inherent overlap in core impairments, the *pervasiveness* of the symptoms or traits described across settings and the *nature* of the problems will help to determine the presence of autism and whether it is "driving the bus," or not. Comprehensive assessment of attentional difficulties for ADHD or manifestations of anxiety can give clarity on diagnoses. Multiple perspectives are also required. It may be that ADHD, anxiety, etc. is present without autistic traits. It is also possible that attention and anxiety are unique or characteristic of autism. Finally, autistic people may have anxiety and attention difficulties in addition to autism that look different from what is most commonly seen in non-autistic populations, requiring a dual diagnosis (Shulman et al., 2020).

ADHD

Prior to the *Diagnostic and Statistical Manual of Mental Disorders*, Fifth Ed. (DSM-5; APA, 2013), an additional diagnosis of ADHD was not allowed if the primary diagnosis was autistic disorder, Asperger's syndrome, or pervasive developmental disorder, not otherwise specified. As of 2013, however, ADHD diagnoses are expected to be listed along with autism spectrum disorder, if indicated. The DSM-5 Text Revision (DSM-5-TR; APA, 2022) allows for both diagnoses when appropriate, but also provides some guidance on distinguishing ADHD without autism. Common features across both include social difficulties such as interrupting, talking too loudly for the setting, and invading personal space. Attention that is easily distracted or overly focused is also characteristic of both. Executive function difficulties are also common in both conditions.

Key factors for distinguishing ADHD *without autism* include qualitative differences in special or intense interests (or absence of an intense interest) and absence of stimming behaviors (APA, 2022). This is even more difficult to tease apart in the case of nuanced autism, including many autistic females, whose special interests are often not obvious because they are seemingly mainstream. Sometimes the special interests become more evident over time (e.g., in adolescence). A strong tendency toward overfocused attention may be evidence of autism in addition to ADHD. We have also noticed that when someone has ADHD, they tend to *forget* to use learned social abilities, whereas autistic people are often bewildered even after social information is explained or they are reminded about social behaviors. Another autistic pattern might be to realize there was a social mistake and try to learn how to act so they blend in. See Chap. 5 for more details on special interests and stimming behaviors and interests and Chap. 7 for executive function.

It is understandable that, by looking only at diagnostic criteria, ADHD seems a more plausible, more readily adopted explanation for attention differences. However, treatment for ADHD alone, though likely to have some benefit, does not affect core autism traits and therefore may not meet all support needs. A careful examination of executive function and autism screeners for evidence of very high scores on transition scales and atypicality—both present to some extent in ADHD—are characteristically higher in autism. Some screeners allow for a comparison of score profiles provided by parents of children with ADHD to help distinguish between the two. Also look for evidence of special interests very carefully, including special interests that were more evident at a young age but are now gone or some that become more evident as the person enters adolescence.

Anxiety and Social Anxiety

Deciding if anxiety is the most relevant and comprehensive diagnosis is one of the most difficult differentiations to make. The best approach we have found is to make sure you have a comprehensive evaluation to provide you with data regarding language differences (more likely autism), early developmental history (look for special interests in autism), and indications of developmental delays in other domains (more likely autism). Executive function may be less likely to be impacted if social anxiety or other anxiety disorders are the core difficulty rather than autism.

Because social anxiety has traditionally been the most common type of anxiety in adolescents (Merikangas et al., 2010), extra caution is necessary in assessment with this population. Autism screening measures alone may not be able to adequately distinguish anxiety (without autism) from autism with anxiety, particularly the Social Responsiveness Scales, second Ed. (SRS-2; Constantino & Gruber, 2012). South et al. (2017) illustrated this for adults, and Capriola-Hall (2021) published similar findings for children and adolescents. Comprehensive assessments of other aspects of autism, including interview and observation, are needed to distinguish social anxiety from autism or identify if autism traits are present in addition to social anxiety. In our experience, social anxiety is worrying about doing something wrong and being judged. The type of anxiety we most often see in autism is worry that they don't know how to do something socially and they can't figure out how everyone else seems to know.

Obsessive-Compulsive Disorder (OCD)

In clinical practice, the crossover of symptoms with autism traits can be confusing to some, but the neurological data actually show consistent differences. For autistic females, OCD may be one of the most complex issues to support. Treatment or reductive approaches that may be helpful generally for OCD are not very helpful when OCD is interfering with an autistic person's quality of life.

Researchers are looking for biological ways to define (and hopefully better support) females with OCD. In a data-driven imaging study, ADHD and OCD consistently clustered together by group according to their data (psychological measures of ADHD or OCD) and imaging results. Autistic females, by contrast, were distributed across all data groups (ADHD, OCD, and autism). Strong evidence exists that there are specific autistic, sex-specific brain structures, and functional connectivity patterns. These patterns are less evident in ADHD and OCD, yet females with these conditions resemble each other by observed and reported traits within groups. Several studies were found showing that children with OCD had "milder alterations at the brain and behavioral level compared to children with ASD or ADHD" (Jacobs et al., 2021, p. 650). This suggests that while OCD can have significant effects on daily life, if there is a complex range of traits in addition to OCD, the likelihood of OCD *with* autism may be high. Consider assessing for autism if there is more than OCD in the referral question.

Bipolar Disorder

Bipolar disorder (BD) has many features that cross over with the characteristics of autism, and prevalence rates are roughly similar (1.5% for BD, 2% for autism). BD symptoms appear to be episodic, which is not true of autism, but camouflaging could possibly hide autism traits to an extent that they may seem to follow the cyclical pattern of BD. There is no significant gender difference in BD prevalence (APA, 2022). While BD can co-occur with autism, particularly with higher language and cognitive levels (6%–21.4%; Vannucchi et al., 2014), it is also possible that BD diagnoses are given when the more accurate diagnosis is autism. There are some differences in etiology and presentation between BD and autism that are helpful in differential diagnoses.

BD onset is typically during adolescence, with mean age of onset for women at 21.5 years (APA, 2022), whereas autism traits are lifelong and begin in early development. Autistic traits in females may have gone unrecognized until adolescence, thus complicating the differential diagnosis, but a detailed developmental history of childhood may still be helpful. In addition to adolescent onset for BD, it is helpful to note that a family history of BD increases risk of BD in autism populations (13%–17%) and BD is slightly less prevalent in autistic individuals with lower language and cognitive performance. Features of BD in autistic people can be confusing, as autistic features (e.g., idiosyncratic thinking, special interests) can be more evident during manic episodes (Vanucchi et al., 2014). If BD is suspected, careful consideration of family history, early development, and extensive interview with the individual and family are required to differentiate BD from autism or confirm the presence of both conditions.

Borderline Personality Disorder

Borderline personality disorder (BPD) diagnoses are sometimes reported by women in their diagnostic journey. One pilot study prior to DSM-5 (APA, 2013) examined female patients in a Swedish outpatient clinic and recommended that autism be considered in patients with BPD if there was a high rate of suicidal thoughts and behaviors, but less substance abuse. Self-hate was also found to be higher in patients with both autism and BPD. Overall function was generally lower in autistic patients with BPD (Rydén et al., 2008). Dudas et al. (2017) found autism traits were highest in an autism + BPD group, slightly lower for autism alone, and lower still for BPD alone. Systemizing or "the drive to analyse or build a system, which itself is defined as any rule-based pattern of information" (p. 2) was similar across autism and BPD groups, suggesting this as the more typical overlap in symptoms. Empathizing traits were measured, but not specified, so differences between groups are not as clear.

In-depth assessment of early developmental history and extensive interviewing of family and the individual may show that BPD traits (including impulsivity, emotional dysregulation, fear of abandonment, and difficulties with relationships) may actually be the effects of autism traits of executive function difficulties, low ability to understand social context, and difficulties recognizing emotions (Fitzgerald, 2005). For clinicians familiar with nuanced autism, these underlying reasons for outward behavior can easily distinguish between BPD and autism. For clinicians unfamiliar with nuanced autism, however, the symptom list may seem inconsistent with classic autism traits and might be dismissed in the differential diagnostic process.

It is obvious that expertise in both BPD and autism should be required when making this differential, particularly if both conditions exist in the family history.

The availability of this dual expertise may not be available, however. In some circumstances, referral to another clinician may not be an option, so clinicians with expertise in only one of the two conditions (or neither) are faced with a dilemma. All parties would like to reach the correct conclusion, and none of the parties wants to go without answers for an extended period of time. Seeking consultation is the ethical course of action for the clinician, as is gathering more comprehensive assessment data based on characteristics that are more unique to autism than BPD and vice versa. More time will be required, but when weighed against a wrong diagnosis and wasted time in ineffective treatment, the additional effort and time would seem the best option for the client. In the meantime, work on supports for the most immediate needs pending diagnosis.

Depression

"But if too many things go wrong, or if we simply become overloaded and exhausted, it morphs into depression right before your very eyes," (Simone, 2012, p. 108)

Among mood disorders, many could describe an autistic person at any single point in time. Meltdowns when routines are disrupted could look like disruptive mood dysregulation disorder (DMDD). Onset of DMDD needs to be before age 10, and if our goal is early identification, it cannot be considered under the developmental age of 6 years, so age/developmental level is the first consideration. There is also a call for looking at trauma in the person's history (in the relevant timeframe).

Depression in autism may also have unique signs. Loss of interest in special or intense interests, changes in sleep patterns, changes in social withdrawal, and changes in sensory sensitivities have all been described in the literature as signs of depression in autistic people. Extensive camouflaging or masking behaviors are also likely to result in depression (Cassidy et al., 2018).

A German study of mood or anxiety disorder (MAD) and autism traits for differential diagnosis in children and adults was reported by Wittkopf et al. in 2021. They found that a combination of communication issues and unusual social overtures facilitates differentiation between autism and mood and anxiety disorders. In general, the autism group scores were higher (more evident) than the MAD group on all domains across measures.

Individual items on the ADOS-G (Rühl et al., 2004) and ADOS-2, Modules 3 and 4 (Poustka et al., 2015), and the ADI-R (Bölte et al., 2006) were examined to see which best differentiated between mood and anxiety that was not related to autism (ADI-R: LeCouteur et al., 2003; ADOS-G: Lord et al., 2000; ADOS-2: Lord et al., 2012). Findings showed that 23%–26% of the MAD sample met the criteria for autism on the ADOS-G or ADOS-2. Subgroups of anxiety (26%), mood disorder (18%), and emotional disorder (15%) were reported as also meeting autism criteria. On the ADI-R, 49% met at least one of the domain thresholds, 20% met two domains, and almost 10% met all three domains (six participants). Of these six, only one met the criteria for autism on both ADOS and ADI-R. *It was uncommon to have both of these autism measures come up positive based only on mood and anxiety disorder, reinforcing the need for comprehensive evaluations and the utility of the ADI-R in conjunction with the ADOS-2 in difficult cases.* None of the MAD group showed special interests and stimming behaviors (RRBIs) on the ADOS Module 3, but in adolescents and young adults (Module 4), the RRBI scores were very similar across MAD and autism groups, indicating more difficulty differentiating adult traits and thus implying that a detailed developmental history would be required. ADI-R scores for the MAD group, however, were similarly low for the RRBI domain on the diagnostic algorithm, which focuses on early childhood (Wittkopf et al., 2021).

Further examination of item scores that clearly distinguished between MAD and autism groups included imitative social play on the ADI-R and speech and language differences associated with autism, reporting of events, and conversation, facial expressions (to the examiner), quality of social overtures, and quality of social response on the ADOS Module 3. For older individuals, the ADOS Module 4 items for conversation; descriptive, conventional, instrumental, or informational gestures; insight; quality of social overtures; quality of social response; and speech abnormalities associated with autism differentiated between MAD and autism groups, with higher scores (more consistent with autism) in the autism group on each of these items. Results pointed to unusual eye contact, offering information, and empathy/comments on other's emotions as discriminating between groups as well. Further analysis of ADI-R items also identified hand and finger mannerisms, unusual preoccupations, reciprocal conversation, interest in children, and group play with peers as discriminating between groups. A third analysis added stereotyped/idiosyncratic use of words or phrases to the list of differences. The authors concluded that in clinical practice, much information beyond scores is gathered. In cases that are difficult to discriminate, including co-occurring or differential mood and anxiety disorders, it can be appropriate to weigh available evidence in congregate rather than focusing on scores and cutoffs. Use of multiple measures is also likely necessary (Wittkopf et al., 2021).

Selective Mutism

Selective mutism, which is somewhat less common than autism (0.2%–1.9% prevalence rates), can be confused with autism by those who don't typically encounter it. Selective mutism is a more likely overall diagnosis if early development did not include delays. Another hallmark of selective mutism is that children develop their own strict rules about which communication strategies they use in which settings. This may look like no spoken language in a classroom, but no problems ordering fast food with spoken language or talking at home. Gestures may be used with friends on the playground to communicate without spoken language, but not in the classroom. Some may use note writing as a substitute for spoken language at a grandparent's house, but may speak freely at a cousin's house.

Selective mutism associated *with* autism is more likely to be associated with anxiety and being overwhelmed rather than connected with a particular setting. It is possible, however, that a particular setting may consistently cause anxiety, and thus it may appear that the setting-dependent nature of selective mutism is present. Social reciprocity is usually more developed in children with selective mutism than in autistic children of similar age, however. Special or intense interests and stimming behaviors are not usually noted for selective mutism alone (APA, 2022). Be sure to assess for both anxiety and speech and language, but also consider rule outs from executive function and autism-specific screeners that may point more to autism.

Direct observation measures may or may not be helpful given refusal to speak. *(Please note that people who do not use spoken language at all can be assessed with direct observation measures, however.)* Conducting an informative ADOS-2 (Lord et al., 2012) may be possible if the individual feels comfortable talking or whispering in the evaluation setting. This is obviously more difficult within school settings in which the student is not speaking, so consider alternate testing locations if possible (e.g., home or other setting in which the person typically speaks). Indirect measures, such as the ADI-R (LeCouteur et al., 2003) or the CARS-2 (Schopler et al., 2010), may be necessary to rule out autism if questions about autism remain following assessment sessions. Parent interview and possibly family videos may be helpful as well.

Supports and Recommendations

Overcoming Clinician-Level Barriers

One of the more frequent barriers to autism identification and effective treatment is that clinicians are not familiar with autism. Beyond just training to gain knowledge, the recommendation is to be mentored by experts in diagnosis and supports. Clinician-level barriers identified by Maddox et al. (2020) included not focusing on practical recommendations (e.g., wanting to talk about processing emotions), not challenging their client to make progress, and not accommodating their client's sensory aversions.

Systems-Level Barriers to Mitigate

Maddox et al. (2020) also reported systems-level barriers to appropriate treatment, including lack of awareness that community mental health centers can also treat autistic people. They further identified the limited connection between developmental disabilities systems and mental health systems as problematic, noting that ability to access the latter would be helpful to mitigate diagnostic overshadowing.

Consideration of Autistic Traits in Therapy: Individualized Treatment

Recommendations from autistic adults in therapy were to incorporate understanding of how autistic clients work best. Using clear and direct language was a primary example. Providing structure and predictability will also help to build a therapeutic relationship. Practical, present-focused therapeutic approaches, showing comfort with silence, and allowing more time for language processing are also requested by autistic clients, as well as focusing on the treatment of the co-occurring conditions, not on changing core autistic traits (Maddox et al., 2020).

Treatment approaches for common co-occurring conditions can be informed by understanding of autistic neurology and should have an evidence base for effectiveness in autistic populations. For example, cognitive behavioral therapy (CBT) is a common approach for supporting improvements in anxiety and depression (Clark, 2011; Hoffman et al., 2012; James et al., 2013). Adaptations of CBT for autistic people are beginning to be established in the scientific literature as well (Spain & Happé, 2020), e.g., *Cognitive Behavioral Therapy for Adults with Autism Spectrum Disorder* (Gaus, 2018).

Dialectical behavior therapy (DBT) has also been shown to have positive effects in autistic people (Huntjens et al., 2020). Therapists should be aware that some negative beliefs may be valid, such as feeling persecuted at work or unable to accomplish certain tasks. It is important to help clients assess the accuracy of such beliefs and cope with truly unchangeable hardships rather than assuming that problems are necessarily due to cognitive distortions. Diagnoses of borderline personality disorder and bipolar disorder should be thoroughly assessed to inform appropriate treatment to ensure that the diagnoses are accurate and that autism diagnoses are not missed and to inform treatment of these conditions given autistic traits in individuals.

Supports for autistic children and adolescents in school settings can be planned in tandem with community supports and as supplementary, introductory, or follow-up to community treatment plans. Working with community providers to create consistent plans for supports and responses to crises and bad days can give students, parents, and school personnel some tools needed to support the student on a daily basis.

School Refusal

School refusal is also a common issue needing support among most conditions in this chapter, typically driven by anxiety. The particular type of anxiety driving the refusal behavior is going to be key to supports for school attendance, however. For example, it is possible that sensory overwhelm may be contributing to anxiety in autistic students. Autistic students are much more likely to have school refusal behavior (SRB) than their neurotypical peers (Munkhaugen et al., 2019). SRB is a multifaceted problem in most cases, with home and family, peers and teachers, and physical and mental health and other environmental factors that may or may not be easily determined. If autism is not yet identified, careful and comprehensive assessment of the underlying causes for school refusal should at least consider autism. A Norwegian study characterized autistic students who were also more likely to have school refusal behavior as having lower social motivation, more difficulties with executive function, more anxiety and depression, more withdrawal, somatic complaints, and thought problems (Munkhaugen et al., 2019). Supporting school attendance will require not just addressing anxiety but also executive function both at home and at school. A collaborative, interdisciplinary approach is key to mitigating school refusal (e.g., Clare School Avoidance Toolkit, TUSLA, 2021, *a UK resource, but applicable elsewhere*):

> *Whether from our peers or teachers, if we are looked at with an unfriendly, intimidating, or threatening eye, we fold. Alone, we are talented, graceful, witty, and smart, but under such circumstances we curl up like hedgehogs....Some of us get backed into a corner and we keep retreating until we are out in the parking lot...then we just keep going. In other words, we quit. Some of us older Aspergirls went from gifted student to high school or college dropout.* (Simone, 2010, p. 31)

In the case of hospitalization, extended day treatment, or residential stays for more intensive support, a transition team from the school can plan for a more successful return to school for students by working closely with the discharge team to continue with effective techniques, communicate if there are setbacks, and monitor progress as the student re-adjusts to school demands and social environments. Because we are focusing on nuanced autism, all supports and plans will need to be individualized to the student's specific needs, which may vary substantially from student to student. A recent review of available transition support programs (Tougas et al., 2022) found eight programs with five consistent themes of support. Key elements across programs were involvement of a multidisciplinary team, implementation of multi-component interventions, development of a reintegration (or transition) plan, gradual transitioning, and prolonged support through frequent contacts between all stakeholders (medical team, school staff, youth, family). Jennifer St. Jude, in a chapter from Sincerely Your Autistic Child (Ballou et al., 2021, pp. 61–69), drafted a table of support needs for autistic girls. A summary of that table includes some of the following issues, organized here to correspond to topics introduced in this chapter (Table 8.2).

Table 8.2 First-person narrative of supports needed for co-occurring conditions

ADHD	Boundaries, cause and effect, frustration, organization, practical, responsibility, safety
Anxiety	Emotions, maturity, meltdowns, OCD and high anxiety, reasoning skills
Depression	Comfort, creativity, seeing the "big picture," sensitive and empathic beings, talents and skills, valued and appreciated
Selective mutism/speech and language issues	Asking for help, expressive and receptive speech, literal, verbal expression vs. monologues
Inclusion	Affection and safe contact, empathy, friends belonging and connections, nurturing
Other	Sensory processing issues and disorder, social cues, etc.

Return to the Case Study

Prompted by the therapist, Jade and their mother began to talk about seeking out further assessment. The difficulty was in finding someone who had experience with young adults AFAB who presented with what the therapist was calling an "atypical" presentation. They were lucky to finally find a psychologist who was available and had experience working with young adults with profiles like Jade's. The psychologist conducted a comprehensive interview with Jade and their parents and spoke with Jade's therapist. This was followed by more conversation and engagement with Jade in person. At the feedback, Jade learned they were autistic. The diagnoses along the way had served to identify presentations of Jade's autism that were most salient during those time periods. The psychologist noted that Jade's anxieties as a child were all centered around mandated social experiences. The attentional concerns appeared most related to Jade's tendency to engage in thinking about their special interests during times of boredom at school. Depressive features appeared related to years of Jade masking (camouflaging) to try to fit in with peers and ultimately being less successful than hoped. Upon receiving this diagnosis and learning more about autism, Jade felt a huge weight "lift off" them. Rather than displaying a menu of neurodevelopmental and mental health challenges, Jade's brain was wired differently from the start. Just getting the diagnosis and learning about how it had presented throughout their life changed Jade's outlook. Although having a diagnosis of autism didn't mean Jade wasn't impacted by any of the features of the previous diagnoses, it is important that Jade, with their psychologist and therapist, explores to what extent autism explained any of the other diagnoses. Had any of the previous evaluators had experience with how autism presents in nuanced presentations and females, Jade may have avoided some of the challenges that arose when interventions for each of the diagnoses were ineffective. With better understanding of themselves, Jade is feeling much more positive about their future. See Table 8.3 for a summary of assessment strategies for co-occuring or differential diagnoses.

Table 8.3 At-a-glance summary for co-occurring and common conditions—differential diagnosis

Domain	Focus	Assessment planning and age ranges
Multiple conditions	Structured interviews for many commonly occurring psychological conditions are helpful, but informal interviews can provide context to differentiate conditions and to provide valuable information for intervention approaches	*Mini International Neuropsychiatric Interview-Adult* (**MINI-Adult**, Sheehan et al., 1998) *Mini International Neuropsychiatric Interview – Adult* (**MINI**) or (**MINI-Kids**) ages *Version 7.0.2 or later for DSM-5* (Sheehan et al., 2010) *Structured Developmental History, Behavior Assessment System for Children* (**SDH, BASC-3**): 2–21 years or older (Reynolds & Kamphaus, 2015)
Multiple conditions	Multi-condition screeners may be a good step to confirm the intensity of traits and behaviors and consistency with diagnostic criteria	*Child and Adolescent Symptom Inventory, Fifth Ed.* (**CASI-5R**): 5–18 years (Gadow & Sprafkin, 2013)
ADHD	Comparison of results with parents of children with ADHD is available for differential diagnosis and confirmation of co-occurring ADHD (Conners-4). Depressed mood and anxious thoughts are also indexed	**Conners-4**: ages 6–18 (Conners, 2022) *Conners Early Childhood* (**Conners-EC**): ages 2–6 (Conners, 2009)
Anxiety	Anxiety symptoms can be mistaken for autism or co-occurring with autism, but need to be addressed to increase quality of life, function, and inclusion. Anxiety measures specific to autism can be helpful in treatment planning	*Anxiety Scale for Children-ASD(c)* (**ASC-ASD**; Rodgers et al. 2016a, b): ages 8–16 *Anxiety Scale for Autism-Adults* (**ASA-A**): ages 18+ (Rodgers et al., 2020)
Depression	Cassidy et al. (2018) found weak evidence to support the BDI-II in an autistic sample. The PHQ-9 and BDI-II were highly rated for the general population	*Beck Depression Inventory, -2nd Ed.* (**BDI-II**): ages 13–80 (Beck et al., 1996) *Patient Health Questionnaire, 9th Ed.* (**PHQ-9**): ages 12+ (Kocalevent et al., 2013)
Depression and anxiety	Depression and Anxiety scales are available on these and other tier 2 social/emotional screeners See also Zhou et al. (2022) for the BASC-3 in autistic populations	*Behavior Assessment Scales for Children, 3rd Ed.* (**BASC-3**): ages 2–25 (Depression and Anxiety subscales) Reynolds & Kamphaus, 2015)
		Child Behavior Checklist (**CBCL**; Achenbach & Rescorla, 2001): ages 6–18 (Depression and Anxiety subscales) and other *Achenbach System of Empirically Based Assessment* (**ASEBA**) measures (Achenbach, 2009)

(continued)

Table 8.3 (continued)

Domain	Focus	Assessment planning and age ranges
School refusal	Anxiety, trauma, and withdrawal associated with school refusal are common across many conditions. Understanding the underlying type of anxiety causing the refusal (separation, performance, social, OCD, etc.) is needed to inform supports	Interview and observation to determine directions for assessment and supports given throughout this chapter
Obsessive-compulsive disorder		*Children's Yale-Brown Obsessive Compulsive Scale* (**CYBOCS**): ages 6–17 (Scahill et al., 1997) *Yale-Brown Obsessive Compulsive Scale* (**YBOCS**): adults (Goodman et al., 1989)

Please see the "References" section in this chapter for additional information on measures. Not all measures and processes listed are available in all settings or appropriate for all cases. Qualification levels apply. Multiple measures in a single domain are not necessary. Some measures can provide data in multiple domains. This is meant to provide a relatively quick reference for assessment planning and implementation, not an endorsement of any particular measure as "best." Emphasis here is on readily available, commonly used measures, but similar measures may also be useful

References

Achenbach, T. M. (2009). *The Achenbach System of Empirically Based Assessment (ASEBA): development, findings, theory, and applications.* University of Vermont, Research Center for Children, Youth, & Families.

Achenbach, T. M., & Rescorla, L. A. (2001). *Manual for the ASEBA school-age forms & profiles.* University of Vermont, Research Center for Children, Youth, & Families.

American Psychiatric Association. (2013). *Diagnostic and Statistical Manual of Mental Disorders (5th ed.).* American Psychiatric Association.

American Psychiatric Association. (2022). *Diagnostic and Statistical Manual of Mental Disorders (5th ed.). Text Revision.* American Psychiatric Association.

Ballou, E. P., da Vanport, S., & Onaiwu, M. G. (Eds.). (2021). *Sincerely, your autistic child.* Beacon Press.

Beck, A. T., Steer, R. A., & Brown, G. K. (1996). *Manual for the Beck Depression Inventory-II.* Psychological Corporation.

Bölte, S., Rühl, D., Schmötzer, G., & Poustka, F. (2006). *ADI-R: Diagnostisches interview für Autismus—Revidiert [ADI-R: Autism Diagnostic Interview – Revised].* Huber.

Capriola-Hall, N. N., McFayden, T., Ollendick, T. H., & White, S. W. (2021). Caution when screening for autism among socially anxious youth. *Journal of Autism & Developmental Disorders, 51*(5), 1540–1549. https://doi.org/10.1007/s10803-020-04642-w

Cassidy, S. A., Bradley, L., Bowen, E., Wigham, S., & Rodgers, J. (2018). Measurement properties of tools used to assess depression in adults with and without autism spectrum conditions: A systematic review. *Autism Research, 11*(5), 738–754. https://doi.org/10.1002/aur.1922

Clark, D. M. (2011). Implementing NICE guidelines for the psychological treatment of depression and anxiety disorders: The IAPT experience. *International Review of Psychiatry, 23*, 318–327. https://doi.org/10.3109/09540261.2011.606803

Conners, K. (2009). *Conners Early Childhood*. Multi-Health Systems, Inc.

Conners, K. (2022). *Conners, 4™*. Multi-Health Systems Inc.

Constantino, J., & Gruber, C. P. (2012). *Social Responsiveness Scale* (2nd ed.). Western Psychological Services.

Cook, B., & Garnett, M. (Eds.). (2018). *Spectrum women: Walking to the beat of Autism*. Jessica Kingsley.

Croen, L. A., Zerbo, O., Qian, Y., Massolo, M. L., Rich, S., Sidney, S., & Kripke, C. (2015). The health status of adults on the autism spectrum. *Autism, 19*(7), 814–823. https://doi.org/10.1177/1362361315577517

Dudas, R. B., Lovejoy, C., Cassidy, S., Allison, C., Smith, P., & Baron-Cohen, S. (2017). The overlap between autistic spectrum conditions and borderline personality disorder. *PLoS One, 12*(9), e0184447. https://doi.org/10.1371/journal.pone.0184447

Duvall, S., Armstrong, K., Shahabuddin, A., Grantz, C., Fein, D., & Lord, C. (2021). A road map for identifying autism spectrum disorder: Recognizing and evaluating characteristics that should raise red or "pink" flags to guide accurate differential diagnosis. *The Clinical Neuropsychologist*, 1–36. Advance online publication. https://doi.org/10.1080/1385404 6.2021.1921276

Fitzgerald, M. (2005). Borderline personality disorder and Asperger syndrome. *Autism, 9*, 452. https://doi.org/10.1177/1362361305056084

Gadow, K. D., & Sprafkin, J. (2013). *Child and Adolescent Symptom Inventory-5*. Checkmate Plus. https://www.checkmateplus.com/casi-5

Gaus, V. L. (2018). *Cognitive behavioral therapy for adults with autism spectrum disorder* (2nd ed.). Guilford Press.

Goodman, W. K., Price, L. H., Rassmussen, S. A., et al. (1989). The Yale-Brown Obsessive-Compulsive Scale (Y-BOCS) Part 1: Development, use and reliability. *Archives of General Psychiatry, 46*(1), 006–1011. https://doi.org/10.1001/archpsyc.1989.01810110048007

Griffin, A. (2016, September 12). *Gender identity issues and females on the spectrum*. #ActuallyAutistic Perspective, Females and Autism. https://the-art-of-autism.com/gender-identity-issues-and-females-on-the-spectrum/

Hendrickx, S. (2015). *Women and girls with autism spectrum disorder: Understanding life experiences from early childhood to old age*. Jessica Kingsley.

Hofmann, S. G., Asnaani, A., Vonk, I. J. J., Sawyer, A. T., & Fang, A. (2012). The efficacy of cognitive behavioral therapy: A Review of meta-analyses. *Cognitive Therapy and Research, 36*, 427–440.

Hossain, M. M., Khan, N., Sultana, A., Ma, P., McKyer, E. L. J., Ahmed, H. U., & Purohit, N. (2020). Prevalence of comorbid psychiatric disorders among people with autism spectrum disorder: An umbrella review of systematic reviews and meta-analyses. *Psychiatry Research, 287*, 112922. https://doi.org/10.1016/j.psychres.2020.112922

Huntjens, A., van den Bosch, L. M. C. W., Sizoo, B., Kerkhof, A., Huibers, M. J. H., & van der Gagg, M. (2020). The effect of dialectical behaviour therapy in autism spectrum patients with suicidality and/ or self-destructive behaviour (DIASS): study protocol for a multicentre randomised controlled trial. *BMC Psychiatry, 20*, 127. https://doi.org/10.1186/s12888-020-02531-1

Jacobs, G. R., Voineskos, A. N., Hawco, C., Stefanik, L., Forde, N. J., Dickie, E. W., Lai, M.-C., Szatmari, P., Schachar, R., Crosbie, J., Arnold, P. D., Goldenberg, A., Erdman, L., & Ameis, S. H. (2021). Integration of brain and behavior measures for identification of data-driven groups cutting across children with ASD, ADHD, or OCD. *Neuropsychopharmacology: Official Publication of the American College of Neuropsychopharmacology, 46*(3), 643–653. https://doi.org/10.1038/s41386-020-00902-6

James, A. C., James, G., Cowdrey, F. A., Soler, A., & Choke, A. (2013). Cognitive behavioural therapy for anxiety disorders in children and adolescents. *Cochrane Database of Systematic Reviews, 6*, CD004690.

Kocalevent, R. D., Hinz, A., & Brähler, E. (2013 Sep-Oct). Standardization of the depression screener patient health questionnaire (PHQ-9) in the general population. *Gen Hosp Psychiatry, 35*(5), 551–555. https://doi.org/10.1016/j.genhosppsych.2013.04.006

Lai, M.-C., Kassee, C., Besney, R., Bonato, S., Hull, L., Mandy, W., Szatmari, P., & Ameis, S. H. (2019). Prevalence of co-occurring mental health diagnoses in the autism population: A systematic review and meta-analysis. *The Lancet Psychiatry, 6*(10), 819–829. https://doi.org/10.1016/S2215-0366(19)30289-5

Le Couteur, A., Lord, C., & Rutter, M. (2003). *Autism Diagnostic Interview-Revised*. Western Psychological.

Lord, C., Charman, T., Havdahl, A., Carbone, P., Anagnostou, E., Boyd, B., Carr, T., de Vries, P. J., Dissanayake, C., Divan, G., Freitag, C. M., Gotelli, M. M., Kasari, C., Knapp, M., Mundy, P., Plank, A., Scahill, L., Servili, C., Shattuck, P., et al. (2022). The Lancet commission on the future of care and clinical research in autism. *Lancet, 399*(10321), 271–334. https://doi.org/10.1016/S0140-6736(21)01541-5

Lord, C., Risi, S., Lambrecht, L., Cook, E. H., Jr., Leventhal, B. L., DiLavore, P. D., Pickles, M., & Rutter, M. (2000). The Autism Diagnostic Observation Schedule—Generic: A standard measure of social and communication deficits associated with the spectrum of autism. *Journal of Autism and Developmental Disorders, 30*, 205–223. https://doi.org/10.1023/a:1005592401947

Lord, C., Rutter, M., DiLavore, P. C., Risi, S., Gotham, K., & Bishop, S. L. (2012). *Autism Diagnostic Observation Schedule* (2nd ed., pp. *1–4*). Western Psychological Services.

Maddox, B. B., Crabbe, S., Beidas, R., Brookman-Frazee, L., Cannuscio, C. C., Miller, J. S., Nicolaidis, C., & Mandell, D. S. (2020). I wouldn't know where to start: Perspectives from clinicians, agency leaders, and autistic adults on improving community mental health services for autistic adults. *Autism, 24*(4), 919–930. https://doi.org/10.1177/1362361319882227

Matsuo, J., Kamio, Y., Takahashi, H., Ota, M., Teraishi, T., Hori, H., Nagashima, A., Takei, R., Higuchi, T., Motohashi, N., & Kunugi, H. (2015). Autistic-like traits in adult patients with mood disorders and schizophrenia. *PLoS ONE, 10*(4). https://doi.org/10.1371/journal.pone.0122711

Mayes, S. D., Calhoun, S. L., Murray, M. J., Ahuja, M., & Smith, L. A. (2011). Anxiety, depression, and irritability in children with autism relative to other neuropsychiatric disorders and typical development. *Research in Autism Spectrum Disorders, 5*(1), 474–485. https://doi.org/10.1016/j.rasd.2010.06.012

Merikangas, K. R., He, J. P., Burstein, M., Swanson, S. A., Avenevoli, S., Cui, L., ... & Swendsen, J. (2010). Lifetime prevalence of mental disorders in US adolescents: Results from the National Comorbidity Survey Replication–Adolescent Supplement (NCSA). *Journal of the American Academy of Child & Adolescent Psychiatry, 49*(10), 980–989. https://doi.org/10.1016/j.jaac.2010.05.017

Miller, J. K. (Ed.). (2015). *Women from another planet? Our lives in the universe of autism*. AuthorHouse.

Munkhaugen, E. K., Torske, T., Gjevik, E., Nærland, T., Pripp, A. H., & Diseth, T. H. (2019). Individual characteristics of students with autism spectrum disorders and school refusal behavior. *Autism: The International Journal of Research and Practice, 23*(2), 413–423. https://doi.org/10.1177/1362361317748619

Nerenberg, J. (2021). *Divergent mind: Thriving in a world that wasn't designed for you*. HarperOne.

Nichols, S. (2009). *Girls growing up on the autism spectrum: What parents and professionals should know about the pre-teen and teenage years*. Jessica Kingsley.

Poustka, L., Rühl, D., Feineis-Matthews, S., Bölte, S., Poustka, F., & Hartung, M. (2015). *ADOS-2: Diagnostische Beobachtungsskala für Autistische Störungen – 2* [ADOS-2: Autism Diagnostic Observation Schedule – 2]. Huber.

Reynolds, C. R., & Kamphaus, R. W. (2015). *Behavior Assessment System for Children* (3rd ed.). Pearson.

Rodgers, J., Wigham, S., McConachie, H., Freeston, M., Honey, E., & Parr, J. (2016a). *Anxiety Scale for Children-Autism Spectrum Disorder (ASC-ASD): Guidelines for use*. Newcastle University. https://research.ncl.ac.uk/neurodisability/leafletsandmeasures/anxietyscaleforchildren-asd/

Rodgers, J., Wigham, S., McConachie, H., Freeston, M., Honey, E., & Parr, J. R. (2016b). Development of the Anxiety Scale for Children with autism spectrum disorder (ASC-ASD). *Autism Research, 9*(11), 1205–1215.

Rodgers, J., Farquhar, K., Mason, D., Brice, S., Wigham, S., Ingham, B., Freeston, M. F., & Parr, J. R. (2020). Development and initial evaluation of the Anxiety Scale for Autism - Adults (ASA-A). *Autism in Adulthood, 2*(1). https://doi.org/10.1089/aut.2019.0044

Rühl, D., Bölte, S., Feineis-Matthews, S., &Poustka F. (2004). *Diagnostische Beobachtungsskala für Autistische Störungen* [Autism diagnostic observation schedule]. Huber.

Rydén, G., Rydén, E., & Hetta, J. (2008). Borderline personality disorder and autism spectrum disorder in females: A cross-sectional study. *Clinical Neuropsychiatry, 5*(1), 22–30. https://psycnet.apa.org/record/2008-07906-004

Scahill, L., Riddle, M. A., McSwiggin-Hardin, M., Ort, S. I., King, R. A., Goodman, W. K., Cicchetti, D., & Leckman, J. F. (1997). Children's Yale-Brown Obsessive Compulsive Scale: Reliability and validity. *J Am Acad Child Adolesc Psychiatry, 36*(6), 844–852. Updated 2007. https://www.mcpap.com/pdf/CYBOCS.pdf

Schopler, E., Van Gourgondien, M. E., Wellmand, G. J., & Love, S. R. (2010). *The Childhood Autism Rating Scales* (2nd ed.). Western Psychological Services.

Sheehan, D. V., Lecrubier, Y., Harnett-Sheehan, K., Amorim, P., Janavs, J., Weiller, E., Hergueta, T., Baker, R., & Dunbar, G. (1998). The Mini International Neuropsychiatric Interview (M.I.N.I.): The development and validation of a structured diagnostic psychiatric interview. *The Journal of Clinical Psychiatry, 59*(Suppl 20), 22–33. http://www.psychiatrist.com/JCP/article/Pages/1998/v59s20/v59s2005.aspx

Sheehan, D. V., Sheehan, K. H., Shytle, R. D., Janavs, J., Bannon, Y., Rogers, J. E., Milo, K. M., Stock, S. L., & Wilkinson, B. (2010). Reliability and validity of the mini international neuropsychiatric interview for children and adolescents (MINI–KID). *The Journal of Clinical Psychiatry, 71*(3), 313–326. https://doi.org/10.4088/JCP.09m05305whi

Shulman, C., Rice, C. E., Morrier, M. J., & Esler, A. (2020). The role of diagnostic instruments in dual and differential diagnosis in autism spectrum disorder across the lifespan. *Child and Adolescent Psychiatric Clinics of North America, 29*(2), 275–299. https://doi.org/10.1016/j.chc.2020.01.002

Simone, R. (2010). *Aspergirls: Empowering females with Asperger syndrome.* Jessica Kingsley.

Simone, R. (2012). *22 things a woman with Asperger's syndrome wants her partner to know.* Jessica Kingsley Publishers.

Snyder, R. (2006). Maternal instincts in Asperger's syndrome. In T. Attwood (Ed.), *Asperger's and girls: World-renowned experts join those with Asperger's syndrome to resolve issues that girls and women face every day!* (pp. 117–146). Future Horizons.

South, M., Carr, A. W., Stephenson, K. G., Maisel, M. E., & Cox, J. C. (2017). Symptom overlap on the SRS-2 Adult self-report between adults with ASD and adults with high anxiety. *Autism Research, 10*, 1215–1220. https://doi.org/10.1002/aur.1764

Spain, D., & Happé, F. (2020). How to optimise cognitive behaviour therapy (CBT) for people with autism spectrum disorders (ASD): A Delphi study. *Journal of Rational-Emotive & Cognitive-Behavior Therapy, 38*(2), 184–208. https://doi.org/10.1007/s10942-019-00335-1

Tougas, A.-M., Houle, A.-A., Leduc, K., Frenette-Bergeron, E., & Marcil, K. (2022). School reintegration following psychiatric hospitalization: A review of available transition programs. *Journal of the Canadian Academy of Child and Adolescent Psychiatry, 31*(2), 75–92. https://www.cacap-acpea.org/wp-content/uploads/School-Reintegration-Following-Psychiatric-Hospitalization.pdf.

Tusla Child and Family Agency. (2021). *Clare school avoidance toolkit: Information for students and parents.* https://www.cypsc.ie/_fileupload/Clare%20CYPSC/uploads/ClareSAT-Final-November%202021%20web.pdf

Vannucchi, G., Masi, G., Toni, C., Dell'Osso, L., Erfurth, A., & Perugi, G. (2014). Bipolar disorder in adults with Asperger's Syndrome: a systematic review. *Journal of Affective Disorders, 168*, 151–160. https://doi.org/10.1016/j.jad.2014.06.042

Wilson, C. E., Murphy, C. M., McAlonan, G., Robertson, D. M., Spain, D., Hayward, H., Woodhouse, E., Deeley, P. Q., Gillan, N., Ohlsen, J. C., Zinkstok, J., Stoencheva, V., Faulkner, J., Yildiran, H., Bell, V., Hammond, N., Craig, M. C., & Murphy, D. G. M. (2016). Does sex influence the diagnostic evaluation of autism spectrum disorder in adults? *Autism, 20*(7), 808–819. https://doi.org/10.1177/1362361315611381

Wittkopf, S., Stroth, S., Langmann, A., Wolff, N., Roessner, V., Roepke, S., Poustka, L., & Kamp-Becker, I. (2021). Differentiation of autism spectrum disorder and mood or anxiety disorder. *Autism, 26*(5), 1056–1069. https://doi.org/10.1177/13623613211039673

Zhou, X., Reynolds, C., & Kamphaus, R. W. (2022). Diagnostic utility of behavior assessment system for children-3 for children and adolescents with autism. *Applied Neuropsychology: Child, 11*(4), 647–651. https://doi.org/10.1080/21622965.2021.1929232

Chapter 9
Guidance for Medical Issues in Female Puberty, Gender Identity, Pregnancy, Parenting and Menopause

Introduction

The focus of assessment is justifiably on the social communication aspects of autism, but clinicians in diagnostic roles may not be as familiar with medical implications and common issues that are reported by autistic females. Perhaps because of the higher number of genetic differences found in autistic females and their mothers (Antaki et al., 2022; Jacquemont et al., 2014; Lawrence et al., 2022; Robinson et al., 2013; Szatmari et al., 2012; Wigdor et al., 2021) and other genetic differences, there is too broad a range of medical issues to address in a single chapter. We can, however focus on experiences of autistic females in terms of reproductive system issues, and parenting and gender identity issues. Medical supports may be necessary to address many of these issues to improve quality of life.

> *Periods are nothing to be feared or dreaded. In fact, I quite enjoy having periods now that I know what to expect each month. It helps me feel grounded and part of the life cycle of this planet and universe. Periods are a routine that I can organize my other life things around.*
> (Balfe, 2021, p. 187)

Case Study—Ana: Autistic Adolescent Distressed by Menstruation

Ana is a 14-year-old autistic girl who started menstruating at age 13. She communicates with scripted and echolalic verbal speech. She has not received any sexuality/health education in her special education classroom or at home. When she sees the blood from her period each month, she cries and says "hurt." At school, a personal care assistant in the classroom helps her with toileting and hygiene, which includes changing her pads during her period. Ana's mother doesn't know how to explain

© The Author(s), under exclusive license to Springer Nature Switzerland AG 2023
T. P. Gabrielsen et al., *Assessment of Autism in Females and Nuanced Presentations*, https://doi.org/10.1007/978-3-031-33969-1_9

Ana's period to her in a way she can understand, and she is concerned that Ana is in a vulnerable position because she relies on others to help with her personal care. She takes Ana to her pediatrician to ask about caring for Ana's needs. During the visit, Ana says, "hello, doctor," repeatedly while holding the pediatrician's hand and following all instructions for her examination. Her mother expresses her concerns to the pediatrician, pointing out that Ana follows instructions from everyone she encounters without question, as she did with the examination. She is worried that Ana may not fully distinguish between medical helpers and other adults, which makes her vulnerable to assault and possible pregnancy. The pediatrician wonders how to counsel Ana's mother and adapt the usual preventive women's healthcare she provides for adolescents for this patient.

Puberty

First Person Narratives

> *Until I had a hysterectomy in my early thirties, I had bloody britches with every period thanks to abnormal uterine bleeding and a propensity to forget it was necessary to change Tampax and a refusal to wear pads that felt like someone was giving me a never-ending wedgie...I think the executive functioning skills were just too weak to plan ahead or have contingency plans beyond turning to a friend or the school nurse.* (Willey, 2012, p. 108)

> *I do not seem to recall the dates or times that are based on the machines or units the world uses to measure the quantity of moments; instead I seem to measure based on the quality of those moments. I never wore a watch, and rarely looked at a calendar. Keeping track of what is called a "period" was impossible. The fact that I was taught about menses or that "special time of the month" did not help at all either. I did not know they both referred to the same thing. I actually was not sure what a period was or even the full use of feminine products until after I had the baby, when they taught me in the hospital.* (Snyder, 2006, p. 123)

> *There are the physical changes that really add to screwing with your head. Periods, which were once predictable, now come early and then eventually change to being late, even up to months at a time. Our bone density declines, with the future prospect of osteoporosis, and unsightly and fast-growing black facial hairs appear as a result of declining levels of estrogen. Oh, and this unpredictability of hormone levels actually matches the unpredictable mood swings--I think there could be a connection there. Barb Cook* (Cook & Garnett, 2018, pp. 39–40)

Puberty is a time of transition for all children, and the principle of preparing autistic children for transition applies here. Changes in body structure, sensory experiences, mood, and cognition occur starting as young as 7 years old in females in the usual biologic progression of puberty (Parent et al., 2003). Some evidence suggests that the body changes of puberty may occur a few months earlier in autistic females compared to neurotypicals (Corbett at al., 2020). Therefore, preparation for the puberty transition and the beginning of sexuality/health education should be ongoing for the young child and be delivered with strategies that autistic individuals find particularly helpful: using pictures, social stories, repetition, and first-person accounts from autistic individuals.

Preparation for these changes is part of sexuality/health education in some states, but practitioners should be aware that some states specifically disallow sexuality/health education at school. Additionally, for many children in special education, sexuality/health education is not provided. Autistic adults report less access to sexuality/health education compared to neurotypical adults and less understanding of the sexuality/health education they received (Joyal et al., 2021; Mehzabin & Stokes, 2011). Practitioners may need to inquire of parents how much education about puberty and sexual health a child has received at home or at school. Many books and websites are available to assist parents with providing sexual education to their autistic child and providing clear explanations and social stories to help answer questions about what to expect and what is expected socially.

Social rules for dating become more important in adolescence, but are often not explicit or nuanced. Social rules that we expect children to pick up on must be made explicit—when and where to expect privacy, what behaviors should only be done in private, what are the social expectations for dating and consent, who can be trusted, and when to tell a trusted adult about another's actions that make a child uncomfortable. Teaching consent for sexual activity is important to protect the individual. Accounts written by autistic girls and young women are available and include sections about their experiences with puberty, receiving sexuality/health education, and figuring out romantic relationships (see books listed in this chapter).

Changes in behavior may signal hormonal or menstrual changes in autistic individuals (Steward et al., 2018). Sensory and executive functioning challenges may make managing menstruation difficult. Mothers of autistic girls report that managing their daughters' menstruation and hygiene is challenging in puberty (Navot et al., 2017). Familiarization with products for managing menstruation should occur in anticipation of the onset of menstruation. Consultation with a medical provider to discuss options for managing and suppressing menstruation may be needed if sensory discomfort, mood changes, or pain with menstruation is distressing to the individual.

As with neurotypical adolescents and young adults, sexual maturation heralds the onset of the need for regular preventive women's health. Guidelines from medical societies recommend vaccines, cancer screening with pap smears, testing for sexually transmitted infections, and contraception if desired for all female patients (Women's Preventive Services Initiative, 2022). In a study of self-reported healthcare access, autistic women received regularly scheduled pap smears less frequently than neurotypicals (Nicolaidis et al., 2013). There are no specific guidelines for autistic females or those with intellectual developmental disabilities, but women's healthcare should not be withheld based on autistic traits or difficulty communicating. If desired, anesthesia (medication for anxiety, pain, amnesia, or sedation) can be arranged for those who cannot tolerate examinations for preventive care due to sensory sensitivities, a history of sexual assault, or lack of understanding. Again, respecting an individual's right to make decisions about their own body and healthcare must be weighed against ensuring equal access to medical care for neurodivergent individuals. Some autistic individuals may need the help of a trusted family member for making medical decisions, and others will make these decisions themselves (Corey & Bulova, 2016).

Gender Identity

Children become aware of societal labels for genders as young as 2 years old and of stereotypical gender roles at 4–5 years old (Perrin, 2002). Practitioners should look beyond communication difficulties, persistent pronoun reversals, literal interpretation of gender as the same as sex, and limited social opportunities, which can give the false sense that autistic children are not aware of or interested in gender identity. Books and pictures that help expose autistic children to facts about their bodies and the bodies of others help them access health education and protect them from the vulnerability induced by naivete (Joyal et al., 2021).

In early puberty, gender identity needs should be addressed if an autistic child is experiencing gender dysphoria. Gender dysphoria is diagnosed when children have persistent identification with a gender identity that differs from that assigned at birth and have significant associated distress (APA, 2022). Children who identify with the opposite gender than their birth-assigned sex or with neither gender were previously pathologized, but now it is the distress associated with societal ostracization that is recognized as the source of depression, anxiety, and suicidality (Lopez et al., 2017; Perrin, 2002).

Gender dysphoria is more common in autism, and access to gender-affirming care is an important aspect of care that should not be denied based on autism diagnosis (Corbett et al., 2023). Recent controversy around whether autistic people are competent to make decisions around gender identity medical care has reinforced the need for equitable care. The higher prevalence of gender dysphoria in autism has been falsely attributed to intense interests, lack of empathy, and indifference to societal norms, leading to movements to exclude autistic people from gender-affirming care. The World Professional Association for Transgender Health (WPATH) guidelines recommend that health professionals caring for adolescents with gender dysphoria develop expertise in autism and acknowledges that autistic individuals qualify for gender-affirming care (Coleman et al., 2022). Timely access to puberty-halting medicine is part of the standard of care for gender dysphoria (Lopez et al., 2017). Gender dysphoria should not be dismissed as a sensory challenge or perseveration if the child's feelings are clear, urgent, pervasive, and persistent and they express a consistent desire to go through a social transition or the opposite puberty (Strang et al., 2018).

Pregnancy and Parenting

First Person Narratives

> *I was still confused, quite literally, as to how I got pregnant. To this day I still believe in divine intervention, even though I also know the physiological aspects now. During the pregnancy I had a shirt made that stated "Kids get in the darndest places." It was a senti-*

ment that was rather funny, and people loved that shirt. I did too, because it explained my confusion without anyone seriously knowing that I was confused. The confusion led to reading as much information as I could get from the doctor. This was the time before the internet. The doctor I had was an amazing person and he seemed to give me extra time to make sure I knew what was going on, as best as he could. - (Snyder, 2006, p. 123)

You sort of fall in love with this child in your head before you've even met them. (Alice) The first time I saw her it was like the most amazing feeling . . . and I looked in her eyes and it was like I'd known her forever . . . I can't even ex[plain], it was beautiful. (Sophie) I didn't have two thoughts to rub together, and that was almost panic inducing. Like, it was like I felt like I was just being taken to pieces. And there was nothing left of me. (Leah). (Dugdale et al., 2021, p. 1980)

When my first baby was born, I soon learned my troubles with vestibular motion went beyond amusement parks and car rides. I could not rock my girls. I could sway, though, and this I did even in my rocking chair. Leaning forward toward the edge or far back into the chair, I would move my body left and right while I patted the babies to quiet their tears. When that made me sick, I would stand and sway, only a few inches in either direction. If that proved to be too much, I walked the floors, bouncing my daughters up and down as I went. My attempts routinely fell short of perfect for my young ones who preferred the wild ride their father could provide them. (Willey, 2014, p. 102)

Supportive Health Care

Autistic women have a higher burden of women's health issues and may be misunderstood when accessing care. In studies directly comparing autistic women to non-autistic women, autistic women report irregular menstruation, painful periods, and polycystic ovarian syndrome at higher rates (Kassee et al., 2020). Pregnancy complications such as preeclampsia and preterm birth also occur more often in autistic women (Sundelin et al., 2018). Depression and postpartum depression have also been found at higher frequency in autistic women (Pohl et al., 2020). Despite similar attendance at prenatal classes and more consistent primary care, autistic women had more health problems during pregnancy (including hypertension, diabetes, and asthma) and felt less often that the process of birth had been explained to them (Pohl et al., 2020; Tint et al., 2021). Sensory experiences during pregnancy, childbirth, and breastfeeding can be challenging for autistic women, and care should be individualized to the person's needs. A qualitative study of eight autistic women found women experienced difficulty processing the new sensations of pregnancy but also the emergence of new sensory sensitivities during pregnancy (Gardner et al., 2016).

In a study asking autistic women about their experiences with parenting, they reported difficulty with the organizational skills and social demands of parenting (Pohl et al., 2020). Compared to neurotypical women, autistic women reported difficulty communicating with professionals about their child and anxiety related to difficulty in communication more often (Pohl et al., 2020). A qualitative analysis of the experience of eight autistic mothers also found that communication difficulty and misunderstandings occurred frequently and interfered with trust in healthcare providers (Dugdale et al., 2021). Self-advocacy skills matched with patience and understanding from healthcare professionals are identified areas of need for autistic parents

> *"Asperger women report the need to feel more empowered about their birthing day and their experience is reliant on three factors including: clear communication, sensory adjustments and change management. (Autism Women Matter)"* (Hendrickx, 2015, p. 184).

See Chapter 12 for more on parenting.

Menopause

First Person Narratives

> *Not knowing you're autistic on the first place – and then suddenly experiencing unprecedented phenomena which don't correlate with 'regular' menopause, so you don't know if it's menopause or not. So you wonder whether you're going nuts, or have some disease, or what.*

> *When I talk about that time, I say, 'My autism broke'. Before that, my autism was working fairly well for me, providing me with good job skills. (P4, Q2)* (Moseley et al., 2020, pp. 1427–1428)

Research is extremely limited about menopause and autism. The little research that does exist suggests that menopausal symptoms are likely to be difficult in the same way that menstruation can be more difficult for autistic females (Groenman et al., 2021). Some see it as a relief; others have more difficulty, particularly with the unpredictability of menopause symptoms; and some women were not aware that their current difficulties were related to menopause (Karavidas & de Visser, 2022). Moseley et al. (2021) reported that some women's inherent autistic traits were amplified during menopause, prompting them to seek assessment and ultimately their autism diagnosis. Moseley et al. (2020) also interviewed women who talked about sensory and executive function differences that were more difficult to cope with during menopause, particularly when menopause came before diagnosis. Difficulties communicating with healthcare providers were some of the biggest barriers reported.

> *"At times I can remember not being able to identify or communicate any of what I was experiencing. P7, Q7"* (Moseley et al., 2020, p. 1428)

Sleep issues were some of the more worrisome symptoms, related to sensory overwhelm (See Table 9.1 for support strategies). See Chap. 4 for more about sleep screening measures.

Table 9.1 At-a-Glance Summary of Supports for Medical Issues in Female Puberty, Gender Identity, Pregnancy, Parenting and Menopause

Domain	Focus
Puberty	Support for transition in identity, sensory experiences, and cognition Some evidence that bodily changes at onset of puberty occur early in autistic females
Menstruation	Counsel parents to prepare with social stories, books, and familiarity with products for menstruation management Medical management and access to contraception should be offered as with neurotypicals and regardless of severity
Gender identity	Develops in young children starting at 2–5 years. Gender dysphoria and non-binary identity are more frequent in autism. Gender-affirming care should not be withheld on the basis of autistic traits
Sexuality/health education	Use literal descriptions and accurate words, and give explicit social rules Be aware of potential lack of sexuality/health education in special education and lack of accessible sexuality/health education in mainstream education Resources: https://www.amightygirl.com/blog?p=14948 https://www.parentcenterhub.org/sexed/ https://www.amazon.com/Autism-Friendly-Guide-Periods-Robyn-Steward/dp/1785923242 Balfe, A. (2021). *A different kind of normal: My real-life completely true story about being unique* Castellon, S. (2020). *The spectrum girl's survival guide: How to grow up awesome and autistic.*
Pregnancy and parenting	Health disparities: increased risk of preeclampsia, giving preterm birth, and receiving elective cesarean delivery for autistic women compared to non-autistic women. More frequent postpartum depression, sensory issues, and communication difficulties with health professionals
Menopause	Consider the possibility of relatively sudden complaints related to mental or physical health as possible signs of menopause. The National Autistic Society addresses menopause with a webpage of first-person accounts and general menopause resources https://www.autism.org.uk/advice-and-guidance/topics/physical-health/menopause
Healthcare communication	Professionals need to accommodate communication differences (e.g., using visuals, written information) and understand that communication may be affected by sensory overwhelm and negative past experiences with healthcare that jeopardizes current care. See more in Chap. 12 on healthcare and aging

References

American Psychiatric Association. (2022). *Diagnostic and statistical manual of mental disorders* (5th ed., text rev.). https://doi.org/10.1176/appi.books.9780890425787

Antaki, D., Guevara, J., Maihofer, A. X., Klein, M., Gujral, M., Grove, J., Carey, C. E., Hong, O., Arranz, M. J., Hervas, A., Corsello, C., Vaux, K. K., Muotri, A. R., Iakoucheva, L. M., Courchesne, E., Pierce, K., Gleeson, J. G., Robinson, E. B., Nievergelt, C. M., & Sebat, J. (2022). A phenotypic spectrum of autism is attributable to the combined effects of rare variants, polygenic risk and sex. *Nature Genetics*. https://doi.org/10.1038/s41588-022-01064-5

Balfe, A. (2021). *A different kind of normal: My real-life completely true story about being unique.* Crown Books for Young Readers/Penguin Random House LLC.

Castellon, S. (2020). *The spectrum girl's survival guide: How to grow up awesome and autistic.* Jessica Kingsley Publishers.

Coleman, E., Radix, A. E., Bouman, W. P., Brown, G. R., de Vries, A. L. C., Deutsch, M. B., Ettner, R., Fraser, L., Goodman, M., Green, J., Hancock, A. B., Johnson, T. W., Karasic, D. H., Knudson, G. A., Leibowitz, S. F., Meyer-Bahlburg, H. F. L., Monstrey, S. J., Motmans, J., Nahata, L., et al. (2022). Standards of care for the health of transgender and gender diverse people, version 8. *International Journal of Transgender Health, 23*(Suppl 1), S1–S259. https://doi.org/10.1080/26895269.2022.2100644

Cook, B., & Garnett, M. (Eds.). (2018). *Spectrum women: Walking to the beat of autism.* Jessica Kingsley Publishers.

Corbett, B. A., Muscatello, R. A., Klemencic, M. E., West, M., Kim, A., & Strang, J. F. (2023). Greater gender diversity among autistic children by self-report and parent-report. *Autism: The International Journal of Research and Practice, 27*(1), 158–172. https://doi.org/10.1177/13623613221085337

Corbett, B. A., Vandekar, S., Muscatello, R. A., & Tanguturi, Y. (2020). Pubertal timing during early adolescence: *Advanced pubertal onset in females with autism spectrum disorder. Autism Research, 13*(12), 2202–2215. https://doi.org/10.1002/aur.2406

Corey, S., & Bulova, P. (2016). Is proxy consent for an invasive procedure on a patient with intellectual disabilities ethically sufficient? Commentary 1. *AMA Journal of Ethics, 18*(4), 373–378. https://doi.org/10.1001/journalofethics.2016.18.4.ecas3-1604

Dugdale, A. S., Thompson, A. R., Leedham, A., Beail, N., & Freeth, M. (2021). Intense connection and love: The experiences of autistic mothers. *Autism: The International Journal of Research and Practice, 25*(7), 1973–1984. https://doi.org/10.1177/13623613211005987

Gardner, M., Suplee, P. D., Bloch, J., & Lecks, K. (2016). Exploratory study of childbearing experiences of women with Asperger syndrome. *Nursing for Women's Health, 20*(1), 28–37. https://doi.org/10.1016/j.nwh.2015.12.001

Groenman, A. P., Torenvliet, C., Radhoe, T. A., Agelink van Rentergem, J. A., & Geurts, H. M. (2021). Menstruation and menopause in autistic adults: Periods of importance? *Autism: The International Journal of Research and Practice, 26*(6), 1563–1572. https://doi.org/10.1177/13623613211059721

Hendrickx, S. (2015). *Women and girls with autism spectrum disorder: Understanding life experiences from early childhood to old age.* Jessica Kingsley Publishers.

Jacquemont, S., Coe, B. P., Hersch, M., Duyzend, M. H., Krumm, N., Bergmann, S., Beckmann, J. S., Rosenfeld, J. A., & Eichler, E. E. (2014). A higher mutational burden in females supports a "female protective model" in neurodevelopmental disorders. *The American Journal of Human Genetics, 94*(3), 415–425. https://doi.org/10.1016/j.ajhg.2014.02.001

Joyal, C. C., Carpentier, J., McKinnon, S., Normand, C. L., & Poulin, M.-H. (2021). Sexual knowledge, desires, and experience of adolescents and young adults with an autism spectrum disorder: An exploratory study. *Frontiers in Psychiatry, 12.* https://www.frontiersin.org/articles/10.3389/fpsyt.2021.685256

Karavidas, M., & de Visser, R. O. (2022). "It's not just in my head, and it's not just irrelevant": Autistic negotiations of menopausal transitions. *Journal of Autism and Developmental Disorders, 52*(3), 1143–1155. https://doi.org/10.1007/s10803-021-05010-y

Kassee, C., Babinski, S., Tint, A., Lunsky, Y., Brown, H. K., Ameis, S. H., Szatmari, P., Lai, M.-C., & Einstein, G. (2020). Physical health of autistic girls and women: A scoping review. *Molecular Autism, 11*(1), 84. https://doi.org/10.1186/s13229-020-00380-z

Lawrence, K. E., Hernandez, L. M., Fuster, E., Padgaonkar, N. T., Patterson, G., Jung, J., Okada, N. J., Lowe, J. K., Hoekstra, J. N., Jack, A., Aylward, E., Gaab, N., Van Horn, J. D., Bernier, R. A., McPartland, J. C., Webb, S. J., Pelphrey, K. A., Green, S. A., Bookheimer, S. Y., … Dapretto, M. (2022). Impact of autism genetic risk on brain connectivity: A mechanism for the female protective effect. *Brain: A Journal of Neurology, 145*(1), 378–387. https://doi.org/10.1093/brain/awab204

Lopez, X., Marinkovic, M., Eimicke, T., Rosenthal, S. M., Olshan, J. S., & Group, on behalf of the P. E. S. T. H. S. I. (2017). Statement on gender-affirmative approach to care from the pediatric endocrine society special interest group on transgender health. *Current Opinion in Pediatrics, 29*(4), 475. https://doi.org/10.1097/MOP.0000000000000516

Mehzabin, P., & Stokes, M. A. (2011). Self-assessed sexuality in young adults with high-functioning autism. *Research in Autism Spectrum Disorders, 5*(1), 614–621. https://doi.org/10.1016/j.rasd.2010.07.006

Moseley, R. L., Druce, T., & Turner-Cobb, J. M. (2020). 'When my autism broke': A qualitative study spotlighting autistic voices on menopause. *Autism: The International Journal of Research and Practice, 24*(6), 1423–1437. https://doi.org/10.1177/1362361319901184

Moseley, R. L., Druce, T., & Turner-Cobb, J. M. (2021). Autism research is 'all about the blokes and the kids': Autistic women breaking the silence on menopause. *British Journal of Health Psychology, 26*(3), 709–726. https://doi.org/10.1111/bjhp.12477

National Autistic Society (n.d.) Menopause. https://www.autism.org.uk/advice-and-guidance/topics/physical-health/menopause

Navot, N., Jorgenson, A. G., & Webb, S. J. (2017). Maternal experience raising girls with autism spectrum disorder: A qualitative study. *Child: Care, Health and Development, 43*(4), 536–545. https://doi.org/10.1111/cch.12470

Nicolaidis, C., Raymaker, D., McDonald, K., Dern, S., Boisclair, W. C., Ashkenazy, E., & Baggs, A. (2013). Comparison of healthcare experiences in autistic and non-autistic adults: A cross-sectional online survey facilitated by an academic-community partnership. *Journal of General Internal Medicine, 28*(6), 761–769. https://doi.org/10.1007/s11606-012-2262-7

Parent, A.-S., Teilmann, G., Juul, A., Skakkebaek, N. E., Toppari, J., & Bourguignon, J.-P. (2003). The timing of normal puberty and the age limits of sexual precocity: Variations around the world, secular trends, and changes after migration. *Endocrine Reviews, 24*(5), 668–693. https://doi.org/10.1210/er.2002-0019

Perrin, E. C. (2002). *Sexual orientation in child and adolescent healthcare.* Kluwer Academic/Plenum Publishers.

Pohl, A. L., Crockford, S. K., Blakemore, M., Allison, C., & Baron-Cohen, S. (2020). A comparative study of autistic and non-autistic women's experience of motherhood. *Molecular Autism, 11*(1), 3. https://doi.org/10.1186/s13229-019-0304-2

Robinson, E. B., Lichtenstein, P., Anckarsäter, H., Happé, F., & Ronald, A. (2013). Examining and interpreting the female protective effect against autistic behavior. *Proceedings of the National Academy of Sciences, 110*(13), 5258–5262. https://doi.org/10.1073/pnas.1211070110

Snyder, R. (2006). Maternal instincts in Asperger's syndrome. In T. Attwood (Ed.), *Asperger's and girls: World-renowned experts join those with Asperger's syndrome to resolve issues that girls and women face every day!* (pp. 117–146). Future Horizons.

Steward, R., Crane, L., Mairi Roy, E., Remington, A., & Pellicano, E. (2018). "Life is much more difficult to manage during periods": Autistic experiences of menstruation. *Journal of Autism and Developmental Disorders, 48*(12), 4287–4292. https://doi.org/10.1007/s10803-018-3664-0

Strang, J. F., Meagher, H., Kenworthy, L., de Vries, A. L. C., Menvielle, E., Leibowitz, S., Janssen, A., Cohen-Kettenis, P., Shumer, D. E., Edwards-Leeper, L., Pleak, R. R., Spack, N., Karasic, D. H., Schreier, H., Balleur, A., Tishelman, A., Ehrensaft, D., Rodnan, L., Kuschner, E. S., et al. (2018). Initial clinical guidelines for co-occurring autism spectrum disorder and gender dysphoria or incongruence in adolescents. *Journal of Clinical Child & Adolescent Psychology, 47*(1), 105–115. https://doi.org/10.1080/15374416.2016.1228462

Sundelin, H. E. K., Stephansson, O., Hultman, C. M., & Ludvigsson, J. F. (2018). Pregnancy outcomes in women with autism: A nationwide population-based cohort study. *Clinical Epidemiology, 10*, 1817–1826. https://doi.org/10.2147/CLEP.S176910

Szatmari, P., Liu, X., Goldberg, J., Zwaigenbaum, L., Paterson, A. D., Woodbury, S. M., Georgiades, S., Duku, E., & Thompson, A. (2012). Sex differences in repetitive stereotyped behaviors in autism: Implications for genetic liability. *American Journal of Medical Genetics Part B: Neuropsychiatric Genetics, 159B*(1), 5–12. https://doi.org/10.1002/ajmg.b.31238

Tint, A., Brown, H. K., Chen, S., Lai, M. C., Tarasoff, L. A., Vigod, S. N., Parish, S., Havercamp, S. M., & Lunsky, Y. (2021). Health characteristics of reproductive-aged autistic women in Ontario: A population-based, cross-sectional study. *Autism: The International Journal of Research and Practice, 25*(4), 1114–1124. https://doi.org/10.1177/1362361320982819

Wigdor, E., Weiner, D., Grove, J., Fu, J., Thompson, W., Carey, C., Baya, N., van der Merwe, C., Mortensen, P. B., Daly, M., Talkowski, M., Sanders, S., Bishop, S., Børglum, A., & Robinson, E. (2021). The female protective effect against autism spectrum disorder. *European Neuropsychopharmacology, 51*, e13–e14. https://doi.org/10.1016/j.euroneuro.2021.07.035

Willey, L. H. (2012). *Safety skills for Asperger women: How to save a perfectly good female life.* Jessica Kingsley Publishers.

Willey, L. H. (2014). *Pretending to be normal: Living with Asperger's syndrome*, Jessica Kingsley.

Women's Preventive Services Initiative. (2022). *Recommendations for well-woman care – A well-woman chart*. ACOG Foundation. Available at: https://www.womenspreventivehealth.org//srv/htdocs/wp-content/uploads/WellWomanChart.pdf. Retrieved February 26, 2023.

Chapter 10
Underlying Autism? Female Eating Disorders, Self-Injury, Suicide, Sexual Victimization, and Substance Abuse

Introduction

Autism as a developmental disorder, by itself, is not typically thought of as life-threatening. The experiences of a neurodivergent person in an environment that can range from unfriendly to intolerable to abusive can, however, result in life-threatening behaviors. It is a mistake to assume that an autistic person doesn't care about social relationships, or is not interested in being accepted by society. These are basic human needs that are shared by all. The presence of crisis events may, unfortunately, be the first signal for identification of autism outside of the family and should be at least considered as part of the evaluation and intake processes. Consideration and consultation with autism specialists, if necessary, can improve the efficacy of treatment strategies and the choice of options best suited to the individual.

> And so, because a lot of my life, because I didn't really know and wasn't pointed out to where I knew how to bring that out in a positive way, it would come out more in a negative way, in the sense of harming myself. So whether it was dealing with my anorexia and the eating disorders I've been dealing with throughout my 20s, whether it had been when I was cutting myself in high school, and when I had nearly lost my life to suicide in 2016-- that was all because it was all built up, that camouflaging, right? And there's a point when it just-- it bursts, right? It just bursts. - Lindsay Nebeker, 2019

Case Study—Rey: Adolescent with an Eating Disorder

Rey is an 18-year-old transgender man with a history of diabetes, anxiety, depression, suicide attempts, and anorexia nervosa who was admitted to the hospital for worsening suicidal ideation. He restricts his diet to a daily calorie limit and wants to lose weight to a specific ideal weight. He also reports suicidal thoughts and does not feel he would be safe from self-harm if he left the hospital. Self-harm is part of a

© The Author(s), under exclusive license to Springer Nature
Switzerland AG 2023
T. P. Gabrielsen et al., *Assessment of Autism in Females and Nuanced Presentations*, https://doi.org/10.1007/978-3-031-33969-1_10

daily routine for him, and he thinks it would be hard to change. This is his sixth admission to the hospital for eating disorder treatment and suicidal ideation. His doctors note that he does not often make eye contact, he has strong likes and dislikes, he refuses to follow others' rules, and he has difficulty socializing with strangers. They call the developmental and behavioral pediatrics team to evaluate him in the hospital for autism, thinking this diagnosis may change their approach to his treatment-refractory eating disorder. Rey tells the developmental and behavioral pediatrician that he has always felt different from other kids his age. He finds conversation with most people difficult, gets confused when people cry when they are not sad, does not have friends but this does not bother him, and rocks in a chair to calm himself. The doctors explain autism and how his traits fit this diagnosis, which could help him understand himself. For his eating disorder, they recommend respecting his texture preferences when reintroducing foods and allowing him to create routines that help him eat enough calories to be safe. For suicidal ideation, they recommend that the treating providers help him make a safety plan with concrete components that he can follow, sensory soothing that he chooses, and someone he feels comfortable calling to talk to when he feels suicidal.

Anorexia Nervosa (AN), Eating Disorders (EDs), and Autism

First Person Narratives

> *It all boils down to the fact that if anyone had connected the dots between autism and eating disorders, if I had found your work earlier, if the professionals who were supposed to be experts in the field had known what autism even looks like in girls or women ... we might have saved Kathryn's life. Rebecca* (O'Toole, 2018, p. 255)

> *Sadly, it is very common for Aspie females to develop eating disorders. This could be related to our obsessive-compulsive nature. It could be our innocent belief that the fashion media's message to be tiny and thin is the message we should follow. Or it could be that our sensory system freaks out when our stomach is too full, a food smells too strongly or tastes too sickening. In my case, it was a bit of a mixture of all the above.* (Willey, 2012, pp. 95–96)

> *Clinicians' attention can be diverted by the presentation of other comorbid mental health conditions in teenage and adult life—conditions such as anorexia and anxiety disorders, which may be part of the autistic profile but may not lead automatically to considering autism as the causal factor... Some research suggests that the cognitive profiles of individuals with anorexia and those with ASD are markedly similar except for differences in empathy scoring* (Oldershaw et al., 2011). *It has been suggested that anorexia is 'the female Asperger's'.* (Hendrickx, 2015, p. 36 and 203)

> *As far as my research shows, no one has looked at a possible connection between eating disorders (ED) and self-injury in autism specifically. However, in my practice experience, they tend to serve similar purposes, which is to foster a barrier to outside and the multilayered pain we experience from the world." - Dena Gassner* (Cook & Garnett, 2018, p. 243)

> *"I do know that to someone like me who has hyposensitive sensory integration dysfunction, self-injury feeds the need to feel, literally and figuratively....without a wake-up call to my sensory system, my body would have shut down. If only this were a safe way to patch things up.* (Willey, 2012, p. 95)

Eating Disorders Related to Autism

As early as 1983, Gillberg suggested that AN might be on the same spectrum as autism, citing familial and chemical study correlations (Gillberg, 1983). Research developments since then suggest that AN may be one way that autism manifests in females who have otherwise not been identified, using the endophenotype framework of social cognition differences to describe phenomena in individuals that are somewhat between genotype and phenotype, thus perhaps obscuring diagnosis and interfering with treatment (Zucker et al., 2007). This grew from Godart et al. (2000) reporting that 75% of individuals with AN described the onset of an anxiety disorder prior to their eating disturbance, with 55% of the sample endorsing social phobia, which may overlap with autism social communication experiences and differences. Koch et al. (2015) examined a Danish national database for familial association in both autism and AN and found a complicated relationship. They first noted that AN was linked with higher association for autism. They also found that in families with autism, there were higher rates of AN. The complication was that in families with AN, there were other co-occurring conditions that also increased the risk of AN, so firm conclusions about the relationship are not yet established, at least in terms of familial (genetic) risk factors.

Tchanturia et al. (2019) tested these theories by comparing autism measures with AN symptomatology. They concluded that autism traits are associated with eating disorder psychopathology behaviorally, but not necessarily physically, i.e., low body weight/BMI. They further concluded that measures of autism traits may slightly decrease with progress in AN treatment, suggesting that the relationship between conditions is possibly bi-directional, but the presence of one likely exacerbates the other. Kerr-Gaffney et al. (2021) looked further into the measurement of traits, finding that special interests and stimming behaviors crossed over with AN, autism, and recovering AN groups. Much like other literature, social response was the distinguishing factor for differentiating between those with autism and those without. This study did not include participants with co-occurring AN and autism, however.

One focus within this research is the relationship of body image and other eating disturbances with autism and eating disorders (EDs) among autistics without intellectual developmental disorder. A Swedish group has studied EDs among autistic populations with the Swedish Eating Assessment for Autism Spectrum Disorders (SWEAA: Karlsson et al., 2013). Their team identified some ED behaviors within autism groups such as hyper-selectivity in eating or food selection, strict routines at mealtime, and not enjoying social aspects of mealtimes. Spek et al. (2020) found that autistic women exhibited more eating disturbances than non-autistic participants and autistic males. Karjalainen et al. (2019) found some of these traits lingered after weight was normalized, suggesting underlying autistic traits that may have been overshadowed by the ED. They questioned whether autism traits were induced by starvation and subsided with weight recovery, but this was not always the case. Because of evidence that autistic traits related to eating may have been present prior to the onset of the ED (Nielsen et al., 2015; Rastam, 1992; Wentz et al., 2005), starvation may have exacerbated autism traits or merely brought them to the attention of clinicians. Other differences in autistic populations include reduced occurrence of self-induced vomiting (purging) in eating disorders, but higher prevalence of binge eating without purging (Numata et al., 2021):

> Standard eating disorder treatment options and settings may need to be modified to better accommodate autistic female individuals. Autistic traits, such as rigid thinking, difficulty communicating thoughts and feelings, and sensory processing abnormalities can hinder traditional approaches to eating disorder treatment. (Brown & Stokes, 2020, p. 735)

Most recently, Nisticò et al. (2022) connected hypersensitivity in the visual domain to higher autistic eating behaviors and levels of ED symptomatology. The rationale behind this connection is that vision contributes to satiety and food intake. Another possible factor is that body image associated with eating disorders could also be mediated by visual perception, including distortion of visual perception of one's own body size. This hypothesis is consistent with extensive first-person accounts of increased sensory sensitivity in autistic females. Brede et al. (2020) proposed a model of ED traits specific to autistic women including sensory sensitivities and difficulties with social interaction, relationship and emotional difficulties, sense of self and identity issues, autistic thinking styles, and need for control and predictability.

A meta-analysis conducted by Sharp et al. (2013) found nutritional deficits associated with autism and feeding difficulties including lower intake of calcium and protein. Unfortunately, the samples included were 83–95% male, but the findings may be even more critical for females if they are similar. Calories for energy and growth were found to be sufficient, but the low levels of calcium and protein are likely to have more significant long-term effects for females' health. Recommendations from the authors included assessment of feeding problems in routine medical evaluations and screening for nutritional deficits or excesses in addition to regularly measuring height and weight. If gluten-free-casein-free (GFCF) or any other elimination diets are in the patient history, closer assessment and counseling of individual long-term nutritional needs is recommended.

Non-suicidal Self-Injury (NSSI) and Self-Injurious Behavior (SIB)

Although self-injurious behaviors (SIB) are a well-documented phenomenon among autistic children with lower cognitive and language performance (Esbensen et al., 2009; Lecavalier, 2006; McClintock et al., 2003), it is possible that the connection between non-suicidal self-injury (NSSI) encountered clinically and potential autism diagnoses may be overlooked. The two conditions look different and occur in different populations (Jacobson & Gould, 2007), but they may nevertheless be a signal that autism should be at least considered.

A 2017 study with a relatively small sample ($n = 84$, half with autism, half neurotypical [NT]) established some data suggesting that adult autistic women had significantly higher rates of history of NSSI than either adolescents with autism or a comparable neurotypical population. Autistic women also showed much higher rates of NSSI (75%) than men with autism (33%). The overall rate of NSSI in the autistic sample was 50%—more than double the rate in the general population and adolescents with autism (Maddox & White, 2013). The authors separated self-injurious behaviors (SIB) associated with restricted and repetitive behaviors (RRBs) that are often a feature in children with autism from the types of NSSI that are more aligned with neurotypical NSSIs such as cutting. Mean age of onset of NSSI was similar to the NT control group (*m* age, 12.7; *SD*, 5.5 years). Although the presence of depression or emotional dysregulation did not predict NSSI in the autism group, there was some relationship between difficulties with emotional dysregulation and sensory seeking behaviors. The most frequent form of NSSI in both autism (15%) and NT (25%) groups was severe scratching or pinching, with other patterns in NSSI fairly consistent between groups. Autistic females in the study were much more likely to report NSSI (72.2%) than males (33.3%). Half of the autistic participants in the study (50%) reported receiving an autism diagnosis after the age of 18 (Maddox et al., 2017).

Suicidality

First Person Narratives

In the fourth grade, I came home from school one day and told my mother that I felt like killing myself. My parents quickly sought help. We shuffled from specialist to specialist, none having any definitive answers until we got to the Child Psychology department at Stony Brook University in New York. At age 11, I was finally diagnosed with a form of autism that used to be known as Asperger's syndrome. Amy Gravino (2021)

The magic was gone. I had somehow been abandoned, left behind, as though childhood had continued without me and left me waiting at the station. I was shut out of this realm forever. This was devastating for me. I wanted to die, and felt very scared because these games helped me shut out everything else and felt threatened by the now very present, outside world. I almost feel I would have tried to kill myself if I had had any concept of suicide. However I soon resigned myself to living in this gray, without magic and with very little purpose. April Masilimani (Cook & Garnett, 2018, p. 167)

For years, I tried to be somebody that I was not, and I was not happy. I felt like I was living a lie every day of my life. Sadly, in my teenage years, I was so unhappy that I thought about committing suicide, but I never had the guts to do it, so I did not try to commit suicide even though deep inside I wanted to. Kayla Smith (Ballou et al., 2021, p. 97)

Despite rampant levels of serious depression, the majority of Aspergirls interviewed have not thought seriously of suicide. Although most of us have contemplated it, few had made any real attempts and most said it was something they could never bring themselves to do. Consideration for loved ones and fear of the unknown stopped us. Although wanting control over ourselves can cause us to contemplate it, not being in control of what happens after we die is an even bigger deterrent. (Simone, 2010, p. 172)

Unexpectedly High Suicidal Thoughts and Behaviors

Unfortunately, the prevalence of suicidality among autistic females is higher than for any of the other comparable groups, except neurotypical males (Hirvikoski et al., 2016; Strang et al., 2021). Prevalence rates for suicidal thoughts and behaviors (STBs) in autistic populations are reported across a very high range: 66% for autistic populations overall (Cassidy et al., 2014); threefold that of neurotypical populations (Kõlves et al., 2021); autistic female risk was 300–400% higher than other groups, including autistic males (Kirby et al., 2019; Kõlves et al., 2021); 10–50% across genders (Segers & Rawana, 2014) and 46% of women with high levels of autism traits with a history of suicide plans (South et al., 2020). Kato et al. (2013) investigated differences among admitted patients in a psychiatric hospital for suicide and found autistic patients were younger, had used more lethal means, were more likely to be single, and were not as likely to have a mood disorder and their attempt was more likely to be in reaction to a more distal event in time than their peers. They also stayed longer in the hospital. Chen et al. (2017) found autism to be an independent risk factor for suicide in a national study in Taiwan.

A very large Swedish population study found the risk of death from other causes was higher for autistic females with lower cognitive and language levels, which is likely consistent with the higher number of genetic differences in females who have been traditionally included in research. Autistic females with higher cognitive and language abilities, however, were strikingly different, with suicide as the most frequent cause of death (Hirvikoski et al., 2016). Common autistic experiences such as trauma and unmet healthcare needs can contribute to premature death from both suicide and physical ailments.

Beyond the statistics, why is the risk of suicide so much higher for autistic females? According to the interpersonal theory of suicide (Joiner et al., 2009), thwarted belongingness, social alienation, and perceived burdensomeness are strongly associated with suicidal thoughts and behaviors. Each of these factors can be considered common features of unsupported autism. Some additional theories include camouflaging associated with thwarted belongingness (Cassidy et al., 2020), autistic burnout (Raymaker et al., 2020), low self-esteem and rumination (Arwert & Sizoo, 2020), and psychiatric co-occurring conditions (Kõlves et al., 2021). (See Chap. 11 for more about burnout and Chap. 8 for co-occurring conditions.) It is also possible that suicide risk might be overshadowed by other concerns and missed by clinicians or that intense anxiety and/or depression might not be communicated effectively by autistic individuals (Crane et al., 2019).

Some researchers have commented that a delayed autism diagnosis (into adulthood) might be a risk factor for suicidal ideation, behaviors, and earlier deaths in autistic individuals (Cassidy et al., 2014). In a predominantly autistic female or non-binary sample with a mean age of diagnosis at about 13 years, when asked what "normal" life was like for them, respondents reported normally feeling "unhappy and depressed; worthless; under strain; unable to overcome their difficulties; unable to face up to problems and lacking in confidence" (Crane et al., 2019, p. 482).

Although virtually all (90%) had sought help from clinical or educational professionals, only 23% thought that services they received were helpful. Supports are likely to be delayed or difficult to navigate or only provided at a crisis point. Many could not tell if their difficulties were attributed to autism or another mental health state or condition. Young women were observed to have more notable difficulties, agreeing that late diagnosis may be a possible cause.

We have noted the importance of clinician expertise in autism throughout this text. South et al. (2021) commented that there are some aspects to this particular barrier to effective treatment. First is that autism may overshadow or confound depression or (possibly more likely) clinicians well-versed in mood and anxiety disorders may miss autism. Either of these factors mean that important elements of treatment approaches will be absent, decreasing the effectiveness of supports.

Sexual Victimization

First Person Narratives

> My first experiences were not willing. I lost my virginity at age 14 to [rape by] my cousin. I misread cues and ended up in situations where dates expected sex and I froze and could not fight them. I got pregnant at age 16 as a result of one of those encounters. Woman with autism (Hendrickx, 2015, p. 174)

> So there I was, biologically an attractive young white lady in my 20s, but socially the level of a pre-school kid.... Once I realized rape was inevitable, I shifted my goal to simply staying alive. Coa (Miller, 2015, p. 279)

> I've been a consultant in far too many cases of rape, domestic abuse, and child custody battles to think courts will be able to really understand the seriousness of our abuse largely because our communication styles tend to be too placid, our pain tolerance oddly high or very low, our eye contact vague, and our body language not intense enough to convince a judge we were significantly damaged. Liane Holliday Willey (Cook & Garnett, 2018, p. 101)

Prevalence of Sexual Assault in Autistic Populations

Experiencing sexual assault may be a point of crisis in a woman's life when autism (even if not yet diagnosed) is definitely not the *cause* of the violence, but is a particular vulnerability before, during, and after the assault. Many hypothesize that autistic female, transgender, and non-binary people are specifically targeted because they are so vulnerable. A French study looked at sexual violence against autistic women and found 88% reported some sort of sexual violence, compared to 30% of allistic women (WHO, 2021), with the majority of events occurring before adulthood (age 18). Only one-third reported their assaults, and when they did, 75% of reports did not result in any action (either medical or legal), and 35% were not believed (Cazalis et al., 2022). This high rate of victimization of autistic females is consistent with Gotby et al.'s (2018) finding of a threefold risk and Weiss and Fardella's (2018) report of seven times the rate of sexual victimization by a peer.

Another aspect of being female and autistic is earlier onset of puberty (averaging 9.5 months earlier; Corbett et al., 2020), which has been found to be a factor in sexual harassment at younger ages (Skoog & Özdemir, 2016). Awareness of these high rates of assault is needed in both assessment and support processes of autistic females already identified (ask about victimization and teach protective strategies). Clinicians should also screen for autism in assault cases if something seems different.

Substance Use

First Person Narratives

> *I was not so much a person abusing drugs, as I was a person trying to self-medicate my way to a life I could manage….my reason for doping was to feel normal, not to be cool getting high or impress friends at a keg party.* (Willey, 2012, p. 95)

> *To me, in a way drinking was actually helping with my social skills. I became less self-conscious when I had a few drinks under my belt. I could start to understand the dynamics of what people were saying, and was never sure if it was my brain slowing down enough to be able to allow more information in or the other people around me slowing down due to their excessive alcohol consumption. Since I was so young and naïve, I never realized just how often I put myself in dangerous situations. Back then I was a tall, blonde, good-looking girl with the insight of a ten-year-old. That is why I called myself a "girl" not a "young woman," as I didn't have the maturity that most women of my age possessed. Being desperate to fit in, I would often take unnecessary risks; the added effects of the alcohol certainly contributed to my poor judgment. Barb Cook* (Cook & Garnett, 2018, pp. 82–83)

> *Drugs did nothing for my social skills. In fact, they made them worse. My mutism episodes and fainting spells increased. Aspergirls and parents be warned—we are far too sensitive mentally and physically to engage in "recreational" drugs.* (Simone, 2010, p. 73)

> *Neurotypical girls survive by "talking out" their feelings and problems to their peers and trusted adults. I could not speak about my emotions or problems to anyone. This involved expressive organized speech, something in which I was weak and completely unpracticed. I also sometimes thought in pictures and emotional snippets, and my feelings had no words. I struggled to find scripts to accomplish expressing my feelings or troubles. But because these conversations are often private and hidden from bystanders, I couldn't watch others or copy them. Without the words to share my pain, and with no connections who could reach in and grab me. I grew silent and turned to drugs to comfort my anguished soul. Jennifer St. Jude* (Ballou et al., 2021, pp. 58–59)

> *I tried drugs for roommates who asked me to "go first" so they could tell how strong the strain was, because, heck, I never said no to a dare—a dare was an act of comradery, ya know? No. No, it wasn't. And neither was it an act of comradery when a few dates easily convinced me that dates ended with things I never suspected, liked, or wanted. Liane Holliday Willey* (Cook & Garnett, 2018, p. 96)

Untrue Assumptions about Substance Use and Abuse in Autism

Studies on substance use in autism are beginning to appear in the scientific literature, but have not yet been reported by gender. Therefore, available data are focused on autistic populations and not specific to any subgroup or gender. A 2019 metaanalysis for substance abuse prevalence in autism groups ranged from 8.3% to 12.9% (Lugo-Marín et al., 2019). Strauss et al. (2021) found substance abuse histories to be eight times higher in autistic youth compared to neurotypical youth in a transgender treatment center. Large population studies have been conducted in national registries, finding higher rates of substance use in autistic individuals (Butwicka et al., 2017), but also suggested that family history of substance use was likely a factor. Huang et al. (2021) expanded on that study with another case-control study in Taiwan with similar findings, but also did not report results by gender. The Taiwan study made a point of looking at youth with mental health system engagement, using access to psychotropic agents as a comparative factor for outcomes. They found lower risk of substance use when youth had access to prescribed psychotropic medication.

Despite the lack of gender-specific scientific data, the first-person literature suggests that substance use may be a source of help in social settings, but that kind of "help" also greatly increased the risk of victimization while impaired or in impaired groups. Consistent with recommendations made for assessing sexual victimization, screen for and/or interview about substance use in autistic females and others with more nuanced autism. It may also be the case that a client or student with emerging or well-established substance use (or possible abuse) who is not responding yet to treatment may need to be screened for autism if the clinician thinks there is something different about their social experiences or understanding (despite average or high cognitive abilities). Substance use in autism is not yet well-studied, and although most studies were conducted in treatment settings, there is very limited information available regarding treatment approaches adapted for neurodiverse populations. A study of healthcare providers in a very large healthcare system discovered that some providers admitted that they did not ask autistic patients about sex, drugs, and alcohol use, assuming that autistic people would not have any needs related to these topics (Zerbo et al., 2015).

Assessment Planning in Mental Health Crises

Interviews and observations are likely to provide at least the same amount of clinical information as standardized instruments, which are typically not yet normed on autistic individuals, particularly females. Interviews of individuals in the client's support system (with the client's permission; e.g., caregiver, roommate, or significant other) are also likely to yield significant data. Camouflaging may be involved at different levels—trying to fit in without recognizing the personal cost or harm or telling the interviewer what they expect to hear. Establishing a safe and secure relationship before interviewing is likely to be the best way to get past camouflaging effects in either case. It is also possible that expressive language differences (even if IQ is high) may interfere with a person's ability to say or effectively tell what they have experienced or are experiencing. Getting to know the person's interests to establish a common "language" is likely to reduce both of these barriers. As always, consider visual supports of some type (which could also be visual *media*) if needed to assist, and remember that concrete, direct approaches are likely to be easiest. Take care to not "dumb" down any of your interviewing, as that may easily backfire. Direct does not mean simple, just open and honest, with evident caring.

Anorexia Nervosa (AN) and Eating Disorders (EDs)

In addition to extensive interviewing, some questionnaires have been used for decades to identify disordered eating. They are often used in research as well as clinical work. There has been little research on eating disorder screening measures and how they perform in autistic populations, however. Measures used in research (e.g., SWEAA: Karlsson et al., 2013) are not yet validated in clinical settings. The Eating Disorder Examination-Questionnaire (EDE-Q; Fairburn & Beglin, 1994) has been used in autistic group studies to determine correlations between the EDE-Q factors and autism traits, but eating disorder screens of autistic clients should be interpreted with caution. The EDE-Q can be viewed online, but should be purchased for commercial use. Training is recommended to properly identify the appropriate version and normative comparisons. If the interview version is used, training is also needed. See Fairburn et al. (2014).

Suicidality, Non-suicidal Self-Injury (NSSI), and Self-Injurious Behavior (SIB)

Jager-Hyman et al. (2020) surveyed clinician perceptions surrounding the assessment of autistic individuals for suicide risk. Clinicians were not as confident in their ability to screen effectively and did not perceive that as many of their autistic clients were suicidal. This perception stands in contrast to the evidence of much higher risk for autistic clients than the general population. This lower rating of self-efficacy is likely related to the lack of measures shown to be valid for autistic clients. It also points to the need for measures validated in autistic populations.

Systematic reviews of the literature for suicide measures used specifically with autistic populations were conducted in 2018 (Cassidy et al., 2018a) and 2020 (Howe et al., 2020), resulting in *no studies that met this criteria*. Subsequently, five measures were identified as being commonly used to assess suicidality in the general population, but their use in autistic populations has not yet been studied:

- Suicide Behavior Questionnaire-Revised (SBQ-R: Osman et al., 2001).
- Beck Scale for Suicidal Ideations (BSS: Beck, 1991).
- Columbia Suicide Severity Rating Scale Clinician Version (C-SSRS: Posner et al., 2008).
- Self-Injurious Thoughts and Behaviors Interview (SITBI: Nock et al., 2007).
- Suicidal Ideation Questionnaire-Junior (SIQ-JR: Reynolds & Mazza, 1999).

These measures were found to have mixed results regarding effectiveness in general populations, but also some promising results across studies. All but the BSS were found to have weak cross-cultural validity, with the BSS showing only moderate cross-cultural application (Cassidy et al., 2018a). Howe et al. (2020) updated the 2018 research for children and youth and found similar results. In addition to the findings for adults, the Suicidal Ideation Thoughts and Behaviors Interview (SITBI: Nock et al., 2007) was used in two or more studies, although Cassidy et al. (2018a) found the SITBI to have weaker evidence for effectiveness in the general population. A revised version of the SITBI, the SITBI-R, has had preliminary validity established in relatively small samples, including online administration instead of interview, with good results, with many sections comparable to the C-SSRS (Fox et al., 2020). The SITBI-R, SITBI, and C-SSRS can be viewed online.

One advantage of validation studies in the general population is that females are represented at parity or above. There is still the issue of asking the same questions in the same manner across neurotypical and autistic populations and not having any evidence yet about how autistic individuals might interpret questions differently and how that might change their responses. The danger of this unknown effect is that autism may interfere with care if their suicidality is actually higher than indicated by their responses compared to typical peers. On the other hand is the possibility that a well-thought-out plan may or may not reflect imminent suicidal behaviors, so criteria for hospitalization may need to be individualized to the person. In the systematic reviews, conclusions are that none of the measures effectively predict suicide and none were evaluated in autistic populations (Cassidy et al., 2018a; Howe et al., 2020), so interpret all results with caution, realizing the risk of differences in responses for autistic clients. More care and time are likely to be necessary for clinicians to learn enough about a client to know if they are asking questions in a way that will produce an accurate measure of suicidality. The SBQ has been specifically adapted for autistic populations, but has been studied in research settings only (SBQ-ASC; Cassidy et al., 2021). Results have been promising, so it may be useful in the future. *See* https://sites.google.com/view/mentalhealthinautism/resources/tools, *University of Nottingham, UK.*

Howe et al. (2020) recommended the following approaches in the absence of autism-adapted measures when assessing for suicidal ideation in autistic children and adolescents:

- Gather both self-report and parent/caregiver report measures.
- Use multiple sources of data and reporting.
- Present questions clearly and concisely with limited use of abstract, hypothetical, or ambiguous language (e.g., "What is the likelihood that you will have thoughts of suicide again in the future?", p. 3473).
- Gather information on restrictive and repetitive behaviors and interests to differentiate suicidal ideation from a special interest in death and/or violence (Howe et al., 2020).

Non-suicidal self-injury measures have also not been validated in autism studies. Some measures that have been validated in the general populations may be useful as part of a clinical assessment, but should not be relied on without extensive data collected from interviews. One measure that has been used in some autism research studies is the Non-Suicidal Self-Injury Assessment Tool (NSSI-AT: Whitlock & Purington, 2013). Conclusions drawn from these studies characterized self-injury as something that may be regarded as positive or neutral by autistic individuals, as NSSI is described by some as a preferred method of reducing suicidal thoughts. Associations of NSSI with suicidal thoughts and behaviors may look different across populations, and there is no proof of causative relationships. NSSI is a significant physical and mental health concern, however (Mosely et al., 2020).

Supports and Recommendations

Cassidy et al. (2018b) explored risk factors for suicidal thoughts and behaviors by interviewing autistic adults. Risk factors unique to this group were camouflaging and unmet support needs. Other risk markers shared with the general population were non-suicidal self-injury, employment issues, and mental health problems. Because these shared factors are more prevalent in the autistic community, they are also important areas for suicide prevention.

Safety Planning Intervention

At the time of writing, large studies of safety planning interventions in autistic populations (SPI-ASD) are being conducted in the United Kingdom (Rodgers et al., 2021) as well as four health systems in the United States (Maddox & Jager-Hyman,

2021). Safety planning interventions (SPI: Stanley & Brown, 2012) and SPI plus follow-up (Stanley et al., 2016, 2018) have been shown to be acceptable and improve engagement in treatment. In a meta-analysis of SPI, Nuij et al. (2021) found that SPI had positive effect, reducing suicidal behaviors, but not necessarily on suicidal ideation. See https://suicidesafetyplan.com/ for details on SPI.

Resources for Crisis Workers

Autistica, an advocacy and support organization in the United Kingdom, has made available an evidence-based guide for crisis workers working with autistic children and young people that can be viewed at https://www.autistica.org.uk/downloads/files/Crisis-resource-2020.pdf. An important note at the beginning of this guide is that not all autistic individuals know about their diagnosis or they may not be able to disclose their diagnosis in crisis, making it critical that crisis workers have enough awareness of autism characteristics to be able to individualize supports (Hughes et al., 2020). Detailed information about how to work with autistic clients is given. Tips for making initial contact, working with parents, alternative communication styles, and creating a positive experience and actions plans are given.

More autism-specific suicide resources, including toolkits, are also available through the American Association of Suicidology https://suicidology.org/resources/autism-resources/.

"Understanding autism and the culture of autistic people, so autistic people do not have to mask/camouflage their autism, is suicide prevention." - Lisa Morgan (2021)

Intensive and Individually Tailored Interventions

Westwood and Tchanturia (2017) reviewed recent studies of AN and autism, concluding that there is still a lot of difficulty in efforts to separate autism traits from AN, but that there is consistently a connection between the traits within individuals. When autism traits are present in AN, more intensive treatment is likely to be required, and intervention techniques will need to be specifically tailored to the individual, suggesting a longer treatment process may be necessary. Female-specific diagnostic tools for autism were one of the recommendations to improve outcomes for autistic females with AN.

Autism Traits May Be Maintaining Factors to Consider in Treatment Approaches

In one study, characteristics common in autism were not shown to affect the outcome of inpatient treatment, but individuals with autistic traits had more severe symptoms of eating disorder and depression and more difficulty with work and social functioning (Tchanturia et al., 2019). In their 2013 study, Tchanturia et al. hypothesized that autistic traits, when present, may be the maintaining factors for eating disorders, naming cognitive rigidity, low mood, and low social motivation or lack of conventional social skills as traits that exacerbate eating disorders, but are not necessarily the cause of disordered eating. This suggests that treatment approaches need to take these traits into consideration regardless of the diagnostic status of the patient regarding autism.

Importance of Support Network to Reduce Stigma

Family and friends are noted to be a strong source of support for mental health. Perceptions of stigma associated with both mental health issues and autism were reported by autistic adults as barriers to supports (Crane et al., 2019).

Sex Education and Consent

> *"Remember that dating will often turn into something interpersonal, so don't underestimate the importance of sex education. Research and read up on sex and intimacy, sexually transmitted diseases, birth control, the urban myths surrounding all the above, and the importance of knowing 'no means no'."* (Willey, 2012, p. 44)

The Organization for Autism Research (OAR) has been proactive for several years to promote sex education for autistic people (2018). Their work is typically featured on their website https://researchautism.org/sexuality-on-the-spectrum/. There are resources, short modules, and podcasts available, featuring Amy Gravino and Peter Gerhardt. Liane Holliday Willey has also specifically addressed issues of sex education and consent. See Willey, L. H. (2012). *Safety skills for Asperger women: How to save a perfectly good female life*. Jessica Kingsley Publishers. See also Debi Brown (2013) *The Aspie Girl's Guide to Being Safe With Men: The Unwritten Safety Rules No-one is Telling You*. Jessica Kingsley Publications. See Table 10.1 for assessment strategies related to mental health issues and crises.

Table 10.1 At-a-Glance Summary for Female Eating Disorders, Self-Injury, Suicide, Sexual Victimization and Substance Abuse

Domain	Focus	Assessment choices and age ranges
Suicidal thoughts and behaviors	Suicidal ideation severity and frequency, stressors, activity levels, support systems From Howe et al. (2020): Gather self-report and parent/caregiver report measures Use multiple sources of data and reporting Present questions clearly and concisely with limited use of abstract, hypothetical, or ambiguous language Gather information on restrictive and repetitive behaviors and interests to differentiate suicidal ideation from a special interest in death and/or violence	**Interpret results with caution; these are commonly used measures, but not validated on autism populations** *Columbia Suicide Severity Rating Scale Clinician Version* **(C-SSRS)**: 11–adult (Posner et al., 2008) *Suicide Behavior Questionnaire-Revised* **(SBQ-R)**: adult (Osman et al., 2001) *Suicide Behavior Questionnaire- Autism Spectrum Condition* **(SBQ-ASC) not yet validated in clinical settings** (Cassidy et al., 2021)
Feeding/eating disorders	Feeding behaviors in early childhood	**History from parent interview**
	Sensory aspects of food and eating	**Client interview** (also see Sensory profile below)
	Nutritional history and analysis	**Healthcare provider individualized tests**
	Underlying mechanisms and types of disordered eating *Not yet validated in autistic populations; interpret results with caution*	*Eating Disorder Examination—Questionnaire* **(EDE-Q) 14+ or EDE** interview (Fairburn et al., 2014) *Training in the EDE-Q is recommended, as there are multiple versions, different community norms, and differences in performance in adolescent populations*
Sensory sensitivity	Sensory interests are reported in most first-person reports, but look for intensity of sensory interests more than the type of interest, which may be mainstream (touch, sound, smell, etc.)	*Sensory Profile 2* (SP2) **SP2 Infant Toddler: 7–35 mos.** **SP2 Child: 3:0–14:11** **SP2 School: 3:0–14:11** **SP2 Short: 3:0–14:11** *Spanish avail.* (Dunn, 2014)

(continued)

Table 10.1 (continued)

Domain	Focus	Assessment choices and age ranges
Compulsions or restrictive and repetitive behaviors	Gather information on special and intense interests; if they relate to eating, suicidal thoughts and behaviors, and self-injury, including rituals associated with OCD traits, further assess for the degree of impact on healthy habits and daily living to better differentiate harmful behaviors from intense interests	**Interviews** with client and caregivers
Self-injury	Interview with straightforward questions	See above explanation of **SITBI** and **SITBI-R** and **NSSI-AT** in this chapter (Cassidy et al., 2018a)
Substance abuse	Interview with straightforward questions. Do not assume that the person would not be involved in substance abuse because they are autistic	*Mini-International Neuropsychiatric Interview-Adult* **(MINI)** (Sheehan et al., 1998) **(MINI-Kids)**: ages 6–17:11 (Sheehan et al., 2010) *Use Version 7.0.2 or later for DSM-5*
Sexual Assault	Interview with straight-forward questions. Do not assume that the person would not be involved in sexual activity because they are autistic	Explore understanding of consent. Changes in behavior are the most likely indicator, but also listen for how interactions with adults and peers are described and changes in the frequency of talk about individuals. Vocabulary differences may be a barrier to clinician awareness, so probing with different questions and taking multiple opportunities for talking about it may be needed
Multiple conditions (all of the above)	Questionnaire to consider at intake	*Child and Adolescent Symptom Inventory, Fifth Ed.* **(CASI-5R)**: 5–18 years (Gadow & Sprafkin, 2013)

Please see the "References" section in this chapter for additional information on measures.
Not all measures and processes listed are available in all settings or appropriate for all cases. Qualification levels apply. Multiple measures in a single domain are not necessary. Some measures can provide data in multiple domains. This is meant to provide a relatively quick reference for assessment planning and implementation, not an endorsement of any particular measure as "best." See above for details. Emphasis here is on readily available, commonly used measures, but similar measures may also be useful

References

Arwert, T. G., & Sizoo, B. B. (2020). Self-reported suicidality in male and female adults with autism spectrum disorders: Rumination and self-esteem. *Journal of Autism and Developmental Disorders, 50*(10), 3598–3605. https://doi.org/10.1007/s10803-020-04372-z

Ballou, E. P., daVanport, S., & Onaiwu, M. G. (Eds.). (2021). *Sincerely, your autistic child.* Beacon Press.

Beck, A. T. (1991). *The Beck Scale for Suicidal Ideation.* Pearson.

Brede, J., Babb, C., Jones, C., Elliott, M., Zanker, C., Tchanturia, K., Serpell, L., Fox, J., & Mandy, W. (2020). "For me, the anorexia is just a symptom, and the cause is the autism": Investigating restrictive eating disorders in autistic women. *Journal of Autism and Developmental Disorders, 50*(12), 4280–4296. https://doi.org/10.1007/s10803-020-04479-3

Brown, D. (2013) *The Aspie girl's guide to being safe with men: The unwritten safety rules no-one is telling you.* Jessica Kingsley Publications.

Brown, C. M., & Stokes, M. A. (2020). Intersection of eating disorders and the female profile of autism. *The Psychiatric Clinics of North America, 43*(4), 735–743. https://doi.org/10.1016/j.psc.2020.08.009

Butwicka, A., Långström, N., Larsson, H., Lundström, S., Serlachius, E., Almqvist, C., Frisén, L., & Lichtenstein, P. (2017). Increased risk for substance use-related problems in autism spectrum disorders: A population-based cohort study. *Journal of Autism and Developmental Disorders, 47*(1), 80–89. https://doi.org/10.1007/s10803-016-2914-2

Cassidy, S., Bradley, P., Robinson, J., Allison, C., McHugh, M., & Baron-Cohen, S. (2014). Suicidal ideation and suicide plans or attempts in adults with Asperger's syndrome attending a specialist diagnostic clinic: A clinical cohort study. *The Lancet Psychiatry, 1*(2), 142–147. https://doi.org/10.1016/S2215-0366(14)70248-2

Cassidy, S. A., Bradley, L., Bowen, E., Wigham, S., & Rodgers, J. (2018a). Measurement properties of tools used to assess suicidality in autistic and general population adults: A systematic review. *Clinical Psychology Review, 62*, 56–70. https://doi.org/10.1016/j.cpr.2018.05.002

Cassidy, S., Bradley, L., Shaw, R., & Baron-Cohen, S. (2018b). Risk markers for suicidality in autistic adults. *Molecular Autism, 9*(1), 42. https://doi.org/10.1186/s13229-018-0226-4

Cassidy, S. A., Gould, K., Townsend, E., Pelton, M., Robertson, A. E., & Rodgers, J. (2020). Is camouflaging autistic traits associated with suicidal thoughts and behaviours? Expanding the interpersonal psychological theory of suicide in an undergraduate student sample. *Journal of Autism and Developmental Disorders, 50*(10), 3638–3648. https://doi.org/10.1007/s10803-019-04323-3

Cassidy, S. A., Bradley, L., Cogger-Ward, H., & Rodgers, J. (2021). Development and validation of the suicidal behaviours questionnaire—Autism spectrum conditions in a community sample of autistic, possibly autistic and non-autistic adults. *Molecular Autism, 12*(1), 1–22. https://doi.org/10.1186/s13229-021-00449-3

Cazalis, F., Reyes, E., Leduc, S., & Gourion, D. (2022). Evidence that nine autistic women out of ten have been victims of sexual violence. *Frontiers in Behavioral Neuroscience, 16.* https://www.frontiersin.org/articles/10.3389/fnbeh.2022.852203

Chen, M. H., Pan, T. L., Lan, W. H., Hsu, J. W., Huang, K. L., Su, T. P., Li, C. T., Lin, W. C., Wei, H. T., Chen, T. J., & Bai, Y. M. (2017). Risk of suicide attempts among adolescents and young adults with autism spectrum disorder: A nationwide longitudinal follow-up study. *The Journal of Clinical Psychiatry, 78*(9), e1174–e1179. https://doi.org/10.4088/JCP.16m11100

Cook, B., & Garnett, M. (Eds.). (2018). *Spectrum women: Walking to the beat of autism.* Jessica Kingsley.

Corbett, B. A., Vandekar, S., Muscatello, R. A., & Tanguturi, Y. (2020). Pubertal timing during early adolescence: Advanced pubertal onset in females with autism spectrum disorder. *Autism Research, 13*(12), 2202–2215. https://doi.org/10.1002/aur.2406

Crane, L., Adams, F., Harper, G., Welch, J., & Pellicano, E. (2019). 'Something needs to change': Mental health experiences of young autistic adults in England. *Autism, 23*(2), 477–493. https://doi.org/10.1177/1362361318757048

Dunn, W. (2014). *Sensory Profile 2*. Pearson.

Esbensen, A. J., Seltzer, M. M., & Lam, K. S. L. (2009). Age-related differences in restricted repetitive behaviors in autism spectrum disorders. *Journal of Autism and Developmental Disorders, 39*(1), 57–66. https://doi.org/10.1007/s10803-008-0599-x

Fairburn, C. G., & Beglin, S. J. (1994). Assessment of eating disorders: Interview or self-report questionnaire? *The International Journal of Eating Disorders, 16*(4), 363–370. https://doi.org/10.1002/1098-108X(199412)16:4<363::AID-EAT2260160405>3.0.CO;2-%23

Fairburn, C., Cooper, Z., & O'Conner, M. (2014). *Eating Disorder Examination*. Edition 17.0D. https://www.corc.uk.net/media/1951/ede_170d.pdf

Fox, K. R., Harris, J. A., Wang, S. B., Millner, A. J., Deming, C. A., & Nock, M. K. (2020). Self-injurious thoughts and behaviors interview-revised: Development, reliability, and validity. *Psychological Assessment, 32*(7), 677–689. https://doi.org/10.1037/pas0000819

Gadow, K. D., & Sprafkin, J. (2013). *Child and Adolescent Symptom Inventory-5*. Checkmate Plus. https://www.checkmateplus.com/casi-5

Gillberg, C. (1983). Are autism and anorexia nervosa related? *The British Journal of Psychiatry, 142*(4), 428. https://doi.org/10.1192/bjp.142.4.428b

Godart, N. T., Flament, M. F., Lecrubier, Y., & Jeammet, P. (2000). Anxiety disorders in anorexia nervosa and bulimia nervosa: Comorbidity and chronology of appearance. *European Psychiatry, 15*, 38–45. https://doi.org/10.1016/s0924-9338(00)00212-1

Gotby, V. O., Lichtenstein, P., Långström, N., & Pettersson, E. (2018). Childhood neurodevelopmental disorders and risk of coercive sexual victimization in childhood and adolescence—A population-based prospective twin study. *Journal of Child Psychology and Psychiatry, 59*, 957–965. https://doi.org/10.1111/jcpp.12884

Gravino, A. (2021, April 22). *I now know what caused my autism, which changes everything—And nothing*. CNN Opinion. https://www.cnn.com/2021/04/21/opinions/my-autism-cause-changes-everything-and-nothing-gravino/index.html

Hendrickx, S. (2015). *Women and girls with autism spectrum disorder: Understanding life experiences from early childhood to old age*. Jessica Kingsley Publishers.

Hirvikoski, T., Mittendorfer-Rutz, E., Boman, M., Larsson, H., Lichtenstein, P., & Bolte, S. (2016). Premature mortality in autism spectrum disorder. *British Journal of Psychiatry, 208*, 232–238. https://doi.org/10.1192/bjp.bp.114.160192

Howe, S. J., Hewitt, K., Baraskewich, J., Cassidy, S., & McMorris, C. A. (2020). Suicidality among children and youth with and without autism spectrum disorder: A systematic review of existing risk assessment tools. *Journal of Autism and Developmental Disorders, 50*(10), 3462–3476. https://doi.org/10.1007/s10803-020-04394-7

Huang, J., Yang, F., Chien, W., Yeh, T., Chung, C., Tsai, C., Tsai, S., Yang, S., Tzeng, N., Shen, M., & Liang, C. (2021). Risk of substance use disorder and its associations with comorbidities and psychotropic agents in patients with autism. *JAMA Pediatrics, 175*(2), e205371. https://doi.org/10.1001/jamapediatrics.2020.5371

Hughes, C., Davies, B., Cassidy, S., Rodgers, J., Kyriakopoulos, M., & Spain, D. (2020). Supporting autistic children and young people through crisis—An Autistica evidence resource on suicide for crisis workers. *AMRC Open Research, 2*(30). https://doi.org/10.21955/amrcopenres.1114928.1

Jacobson, C. M., & Gould, M. (2007). The epidemiology and phenomenology of non-suicidal self-injurious behavior among adolescents: A critical review of the literature. *Archives of Suicide Research, 11*(2), 129–147. https://doi.org/10.1080/13811110701247602

Jager-Hyman, S., Maddox, B. B., Crabbe, S. R., & Mandell, D. S. (2020). Mental health clinicians' screening and intervention practices to reduce suicide risk in autistic adolescents and adults. *Journal of Autism and Developmental Disorders, 50*(10), 3450–3461. https://doi.org/10.1007/s10803-020-04441-3

Joiner, T. E., Van Orden, K. A., Witte, T. K., & Rudd, M. D. (2009). *The interpersonal theory of suicide: Guidance for working with suicidal clients*. American Psychological Association.

Karjalainen, L., Råstam, M., Paulson-Karlsson, G., & Wentz, E. (2019). Do autism spectrum disorder and anorexia nervosa have some eating disturbances in common? *European Child & Adolescent Psychiatry, 28*(1), 69–78. https://doi.org/10.1007/s00787-018-1188-y

Karlsson, L., Råstam, M., & Wentz, E. (2013). The Swedish Eating Assessment for Autism spectrum disorders (SWEAA)—Validation of a self-report questionnaire targeting eating disturbances within the autism spectrum. *Research in Developmental Disabilities, 34*(7), 2224–2233. https://doi.org/10.1016/j.ridd.2013.03.035

Kato, K., Mikami, K., Akama, F., Yamada, K., Maehara, M., Kimoto, K., Kimoto, K., Sato, R., Takahashi, Y., Fukushima, R., Ichimura, A., & Matsumoto, H. (2013). Clinical features of suicide attempts in adults with autism spectrum disorders. *General Hospital Psychiatry, 35*(1), 50–53. https://doi.org/10.1016/j.genhosppsych.2012.09.006

Kerr-Gaffney, J., Hayward, H., Jones, E. J. H., Halls, D., Murphy, D., & Tchanturia, K. (2021). Autism symptoms in anorexia nervosa: A comparative study with females with autism spectrum disorder. *Molecular Autism, 12*(1), 47. https://doi.org/10.1186/s13229-021-00455-5

Kirby, A. V., Bakian, A. V., Zhang, Y., Bilder, D. A., Keeshin, B. R., & Coon, H. (2019). A 20-year study of suicide death in a statewide autism population. *Autism Research, 12*(4), 658–666. https://doi.org/10.1002/aur.2076

Koch, S. V., Larsen, J. T., Mouridsen, S. E., Bentz, M., Petersen, L., Bulik, C., Mortensen, P. B., & Plessen, K. J. (2015). Autism spectrum disorder in individuals with anorexia nervosa and in their first- and second-degree relatives: Danish nationwide register-based cohort-study. *The British Journal of Psychiatry, 206*(5), 401–407. https://doi.org/10.1192/bjp.bp.114.153221

Kõlves, K., Fitzgerald, C., Nordentoft, M., Wood, S. J., & Erlangsen, A. (2021). Assessment of suicidal behaviors among individuals with autism spectrum disorder in Denmark. *JAMA Network Open, 4*(1). https://doi.org/10.1001/jamanetworkopen.2020.33565

Lecavalier, L. (2006). Behavioral and emotional problems in young people with pervasive developmental disorders: Relative prevalence, effects of subject characteristics, and empirical classification. *Journal of Autism and Developmental Disorders, 36*(8), 1101–1114. https://doi.org/10.1007/s10803-006-0147-5

Lugo-Marín, J., Magán-Maganto, M., Rivero-Santana, A., Cuellar-Pompa, L., Alviani, M., Jenaro-Rio, C., Díez, E., & Canal-Bedia, R. (2019). Prevalence of psychiatric disorders in adults with autism spectrum disorder: A systematic review and meta-analysis. *Research in Autism Spectrum Disorders, 59*, 22–33. https://doi.org/10.1016/j.rasd.2018.12.004

Maddox, B. B., & Jager-Hyman, S. (2021). *A comparison of two brief suicide prevention interventions tailored to youth on the autism spectrum [Study]*. https://www.pcori.org/research-results/2021/comparison-two-brief-suicide-prevention-interventions-tailored-youth-autism-spectrum

Maddox, B. B., & White, S. W. (2013, November 22). Perspectives on repetitive behavior in ASD: Core, secondary, or something else? In *Repetitive behaviors across the disorders: A transdiagnostic framework*. Symposium presented at the meeting of the Association for Behavioral and Cognitive Therapies (chair Richey, JA), Nashville, TN.

Maddox, B. B., Trubanova, A., & White, S. W. (2017). Untended wounds: Non-suicidal self-injury in adults with autism spectrum disorder. *Autism, 21*(4), 412–422. https://doi.org/10.1177/1362361316644731

McClintock, K., Hall, S., & Oliver, C. (2003). Risk markers associated with challenging behaviours in people with intellectual disabilities: A meta-analytic study. *Journal of Intellectual Disability Research, 47*(6), 405–416. https://doi.org/10.1046/j.1365-2788.2003.00517.x

Miller, J. K. (Ed.). (2015). *Women from another planet? Our lives in the universe of autism.* Author House.

Morgan, L. (2021). *Warning signs of suicide and crisis supports for autistic people AUCD webinar series [powerpoint slides]*, April 28, 2022. https://www.aucd.org/docs/webinars/4.28%20Webinar%20Slides.pdf

Moseley, R. L., Gregory, N. J., Smith, P., & Baron-Cohen, S. (2020). Links between self-injury and suicidality in autism. *Molecular Autism, 11*(14). https://doi.org/10.1186/s13229-020-0319-8

Nebeker, L. (Guest) (2019). *It's different for girls: A conversation with four women on the spectrum (No. 5) in Inspiring Change Podcast [audio podcast recording from OCALICON 2019]*. https://www.ocali.org/project/inspiring-change-podcast#ep5

Nielsen, S., Anckarsäter, H., Gillberg, C., Gillberg, C., Råstam, R., & Wentz, E. (2015). Effects of autism spectrum disorders on outcome in teenage-onset anorexia nervosa evaluated by the Morgan-Russell outcome assessment schedule: A controlled community-based study. *Molecular Autism, 6*, 14. https://doi.org/10.1186/s13229-015-0013-4

Nisticò, V., Faggioli, R., Tedesco, R., Giordano, B., Priori, A., Gambini, O., & Demartini, B. (2022). Brief report: Sensory sensitivity is associated with disturbed eating in adults with autism spectrum disorders without intellectual disabilities. *Journal of Autism and Developmental Disorders*. https://doi.org/10.1007/s10803-022-05439-9

Nock, M. K., Holmberg, E. B., Photos, V. I., & Michel, B. D. (2007). Self-injurious thoughts and behaviors interview: Development, reliability, and validity in an adolescent sample. *Psychological Assessment, 19*(3), 309–317. https://doi.org/10.1037/1040-3590.19.3.309

Nuij, C., van Ballegooijen, W., de Beurs, D., Juniar, D., Erlangsen, A., Portzky, G., et al. (2021). Safety planning-type interventions for suicide prevention: Meta-analysis. *The British Journal of Psychiatry, 219*(2), 419–426. https://doi.org/10.1192/bjp.2021.5

Numata, N., Nakagawa, A., Yoshioka, K., Isomura, K., Matsuzawa, D., Setsu, R., Nakazato, M., & Shimizu, E. (2021). Associations between autism spectrum disorder and eating disorders with and without self-induced vomiting: An empirical study. *Journal of Eating Disorders, 9*(1), 1–9. https://doi.org/10.1186/s40337-020-00359-4

O'Toole, J. C. (2018). *Autism in heels: The untold story of a female life on the spectrum*. Skyhorse Publishing.

Oldershaw, A., Treasure, J., Hambrook, D., Tchanturia, K., & Schmidt, U. (2011). Is anorexia nervosa a version of autism spectrum disorders? *European Eating Disorders Review, 19*(6), 462–474. https://doi.org/10.1002/erv.1069

Organization for Autism Research. (2018). *Sexuality on the spectrum*. https://researchautism.org/sexuality-on-the-spectrum/

Osman, A., Bagge, C. L., Gutierrez, P. M., Konick, L. C., Kopper, B. A., & Barrios, F. X. (2001). The Suicidal Behaviors Questionnaire-Revised (SBQ-R): Validation with clinical and nonclinical samples. *Assessment, 8*(4), 443–454. https://doi.org/10.1177/107319110100800409

Posner, K., Brent, D., Lucas, C., Gould, M., Stanley, B., Brown, G., Fisher, P., Zelazny, J., Burke, A., Oquendo, M., & Mann, J. (2008). *The Columbia Suicide Severity Rating Scales*. The Research Foundation for Mental Hygiene, Inc.

Råstam, M. (1992). Anorexia nervosa in 51 Swedish adolescents: Premorbid problems and comorbidity. *Journal of the American Academy of Child and Adolescent Psychiatry, 31*(5), 819–829. https://doi.org/10.1097/00004583-199209000-00007

Raymaker, D. M., Teo, A. R., Steckler, N. A., Lentz, B., Scharer, M., Delos Santos, A., Kapp, S. K., Hunter, M., Joyce, A., & Nicolaidis, C. (2020). "Having all of your internal resources exhausted beyond measure and being left with no clean-up crew": Defining autistic burnout. *Autism in Adulthood, 2*(2), 132–143. https://doi.org/10.1089/aut.2019.0079

Reynolds, W. M., & Mazza, J. J. (1999). Assessment of suicidal ideation in inner-city children and young adolescents: Reliability and validity of the Suicidal Ideation Questionnaire-JR. *School Psychology Review, 28*(1), 17–30. https://doi.org/10.1080/02796015.1999.12085945

Rodgers, J., Cassidy, S., Heslop, P., Kassim, A., O'Connor, R., Ramsay, S., Townsend, L., & Vale, L. (2021). *Autism adapted safety plans*. https://sites.google.com/nihr.ac.uk/safetyplanstudy/home

Segers, M., & Rawana, J. (2014). What do we know about suicidality in autism spectrum disorders? A systematic review. *Autism Research, 7*(4), 507–521. https://doi.org/10.1002/aur.1375

Sharp, W. G., Berry, R. C., McCracken, C., Nuhu, N. N., Marvel, E., Saulnier, C. A., Klin, A., Jones, W., & Jaquess, D. L. (2013). Feeding problems and nutrient intake in children with autism Spectrum disorders: A meta-analysis and comprehensive review of the literature. *Journal of Autism and Developmental Disorders, 43*, 2159–2173. https://doi.org/10.1007/s10803-013-1771-5

Sheehan, D. V., Lecrubier, Y., Harnett-Sheehan, K., Amorim, P., Janavs, J., Weiller, E., Hergueta, T., Baker, R., & Dunbar, G. (1998). The Mini International Neuropsychiatric Interview (M.I.N.I.): The development and validation of a structured diagnostic psychiatric interview. *The Journal of Clinical Psychiatry, 59*(suppl 20), 22–33. http://www.psychiatrist.com/JCP/article/Pages/1998/v59s20/v59s2005.aspx

Sheehan, D. V., Sheehan, K. H., Shytle, R. D., Janavs, J., Bannon, Y., Rogers, J. E., Milo, K. M., Stock, S. L., & Wilkinson, B. (2010). Reliability and validity of the Mini International Neuropsychiatric Interview for children and adolescents (MINI–KID). *The Journal of Clinical Psychiatry, 71*(3), 313–326. https://doi.org/10.4088/JCP.09m05305whi

Simone, R. (2010). *Aspergirls: Empowering females with Asperger syndrome*. Jessica Kingsley.

Skoog, T., & Özdemir, S. B. (2016). Explaining why early-maturing girls are more exposed to sexual harassment in early adolescence. *Journal of Early Adolescence, 36*, 490–509. https://doi.org/10.1177/0272431614568198

South, M., Beck, J. S., Lundwall, R., Christensen, M., Cutrer, E. A., Gabrielsen, T. P., Cox, J. C., & Lundwall, R. A. (2020). Unrelenting depression and suicidality in women with autistic traits. *Journal of Autism and Developmental Disorders, 50*(10), 3606–3619. https://doi.org/10.1007/s10803-019-04324-2

South, M., Costa, A. P., & McMorris, C. (2021). Death by suicide among people with autism: Beyond zebrafish. *JAMA Network Open, 4*(1). https://doi.org/10.1001/jamanetworkopen.2020.34018

Spek, A. A., van Rijnsoever, W., van Laarhoven, L., & Kiep, M. (2020). Eating problems in men and women with an autism spectrum disorder. *Journal of Autism and Developmental Disorders, 50*(5), 1748–1755. https://doi.org/10.1007/s10803-019-03931-3

Stanley, B. S., & Brown, G. K. (2012). Safety planning intervention: A brief intervention to mitigate suicide risk. *Cognitive and Behavioral Practice, 2012*(19), 256–264. https://doi.org/10.1016/j.cbpra.2011.01.001

Stanley, B. S., Chaudhury, S. R., Chesin, M., Pontoski, K. P., Bush, A. M., Knox, K. L., & Brown, G. K. (2016). An emergency department intervention and follow-up to reduce suicide risk in the VA: Acceptability and effectiveness. *Psychiatric Services, 67*, 680–683. https://doi.org/10.1176/appi.ps.201500082

Stanley, B. S., Brown, G. K., Brenner, L. A., Hanga, G. C., Currier, G. W., & Knox, K. (2018). Comparison of the safety planning intervention with follow-up vs usual care of suicidal patients treated in the emergency department. *JAMA Psychiatry, 75*, 894–900. https://doi.org/10.1001/jamapsychiatry.2018.1776

Strang, J. F., Anthony, L. G., Song, A., Lai, M.-C., Knauss, M., Sadikova, E., Graham, E., Zaks, Z., Wimms, H., Willing, L., Call, D., Mancilla, M., Shakin, S., Vilain, E., Kim, D.-Y., Maisashvili, T., Khawaja, A., & Kenworthy, L. (2021). In addition to stigma: Cognitive and autism-related predictors of mental health in transgender adolescents. *Journal of Clinical Child & Adolescent Psychology, 52*(2), 212–229. https://doi.org/10.1080/15374416.2021.1916940

Strauss, P., Cook, A., Watson, V., Winter, S., Whitehouse, A., Albrecht, N., Wright Toussaint, D., & Lin, A. (2021). Mental health difficulties among trans and gender diverse young people with an autism spectrum disorder (ASD): Findings from trans pathways. *Journal of Psychiatric Research, 137*, 360–367. https://doi.org/10.1016/j.jpsychires.2021.03.005

Tchanturia, K., Smith, E., Weineck, F., Fidanboylu, E., Kern, N., Treasure, J., & Baron-Cohen, S. (2013). Exploring autistic traits in anorexia: A clinical study. *Molecular Autism, 4*, 44. https://doi.org/10.1186/2040-2392-4-44

Tchanturia, K., Adamson, J., Leppanen, J., & Westwood, H. (2019). Characteristics of autism spectrum disorder in anorexia nervosa: A naturalistic study in an inpatient treatment programme. *Autism: The International Journal of Research and Practice, 23*(1), 123–130. https://doi.org/10.1177/1362361317722431

Weiss, J. A., & Fardella, M. A. (2018). Victimization and perpetration experiences of adults with autism. *Frontiers in Psychiatry, 9*, 203. https://doi.org/10.3389/fpsyt.2018.00203

Wentz, E., Lacey, J. H., Waller, G., Råstam, M., Turk, J., & Gillberg, C. (2005). Childhood onset neuropsychiatric disorders in adult eating disorder patients: A pilot study. *European Child & Adolescent Psychiatry, 14*, 431–437. https://doi.org/10.1007/s00787-005-0494-3

Westwood, H., & Tchanturia, K. (2017). Autism spectrum disorder in anorexia nervosa: An updated literature review. *Current Psychiatry Reports, 19*(7), 41. https://doi.org/10.1007/s11920-017-0791-9

Whitlock, J., & Purington, A. (2013). *Assessment of Nonsuicidal Self Injury Assessment Tool.* The Cornell Research Program on Self-Injury and Recovery. selfinjury.bctr.cornell.edu/perch/resources/fnssi.pdf

Willey, L. H. (2012). *Safety skills for Asperger women: How to save a perfectly good female life.* Jessica Kingsley Publishers.

World Health Organization (WHO). (2021, March 9). *Violence against women [Fact sheet].* https://www.who.int/news-room/fact-sheets/detail/violence-against-women

Zerbo, O., Massolo, M. L., Qian, Y., & Croen, L. A. (2015). A study of physician knowledge and experience with autism in adults in a large integrated healthcare system. *Journal of Autism and Developmental Disorders, 45*, 4002–4014. https://doi.org/10.1007/s10803-015-2579-2

Zucker, N. L., Losh, M., Bulik, C. M., LaBar, K. S., Piven, J., & Pelphrey, K. A. (2007). Anorexia nervosa and autism spectrum disorders: Guided investigation of social cognitive endophenotypes. *Psychological Bulletin, 133*, 976–1006. https://doi.org/10.1037/0033-2909.133.6.976

Chapter 11
Autism Diagnosis in Adult Females: Post-secondary Education, Careers, and Autistic Burnout

Introduction

Another "hidden" experience that should be explored in assessment is the degree of burnout among people who appear to be highly confident and competent in their field or educational career, but who are suffering from the incessant demand and effort of trying to fit in and be accepted. In our clinical experience, people are fairly open and articulate about discussion and acknowledgement of their daily workload in impression management if asked.

> *"You need enough balloons to manage the weight of the rocks."* (Mantazalas et al., 2022, p. 52).

> *A lot of people who know me superficially express surprise that I am autistic. I don't take it as a compliment and I often want to respond with 'Do you realise how much damn hard work it is to seem this normal?' - Transgender female, diagnosed, aged 41–50 years* (Livingston et al. 2019, p. 772)

Case Study—Britta: College Graduate, Ever-Changing Schedule, Limited Break Time, and Struggles with Anxiety

Britta is a recent college graduate. She majored in psychology, which allowed her to focus time on her intense interests of exploring dynamics between others while better understanding her own brain. While she did well in her coursework, she struggled with other aspects of her college experience. When she wasn't in class, she spent most of her time in her room, headphones on. She often wore her headphones during mealtimes and walking between classes because, as she put it, it gave her "a way to avoid accidental conversations." Britta has experienced anxiety in the past, but the flexibility in her schedule allowed Britta frequent breaks from forced

T. P. Gabrielsen et al., *Assessment of Autism in Females and Nuanced Presentations*, https://doi.org/10.1007/978-3-031-33969-1_11

interaction and productivity. This helped her in managing her anxiety. Britta would eventually like to attend graduate school, but she decided it made sense to get a job (and take a break from school) while figuring out her next steps. Britta was thrilled to land her first job out of college working in another university's child development research lab, but she is struggling to keep up with expectations. Britta is required to attend weekly lab meetings and bi-weekly supervisor meetings, call families to schedule appointments, prepare materials for each research visit, and work with families to establish consent and coordinate follow-up services. Her schedule is different every day, and she doesn't even have time for a break some days. Britta would love to use her lunch time to decompress alone, but her supervisor often calls impromptu meetings during that hour to trouble-shoot scheduling issues. Britta struggles to remain flexible and "on" during every interaction with families and colleagues in an ever-changing schedule. When Britta is not working, she spends most of her time alone in her room. Her anxiety, which she was able to manage during college because of the inherent flexibility in her schedule, is starting to become unmanageable. She has received really good reviews from her supervisor, but Britta is now second-guessing her career plans.

Burnout

The term "burnout" implies not just a phenomenon, but its possible outcome. It is likely to occur on a daily basis to some extent, depending on the daily demands, but when demands increase, the burnout can escalate to become a crisis if not addressed or supported.

> *Autistic burnout is a syndrome conceptualized as resulting from chronic life stress and a mismatch of expectations and abilities without adequate supports. It is characterized by pervasive, long-term (typically 3+ months) exhaustion, loss of function, and reduced tolerance to stimulus.* (Raymaker et al., 2020)

Interviews conducted by Raymaker et al. (2020) indicated that life stressors added to the cumulative load of independent living—without access to adequate support—create a situation in which expectations outweigh abilities in autistic adults. We have also heard this referred to as "crashing." The acronym BIMS is also present in the literature, representing burnout, inertia, meltdown, and shutdown (Phung et al., 2021). Raymaker's interviewees reported health issues, reduced independent living and quality of life, and suicidal thoughts and behaviors. Contributing factors to burnout include lack of empathy from neurotypical people, the need for camouflaging/masking (Mandy, 2019), gaslighting (making the person question his or her own sense of reality), and dismissal of the problem as their fault or not a real problem (Raymaker et al., 2020).

First Person Narratives

I am so low on energy, I can't cope with anything right now. I shut down after only little stimuli. I don't know how to cook, how to clean the house, can't go to the store. . . I shut down so badly I don't dare to drive anymore (too dangerous). I don't enjoy my special interests anymore, and feel mentally stupid. (WP59) . . . Stimming is the autistic way of dealing with stress. Even a few minutes here and there in the bathroom could be of help. (WP9; Mantzalas et al., 2022, p. 59)

People who don't understand autism are seeing behaviours that they assume are mental health problems. Confusing burnout for depression, seeing meltdowns and only seeing it as inappropriate negative behaviour, not sensory overwhelm. Using restraints, drugs and ineffective therapy. (T290; Mantzalas et al., 2022, p.58)

I needed solitude and I needed to remove as much sensory stimuli as possible. It was not possible for me to talk to people or to have them around. The only exception was my brother because he spoke to me very quietly and calmly and slowly and directly so that I could clearly understand what he was saying and I did not have to spend energy interpreting or trying to understand his words. (WP93; Mantzalas et al., 2022, p. 59)

Camouflaging

The emotional toll of camouflaging (also known as masking or passing as normal) to gain social acceptance over time can be a key factor in autistic burnout. This suggests that although there are perceived benefits to camouflaging to achieve social success, the ultimate cost may be very high and may actually subvert long-term achievement (Mandy, 2019). Camouflaging behaviors have been reported in up to 70% of autistic adults (Cage & Troxell-Whitman, 2020), suggesting that autistic burnout is likely at some point for a significant majority of autistic adults in the workplace, in college, in adult relationships, or just living independently. Camouflaging is not likely a choice, but more of an obligation, not only to avoid ostracism but also to avoid attack, threats, and bullying (Mandy, 2019). Pearson and Rose (2021) also describe camouflaging as a self-protective mechanism requiring effort and energy to resolve cognitive dissonance and resulting distress. Mental health issues associated with camouflaging have also been described as a third variable, which is the lived experience of being autistic in an inhospitable environment (Mandy, 2019). For more detailed information on camouflaging, please see Chap. 5.

Compensation

Another term related to autistic adult life is compensation, defined as adaptations to show fewer autistic traits, even though underlying cognitive difficulties may still exist (i.e., not understanding the full context or subtlety of social interaction in the same way a neurotypical person might). Compensation is different from camouflaging or masking in that compensation involves generating new behaviors (more or less of a certain behavior) to meet expectations, whereas masking may be understood by some to be blending into the background, which is less effective in engaging in social interaction (masking is also something that neurotypical people may do when necessary). Compensation can be shallow (not as flexible or effective) or deep (finding an alternative route to social cognition, more flexible, enduring, and effective). The appearance generated by compensation in an adult is likely to under-estimate the perception of need for supports in educational and workplace settings (Livingston et al., 2019). See Fig. 11.1. Compensation strategies are specifically mentioned in the DSM-5-TR (APA, 2022) in the context of adult autistic women.

Mantzalas et al. (2022) scraped data from social media posts for analysis of comments about autistic burnout in adults, identifying several themes about the experience. Factors that contribute to burnout include systemic, pervasive lack of autism awareness in people who are in a position to help, discrimination and stigma, and *living with chronic or recurrent medical conditions*. Direct impacts on health and

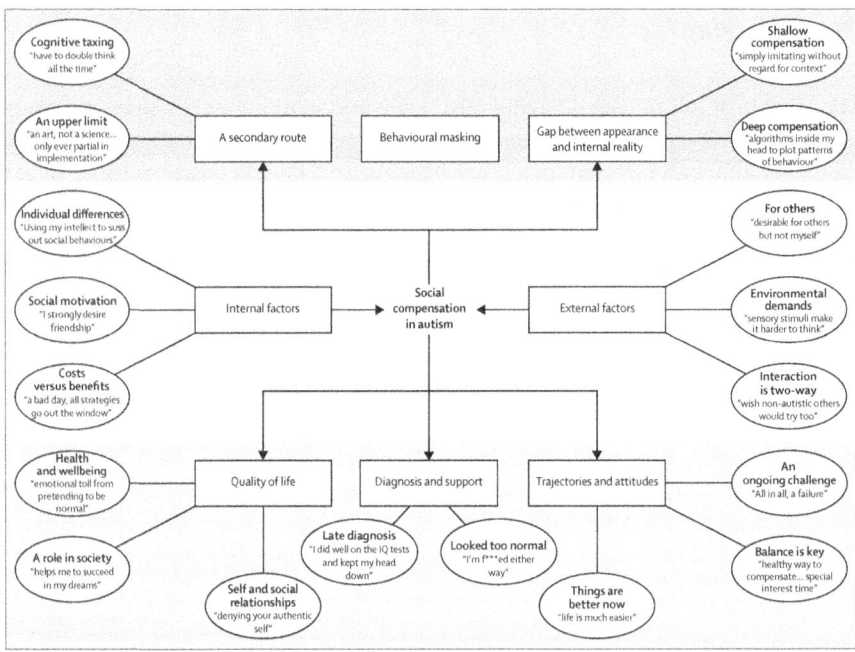

Fig. 11.1 Thematic map of the eight themes (rectangular) and 18 subthemes (oval) in social compensation in autism (Livingston et al. 2019)

well-being and feelings of a life unlived were identified. Mitigating factors were the possibility of burnout as a blessing in disguise (something that helps you to take a break or break away from a bad situation), self-awareness, and personal control. Camouflaging was specifically mentioned as a "Damned if you do, damned if you don't" proposition that is necessary and also hurtful. Ideas for support included asking the experts (autistic peers) and seeking an autistic community to strengthen each other.

Given the competitive and demanding nature of post-secondary education or training and establishing a career trajectory, the need for accommodation of autistic traits is critical, but not all college and career environments have adapted. See later sections for examples of programs taking the lead in valuing autistic students and employees by offering accommodations to increase the likelihood of success (and reducing the impact of burnout).

College/Post-secondary/University

First Person Narratives

My parents decided it was time for me to become more independent. That meant going away to college. This was traumatic to put it mildly. On the drive to the campus I had an out of body experience, I was that terrified. I crashed regularly throughout college. Reaching a state of overload, which resulted in an intense emotional meltdown, followed by extreme fatigue, was a pattern that repeated itself often. - Susan Golubuck (Miller, 2015, p. 171–172)

I was constantly on the outside, more like a satellite on friendship groups, so there was this pervasive feeling of loneliness. Naomi (Goddard & Cook, 2022, p. 2705)

I've been quite lucky to find a nice little friendship group who are all quite quiet and have anxiety issues as well and social issues, but it's quite hard to integrate with other people on the course. Rosie (Goddard & Cook, 2022, p. 2705)

My first burnout was in school. The lights, sounds, business of a full 8 hour day was too much. I was physically sick from it. T369. . . How do I survive autistic burn-out if neither my doctor, nor University, nor psychologist allow me to take the rest I need in order to function? (T231; Mantzalas et al., 2022)

I can only enjoy and fully apply myself to those things in which I have an interest. The list of such things does not include idle chitchat, trading personal information with acquaintances, or discussing clothes, hair, weight, relationships, etc. Over the course of my adult life, I have learned how to redefine many topics in order to make them interesting to me. I did this partly by nature (I home in on the little flakes of interesting-to-me material buried within what everyone else considers a different subject altogether) and partly on purpose.... School/university was a prime example. I needed to be interested in the courses I took or else I would fail them. So I would delve into the material presented until I could dig out the interesting-to-me elements. Either that or I would "re-invent" the material, interpreting it into something I could use to hold my interest. - Jane (Miller, 2015, p. 61)

Adult Transition and First Diagnosis

College students can request accommodations for disabilities in post-secondary education, but there are several caveats, the most important being that they must initiate access to services on their own, which can be problematic given social communication differences, executive function difficulties, and lack of confidence. Accessing accommodations is impossible if the person does not know about or cannot document their disability.

There is much in the college or post-secondary environment that is more difficult to navigate with autism until systems and supports are accessed. This is often the first time away from home without support and programmed education. The amount of choice and freedom is suddenly exponentially larger, but so are the challenges, including sensory intrusions, rigid expectations, and unfamiliar places, people, and environments. New routines take time to develop. Difficulty understanding the unwritten rules of how to be successful may derail an academic career. The social environment is intensified with adulthood, including sexuality, drinking, and exposure to a much broader world away from home. Even for students living at home, the executive function demands of post-secondary work can still become a formidable obstacle to success. Online options can eliminate sensory and social demands, but many other difficulties remain, including executive function challenges and pressure to meet deadlines and prepare for exams. Without familiar support systems, or in the case of someone not yet identified as autistic, the burnout or crash can be a devastating failure that is hard to recover from on your own. This unexpected failure in a highly capable person, and the associated depression and anxiety, may prompt an evaluation as parents and students seek help understanding what has happened.

The transition away from consistent executive function supports (parents) is felt by all college freshmen, but it can be a significant barrier for a neurodivergent freshman, and help is not always welcomed or perhaps stigmatized (Anderson & Butt, 2017). In some studies, the only difference found among autistic freshmen and their peers was lower social self-confidence (Baczewski et al., 2022). Perhaps the most surprising finding was that autistic students have not only more mental health needs in college but more overall physical healthcare needs, including chronic illness, which may contribute to lower graduation rates (Fernandes et al., 2021):

Careers/Workplace

First Person Narratives

> *Work is probably the single greatest challenge for women with autism due to the long-term nature of the social relationships that are developed - you have to see that same people every day - and the sheer effort of having to be somewhere, often surrounded by people* (Hendrickx, 2015, p. 213)

I was dismissed from my last job after I went through autistic burnout and disclosed my autism. They weren't willing to make the necessary accommodations: too burdensome. It's the first time I've ever been fired. T70 (Mantzalas et al., 2022, p. 57–58)

Recovered a bit, but I worry I will never be whole again. It ate part of me. (T355) . . . Autism only gives me so much energy to work with and if I overstretch myself, I'll be prone to melt-down and burnout. (T427) (Mantzalas et al., 2022, p. 57–58).

Barriers to gaining suitable employment: disruptions from moving through the transition points, anxiety, discrimination, exclusion, difficulties understanding work hierarchies, sen-sory issues, difficulties understanding "unwritten rules" and expectations which neurotypi-cal employees seem to know intuitively. Jeannette Purkis (Cook & Garnett, 2018, p. 136)

It seems like if you have a job and live alone, no-one thinks you might still need help. In my experience, you cannot access help until you reach rock bottom. I was only able to get sup-port when I had such crippling anxiety that I could not go shopping or even leave the house. If they had given me support earlier it would have been easier to get back on track again. (Baldwin & Costley, 2016, p. 491)

The world of ordinary work is often unkind to us, especially undiagnosed, unsupported Aspies. Every time we start a job, it isn't long before people, not the actual tasks, make things complicated. If work was just about work, she'd be fine. But it is a social situation, one that she probably has little control over. (Simone, 2012, p. 70)

But then there was also really a profound sense of regret that I couldn't have been diag-nosed, that I was born too early to get diagnosed as a young person so that I could get appropriate career, work, and guidance. And have had a career in something that I was actually suited to instead of struggling along in a lot of jobs where the best I could do was get along. L4. (Johnson & Joshi, 2016, p. 432)

There are specific situations in some workplaces where women are generally expected to take on certain roles without question. Women with autism may not naturally step into this role or even know that it is expected of her. We are often gender-blind in this respect and expect everyone to be treated equally, not seeing invisible gender expectations. (Hendrickx, 2015, p. 215)

I am at a school for children with autism which is very entertaining, because I swear to you I see these kids do the things that I do, and i think, 'Why are you doing? Oh, no wait, dang it! I do that on an adult level.'...I got really lucky that I fell into a job that was exactly my niche. When I first started, I still had very poor self-esteem and then people would talk to me and say, you know, you are so good at this, this is so amazing, we love having you here, and that I had never ever been told in any job that I've ever had. . . . but now because I've experienced what it feels like to be appreciated for what I can do, I am good with it, I am good becoming this person, I am good finding out who this person is. . . it's weird because I will tell people and they're like, like, you don't have Aspergers, . . .and it gives me sort of a two-fold answer, like first of all, I feel like I should say, "Oh, thank you, I've worked really really hard," and then the other part of me just wants to say, "What's wrong with having it?" - *Nancy Rountree* (Sparks, 2017)

In an Australian study, 62% of autistic women not in college had a paid job, compared to 95% of all Australian women in similar circumstances in the same year, with only 41% of the autistic working group working full time. Over half (51%) of those employed were underemployed, meaning that their educational qualifications exceeded the requirements of the job. By comparison, in the general population, 24% of women were underemployed. Despite high levels of skills, the environment of the workplace was full of barriers to success. Being locked into systems that weren't flexible, being treated as if they were "idiots," and not being able to make it through interviews for higher-level jobs were listed by participants in the study as examples of barriers to more satisfying employment. Social communication stressors were mentioned by 61% of autistic women as one of the top factors interfering with job satisfaction (Baldwin & Costley, 2016).

Earlier identification of autism can benefit lifelong career trajectories. When autism identification was established early in life, or the type of work had a lower social demand, or the organization supported a neurodiverse workforce, disclosure of autism was seen as an advantage to gain support without stigma. If none of these conditions were true, however, the overwhelming number of autistic adults is likely to choose nondisclosure in the workplace. Fear of stigma and being treated as somehow less than their peers prevented most from disclosing and/or accepting accommodations in the workplace. (Johnson & Joshi, 2016). For those diagnosed later in life, the need for privacy and fear of stigma were stronger, reinforcing the need for earlier identification. Three indicators of workplace well-being were explored in the study—perceived discrimination, state anxiety (emotional responses to work stressors), and organization-based self-esteem. **As age of diagnosis increased, discrimination and anxiety increased and self-esteem decreased** (Johnson & Joshi, 2016).

One solution to these issues may be to offer autism-friendly accommodations (e.g., sensory breaks, explicit instructions, and modeling) to anyone who wishes to benefit from them, regardless of disclosure of diagnosis. Johnson and Joshi (2016) also proposed beneficial support through the informal fabric of the organization, with tacit but inclusive norms and work relationships.The double empathy problem (Milton et al., 2022) applies here. The need for employees to adapt to the work environment should be matched by the work environment adapting to the needs of the employees. This is consistent with Milton's description of communities that are well-suited among themselves in terms of language, communication norms, expectations, etc., but each community may not be able to translate language, communication norms, expectations, etc. to their interactions with people in other communities. The problem is not with the autistic community. The problem is a breakdown in reciprocity and mutual understanding when people have very different ways of experiencing the world.

Disclose or Not Disclose?

Huang et al. (2022) asked this question of adults in Australia. While almost all (98.2%) had disclosed their autism identity to at least one person (usually a friend) to seek understanding and help, not all were satisfied with the outcome of disclosure. Some encountered dismissal. Half of the participants in the study did not disclose in college (males were more likely to disclose than females, perhaps due to earlier diagnoses), and about 67% disclosed in the workplace. Fear of discrimination and prejudice was a primary factor in disclosure decisions.

There are positive outcomes for disclosure in terms of building autistic community, awareness, and interpersonal understanding, but disclosure has also been described as a balancing act between these laudable outcomes and the personal cost of exposure to stigma (Davidson & Henderson, 2010). In a college setting, disclosure to the disabilities or accessibility office is usually kept confidential and therefore safer. Disclosure to professors, peers, employers, and colleagues may feel riskier. Autistic people should be aware that others are likely to make up their own interpretations for the differences they're observing (e.g., assuming that the autistic person is hostile or unmotivated) and those assumptions may be more stigmatizing than an autism label.

First Person Narratives

> *I have not been able to acquire the accommodations that I need in the work environment. In fact, asking for accommodations has usually angered my employers, who don't understand me, don't understand autism and actually seem to resent my asking. Woman with autism.* (Hendrickx, 2015, p. 216)

> *I have discovered that disclosing my diagnosis (for the purpose of getting a reasonable accommodation for the interview process) results in the presumption of incompetence and the underestimating of my abilities, which results in a lack of opportunities from potential employers or volunteer organizations. I am a lot more capable than people are willing to give me credit for once they become aware of my diagnosis. I believe that this is due to the fact that the general public is still too uninformed about the entire autism spectrum, so when they hear the word "autism" they automatically think of the misinformation and rhetoric... So in effect, I am "handicapped" by the rhetoric and stigma because it interferes with my ability to find work or volunteer positions at an appropriately challenging level for my abilities, so I am confined to underemployment (if I am fortunate enough to find employment at all). - Michelle.* (Kaim, 2017, p. 45)

Considerations in Assessment Planning

As part of adult assessments for autism, interview specifically about work history. Ask about job interviews as well as jobs held. Listen for a history of changing jobs frequently or having difficulty landing or keeping an appropriate job. Many autistic women may turn to sole proprietor businesses (e.g., selling online or writing) with varying levels of success. For some, job-seeking may be extremely aversive. Listen also for high levels of training in a career with either limited success in the field or evidence of success that may include significant personal cost (burnout). It is also possible that an adult may choose not to have a career if they have means to live without their own income. Comparison of ability (e.g., education level, experience, and training) with outcomes (job history) may be an indicator of the gap between cognitive and adaptive skills that has been discussed earlier as a signal of neurodivergence.

Assessment of college students can be more nuanced. Listen for evidence of difference between her abilities (high school performance, test scores, etc.) and her capacity to navigate the executive function demands of schooling plus independent living, particularly if she is not living at home. Prior diagnoses of ADHD may provide students with helpful accommodations if autism is not yet identified. Anxiety is likely to be a limiting factor, particularly as each semester comes to a close and the pressure to deliver work under deadlines becomes overwhelming. Also ask specifically about experiences in group work, social life, and managing activities such as shopping, cooking, laundry, etc. to get a sense of executive function and social barriers to success as a student in her chosen field.

Always ask explicitly about burnout or crashing. Bringing it up specifically (if she has not already mentioned it) will likely make it easier to talk about when it is likely to happen, will provide information about what helps her to recover, and will give clues as to how to structure accommodations to prevent or reduce burnout in academic settings. Also ask about sensory overload, which is almost universally missed in anxiety assessment but is critical to a support and accommodations plan.

Supports and Recommendations

Burnout

Autistic adults reported that acceptance of their neurodiversity, social support, time off or reduced expectations, and the freedom to accomplish tasks/do things in an unmasked, autistic way were helpful for recovery from autistic burnout (Raymaker et al., 2020). Mantzalas et al. (2022) added that online communications can help during recovery.

Awareness of autistic burnout as a phenomenon different from neurotypical burnout in college or the workplace (or clinical depression) would allow for recognition, relief, and prevention in work, educational, and social circles, including families. This is critical for the reduction of discrimination and stigma related to neurodiversity and autism (Raymaker et al., 2020). Clinicians need to understand that the toll of burnout is *cumulative*. It is also important for professionals to consider the stamina required for an autistic person to function in a stressful environment. In order to reduce or prevent burnout, long-term, systemic changes need to be considered (Mantzalas et al., 2022).

The toll of burnout is cumulative. Clinicians need to understand that stamina for functioning in stressful environments is critical for the prevention and/or reduction of burnout (Mantzalas et al., 2022).

It is critical that suicide prevention efforts and programming be aware of autistic burnout and engage in creating supports for the prevention of suicidal crises (Raymaker et al., 2020). Allowances for stimming or breaks for stimming out of public view are described as helpful for managing stress and mitigating burnout. Likewise, talking about special interests instead of current problems may be a good strategy for stabilizing in an escalating crisis situation.

Adjusting communication speed and allowing for additional time to digest instructions is also helpful. Other helpful strategies are finding autistic community, which empowers a person to form a positive autistic identity. This further allows for positive career and lifestyle changes to improve self-esteem and increase confidence and develop the courage to advocate for accommodations. Autistic adults have identified the need for teaching autistic children to cope with stressors (especially as they transition across systems) to help them avoid autistic burnout before it becomes established (Mantzalas et al., 2022).

Some accommodation strategies generated from interviews by Livingston et al. (2019) include the following:

- Play to your strengths (e.g., humor, wit, intelligence).
- Be helpful (social differences may be forgiven).
- Seek neurodivergent others (who are accepting of differences).
- Find accommodating employment (e.g., highly skilled, academia; conventional social skills are not highest value).
- Disclose difficulties (a personal social story—"This is how I work best... this is what I have a hard time with...") See Chapter 13 for more about personal social stories (Table 11.1).

College and Post-secondary

At the time of this writing, US colleges and universities were engaged in intensive efforts generally named Diversity, Inclusion, Equity, and Belonging (or similar) to improve relations and equity across groups, which has created some benefit for neurodiverse groups as well. Advice for this process was given by autistic researchers in Gillespie-Lynch et al. (2021). To conduct training in neurodiversity, the most important element to include is the interpersonal element. Neurotypical people

Table 11.1 Support Strategies for Burnout (adapted from Raymaker et al., 2020, p. 138–39)

Domain	Strategy
Acceptance and social support	Individual, community, and peer supports
Being autistic	Attending to autistic needs, unmasking, using autistic strengths
Formal supports	Reasonable accommodations, instrumental support, mental health supports
Reduced load	Time off/breaks, social withdrawal, reduced activity
Self-advocacy and health	Setting boundaries, asking for help, being healthy
Self-knowledge	Early recognition, autism diagnosis, understanding patterns, and making strategic decisions

learning about autistic people in terms of their own (NT) biases and misconceptions is valuable and fosters empathy. Accessibility is also key to training. Long stretches of text, for example, are hard to attend to. Inclusion of more visuals and interactive exercises in trainings were requested. Breaking up main ideas into shorter modules with common formatting and structure was also recommended. Clarity (not repetition) was requested (e.g., compressing a slide full of text into a video or diagram). The level of detail should suit the audience.

Preparation for college experiences described by families include preparation beyond academics (robust high school transition process, addressing autistic challenges such as social issues, realistically evaluating readiness for college transition, and addressing stresses related to transition in advance). The next key to success is to find the right fit in terms of college location, culture, size, and flexibility, including part-time options. Consideration of disability services offered in terms of benefits, limits (e.g., requiring student initiation and communication with professors), and additional options for support were important. Finally, families reported that the availability of family support (and consideration of the limits allowed) was a major consideration (Anderson & Butt, 2017).

Advocacy

We are beginning to see more neurodiversity supports in colleges and universities. Some are organized as clubs, student-led support groups, guides, or mentors. In most cases, the university accessibility or disability centers will have access to information about these supports. Contacting the accessibility/disability center is often a good first step prior to arrival on campus. Students are expected to initiate this contact, as federal privacy laws generally don't allow parents to discuss confidential issues without the student's written release.

The Autistic Self Advocacy Network (ASAN)

ASAN is a national grassroots disability rights organization for the autistic community run by and for autistic people. It sponsors an Autism Campus Inclusion (ACI) Leadership Academy for college students (https://autisticadvocacy.org/aci/). ACI helps autistic students learn to make their college campuses better for people with disabilities. ACI participants learn about making student groups, understanding disability policy, and talking to people in power. During ACI, all participants go to the US Capitol to talk to their Senators and Representatives about policies important to the disability community. After the Academy, students get help from ASAN to meet their advocacy goals at their college.

Careers

Many large corporations are leading the change to valuing neurodiversity in the workplace. Many are in the tech sector (e.g., Microsoft Neurodiversity Hiring Program, SAP Autism at Work Program). Others are in the financial (e.g., Freddie Mac Autism Internship Program, Ernst and Young Center of Excellence) and automotive (Ford Inclusive Works) sectors. Retail is also represented (e.g., Walgreens' REDI, The Home Depot, and CVS, with support for disabilities—specifically autism). Specialisterne, Auticon, and Ultranauts are other businesses with a mission to match autistic talent with employer needs. The ability to recruit and retain neurodiverse employees is beginning to be recognized as a competitive advantage (Austin & Pisano, 2017). Although too early for conclusive research, there is the possibility that the aftereffects of the COVID-19 pandemic may provide more universal accommodations for workplace stress than were offered in prior years. Additionally, the ranks of prominent employers with neurodivergent hiring practices and support programs is rapidly growing. Experiences of autistic employers in the post-pandemic era are likely to be less restrictive and stigmatized than prior research may suggest.

Return to the Case Study

When Britta reached a breaking point, where she could no longer keep up the pretense of remaining "on" for all the duties she had in a day, she began to withdraw. Her supervisor tried to talk with her, but Britta wasn't sure what to say or how to say it, and she was afraid her supervisor would think less of her if she disclosed her struggles keeping up with the frenetic pace in the lab. After considering her options, including the possibility of quitting, Britta decided to meet with her supervisor to disclose her diagnosis of autism and to request accommodations. Britta prepared for this meeting by making a list of things she found rewarding about her job and those she found challenging. Then she brainstormed how to transform some of those challenges into the situations she found more rewarding. Through this process, she was able to come up with a list of potential accommodations that would be helpful in relieving some of her anxiety while maximizing her performance. Some of the accommodations included brief breaks built into her day that would not be co-opted for impromptu meetings, a more predictable schedule with regard to lab and supervisor meetings, and the ability to take daily lunch without any required meetings. Britta's conference with her supervisor went very well. Her supervisor appreciated the open communication and the ideas Britta brought to the table. While not all of Britta's requests were easily met within this setting, most of them were incorporated into Britta's job description. Once her supervisor saw how effective these changes were for Britta's productivity and sense of well-being, she began to apply a few of these ideas to the wider lab team, including minimizing back-to-back scheduling and providing a more consistent structure to the day. This had positive effects on job satisfaction and productivity for several other team members (See Table 11.2 for a summary of assessment strategies related to burnout for college and work settings).

Table 11.2 At-a-glance summary post-secondary education, careers, and autistic burnout

Domain	Focus	Assessment planning
Work	Job history—no history in adults, sporadic history in adults, success at great personal cost or in an accommodating position (had to leave a job for sense of justice or to maintain their own moral code)	Client interview
Work	Job history—no history in adolescents or grand plans that don't pan out (e.g., internet businesses)	Client interview, parent interview
Work	Job interviewing history difficulties	Client interview
Work	Communication difficulties with employers (little understanding of why they were let go)	In-depth interview **ADOS module 4** (Lord et al., 2012), questions about employment and getting along with others
College	Connectedness and access to supports	Interview, review of records
College	Physical and mental health	Interview, history
Burnout	Relationship between load, access to support, expectations, and abilities	Interview, history

References

American Psychiatric Association. (2022). *Diagnostic and Statistical Manual of Mental Disorders, Fifth Ed., Text Revision.* Author.

Anderson, C., & Butt, C. (2017). Young adults on the autism spectrum at college: Successes and stumbling blocks. *Journal of Autism and Developmental Disorders, 47*(10), 3029–3039. https://doi.org/10.1007/s10803-017-3218-x

Austin, R. D., & Pisano, G. P. (2017). Neurodiversity as a competitive advantage. *Harvard Business Review, 95*(3), 96–103. https://hbr.org/2017/05/neurodiversity-as-a-competitive-advantage

Baczewski, L. M., Pizzano, M., Kasari, C., & Sturm, A. (2022). Adjustment across the first college year: A matched comparison of autistic, attention-deficit/hyperactivity disorder, and neurotypical students. *Autism in Adulthood: Challenges and Management, 4*(1), 12–21. https://doi.org/10.1089/aut.2021.0012

Baldwin, S., & Costley, D. (2016). The experiences and needs of female adults with high-functioning autism spectrum disorder. *Autism, 20*(4), 483–495. https://doi.org/10.1177/1362361315590805

Cage, E., & Troxell-Whitman, Z. (2020). Understanding the relationships between autistic identity, disclosure, and camouflaging. *Autism in Adulthood, 2*(4), 334–338. https://doi.org/10.1089/aut.2020.0016

Cook, B., & Garnett, M. (Eds.). (2018). *Spectrum women: Walking to the beat of autism.* Jessica Kingsley Publishers.

Davidson, J., & Henderson, V. L. (2010). 'Coming out' on the spectrum: Autism, identity and disclosure. *Social & Cultural Geography, 11*(2), 155–170. https://doi.org/10.1080/14649360903525240

Fernandes, P., Haley, M., Eagan, K., Shattuck, P. T., & Kuo, A. A. (2021). Health needs and college readiness in autistic students: The freshman survey results. *Journal of Autism and Developmental Disorders, 51*(10), 3506–3513. https://doi.org/10.1007/s10803-020-04814-8

Gillespie-Lynch, K., Bisson, J. B., Saade, S., Obeid, R., Kofner, B., Harrison, A. J., Daou, N., Tricarico, N., Delos Santos, J., Pinkava, W., & Jordan, A. (2021). If you want to develop an effective autism training, ask autistic students to help you. *Autism: The International Journal of Research & Practice, 1.* https://doi.org/10.1177/13623613211041006

Goddard, H., & Cook, A. (2022). "I spent most of freshers in my room" – A qualitative study of the social experiences of university students on the autistic spectrum. *Journal of Autism and Developmental Disorders, 52*(6), 2701–2716. https://doi.org/10.1007/s10803-021-05125-2

Hendrickx, S. (2015). *Women and girls with autism spectrum disorder: Understanding life experiences from early childhood to old age.* Jessica Kingsley Publishers.

Huang, Y., Hwang, Y. I., Arnold, S. R. C., Lawson, L. P., Richdale, A. L., & Trollor, J. N. (2022). Autistic adults' experiences of diagnosis disclosure. *Journal of Autism and Developmental Disorders, 52*, 5301–5307. https://doi.org/10.1007/s10803-021-05384-z

Johnson, T. D., & Joshi, A. (2016). Dark clouds or silver linings? A stigma threat perspective on the implications of an autism diagnosis for workplace well-being. *Journal of Applied Psychology, 101*(3), 430–449. https://doi.org/10.1037/apl0000058

Kaim, N. (Ed.) (2017). *In our own words: Women with Asperger/Autism profiles share their life stories.* Autism Asperger's Network. https://www.aane.org/wp-content/uploads/2017/03/20-Womens-Stories.pdf

Livingston, L. A., Shah, P., & Happé, F. (2019). Compensatory strategies below the behavioural surface in autism: A qualitative study. *Lancet Psychiatry, 6*, 766–777. https://doi.org/10.1016/S2215-0366(19)30224-X

Lord, C., Rutter, M., DiLavore, P. C., Risi, S., Gotham, K., & Bishop, S. L. (2012). *Autism Diagnostic Observation Schedule* (2nd ed., pp. 1–4). Western Psychological Services.

Mandy, W. (2019). Social camouflaging in autism: Is it time to lose the mask? *Autism, 23*(8), 1879–1881. https://doi.org/10.1177/1362361319878559

Mantzalas, J., Richdale, A. L., Adikari, A., Lowe, J., & Dissanayake, C. (2022). What is autistic burnout? A thematic analysis of posts on two online platforms. *Autism in Adulthood, 4*(1), 52–65. https://doi.org/10.1089/aut.2021.0021

Miller, J. K. (Ed.). (2015). *Women from another planet? Our lives in the universe of autism.* AuthorHouse.

Milton, D., Gurbuz, E., & López, B. (2022). The 'double empathy problem': Ten years on. *Autism, 26*(8), 1901–1903. https://doi.org/10.1177/13623613221129123

Pearson, A., & Rose, K. (2021). A conceptual analysis of autistic masking: Understanding the narrative of stigma and the illusion of choice. *Autism in Adulthood, 3*(1), 52–60. https://doi.org/10.1089/aut.2020.0043

Phung, J., Penner, M., Pirlot, C., & Welch, C. (2021). What I wish you knew: Insights on burnout, inertia, meltdown, and shutdown from autistic youth. *Frontiers in Psychology, 12*. https://doi.org/10.3389/fpsyg.2021.741421

Raymaker, D. M., Teo, A. R., Steckler, N. A., Lentz, B., Scharer, M., Delos Santos, A., Kapp, S. K., Hunter, M., Joyce, A., & Nicolaidis, C. (2020). "Having all of your internal resources exhausted beyond measure and being left with no clean-up crew": Defining autistic burnout. *Autism in Adulthood, 2*(2), 132–143. https://doi.org/10.1089/aut.2019.0079

Simone, R. (2012). *22 things a woman with Asperger's syndrome wants her partner to know.* Jessica Kingsley Publishers.

Sparks, P. K. (Producer) (2017) *On the spectrum* [Film]. KUED, University of Utah (now PBS Utah). https://video.pbsutah.org/video/utah-issues-spectrum/

Chapter 12
Adult Autism and Social Connections: Living Authentically, Sexuality, Partnering, Parenting, and Vulnerabilities

Introduction

Our goal with this work is to raise awareness and educate about nuanced autism, especially in females. In future, we hope that autism is identified early enough to provide supports to improve quality of life and outcomes. For those who are already in adulthood, it is not too late. Some women with "late" diagnoses reflect on the pain that could have been avoided had they known about their autism earlier in life. Others consider their early years without supports as shaping them into the adult they are today in positive ways. Regardless, identification of autism at any age is seen as helpful in adult development.

> *Shortly after Pretending to be Normal was released, I received my own official diagnosis of Asperger's Syndrome. Like many adults who don't find they have AS until they've spent decades practically doing the hokey pokey with the so-called normal world, I was happy to hear a trusted psychologist tell me there was a neurobiological reason behind the heedless, anxious, confused and often sick-to-my-stomach days. The words yes, you have Asperger's syndrome gave me hope and immediately took away the growing fear I was going mad.* (Willey, 2014, pg. 131)

> *Any early intervention/help may ultimately have hindered my development into the adult I've become - I believe I'm stronger through having struggled at times and am far more prepared for the nature of adult life than some people who have had support for years (Woman with autism)* (Hendrickx, 2015, p. 124)

Case Study—Carmen: Late Diagnosis, Parenting, and Communication Struggles

Carmen was in her 40s when she received a diagnosis of autism. Communication with her partner had always been challenging for Carmen, and she struggled to understand her partner's needs. She always felt like she was guessing incorrectly at what he wanted and meant, and their relationship suffered as a result. As a new parent in her early 30s, Carmen struggled to manage the multiple demands of caring for her child, her partner, her home, and herself. After having much more difficulty than she felt she should be and realizing she was not finding joy where other parents seemed to find joy, she sought out therapy. She tried four different therapists over 5 years. Despite putting in the effort and trying the recommendations made by each therapist, Carmen felt she was no better off than when she started. In fact, she felt even worse because she felt like she was "failing" as a partner, a parent, and a person. Around this time, her 7-year-old daughter was referred for testing in the schools because of "social and communication challenges." During the assessment process, Carmen began to hear echoes of her childhood self in the observations school staff made of her daughter. With each new recognition, Carmen marveled at how her daughter's differences mirrored her own. When her daughter was found eligible for school services under the category of autism, Carmen was prompted to begin the long process of finding a specialist who could help her explore the possibility she might be autistic as well. It took two different specialists and several years before Carmen found someone who took the time to listen and understand Carmen's experiences from her own point of view. When the diagnosis finally came, Carmen's overwhelming feeling was one of relief. After years of struggling to manage others' expectations of herself and always feeling she was falling short, Carmen was finally able to embark upon a journey that allowed her to better understand herself and therefore help others better understand her.

Vulnerability and Victimization

First Person Narratives

Had I known about Asperger's, I think I'd have known that I'm more suggestible... and I might not have ended up in the situations that I did. (P14) [I was] gradually being pestered... Because we don't sense danger and can't. That's one reason, I think you not reading people to be able to tell if they're being creepy, you're that desperate for friends and relationships that if someone is showing an interest in you, you kind of go with it and tend not to learn from others' safety skills. (P07) (Barigela et al., 2016, p. 3286, 3288)

I am the same with getting the terminology that came with autism, getting the terminology that came with the relationship abuse. It's really important to be able to put names to the concepts and things. (Jasmine)... I didn't really know how to talk about it. I didn't have the right words and I just felt stupid. (Yvonne)... It takes a long time to process what happened and an even longer time to process how to feel and react. (Norma)... Angry, I guess. Wondering why I didn't realize what was happening. (Jamie) (Pearson et al., 2023, p. 506)

It [support] would be community-based, like support groups with other autistic people where we can relate to each other, validate each other, and figure out ways to face the world together, because I don't believe victimization ends for us. It's kind of an ongoing thing in a neurotypical world. The idea that trauma is just one event you can recover from and one day feel safe again is not really relevant when the world is not built for you, and in many cases, is actively built to harm you. (Luna) (Pearson et al., 2023 p. 507)

Autistic only spaces are desperately needed more than anything else right now . . . realising the problem was never us just for existing it was always other people making us feel like we don't belong, but we do. (Leigh) (Pearson et al., 2023, p. 506)

Unfortunately, victimization rates are higher in autistic adults, particularly females. The rates of sexual violence victimization among autistic college students are high similar to neurotypical students, but in the cases of autistic students, the effects of the violence negatively impacted their academic progress more often. In addition, autistic US college students experience more physical and emotional aggression than their peers (Rothman et al., 2021). Please see Chap. 10 for more on victimization.

Pearson et al. (2023) conducted a qualitative study with autistic adults (64% identifying as female) about their experiences with interpersonal victimization. They described a complex relationship whereby trauma contributed to masking, masking contributed to burnout, and burnout contributed to being unable to mask further. Their comments aligned with the following themes:

1. "Autism as usual," or expectations of being victimized, of being othered because they are autistic.
2. "Personhood revoked," meaning the cost of being part of a neurominority includes trauma, masking, and burnout.
3. "Unpacking the baggage" or the emotional impact as a separate thing from burnout.
4. They described the structural inequalities and power dynamics in their communities as **"If you want to make an apple pie from scratch, you have to invent the universe first."** - attributed to Carl Sagan (Sagan et al., 2000).

Adults in the study also had ideas about how to make things better, primarily by finding a community and spaces. The authors also stressed the importance of ensuring good-quality training for the professional community (ideally developed and delivered with/by autistic/neurodivergent people) and continued professional development for those who might encounter autistic (and otherwise neurodivergent) victims within their line of work. Maddox et al. (2020) gave similar recommendations.

Sexuality

First Person Narratives

> *Before I turned sixteen years old I became sexually active. Had anyone asked me if I were, I probably would have said no, only because I did not comprehend what the term "sexually active" meant. I now can comprehend the term, but not always the degree of "activity" that accurately defines "sexually active."…I now believe that one of my school counselors knew I was sexually active, or at least strongly suspected it. If we could take that same situation now, knowing what we know about autism, the entire situation could have been managed much better. My life as well as many others' lives could have been affected in a more positive manner.* (Snyder, 2006, pp. 121–122)

> *It may be that they had missed signs of attraction or had not felt strong attraction to anyone themselves. What is known is that gender, sexuality and libido may be experienced differently for those with ASD and that norms in these areas should not be applied. The biggest issue for the women who had no established relationships was often a feeling of failure in an NT sense; that they had not managed to achieve what other people had in terms of finding someone who chose them as their exclusive partner. This is a very visible aspect of adult life; people around you know if you are single. Being single is often seen negatively in our society: 'no-one loves you, therefore you are unlovable'. We know that women with autism want to fit in, be accepted and be invisible. For some, not having a partner is the ultimate sign to the world that you are just no good.* (Hendrickx, 2015, p. 170)

> *Support networks in general can include both men and women. But for questions related to boyfriends and sex, you may want to pick a woman out of your support network to discuss this with. Yes, it is hugely embarrassing. But this is a matter of your safety, which is so much more important than your embarrassment.* (Brown, 2013, p. 26)

> *For example, I am emotionally still pretty young, although I am technically an adult. Emotionally, I think I might be around age 12 and, particularly when I am scared or upset, I often need exactly what a 12-year-old would need. Often, what I most need is a parent— not necessarily my actual parents, but support people who take on that role.* (Brown, 2013, p. 30)

Adolescents

Autistic adolescents experience sexual feelings and behaviors including solo and partnered sexual behaviors much like their peers (Hancock et al., 2020; Pecora et al., 2016), with a later average age of first sexual experience (22; Pecora et al., 2016, 2020). Autistic adolescents receive less school-based sex education (28%) than students with intellectual developmental disorders (43%; National Longitudinal Transition Study-2: Harris & Udry, 2000), however. In an updated survey about sexuality conducted by Holmes et al. (2020), parents indicated that only 40–60% of their autistic youth had received sex education. Autistic youth express sexual attraction (68.5%) and desire for relationships (58.4%) that increases with age. Girls are more likely to have a relationship than boys. Girls are more sensitive to negative experiences in relationships (Pecora et al., 2016). About 6.4% of all autistic youth had been sexually abused, and 14% had been bullied for their lack of information about sexual slang and social norms around sex, and about 20% had engaged in some socially transgressive sexual behavior. Autistic girls' risk of known sexual abuse (9%) was three times that of boys (Holmes et al., 2020).

Parents were aware of same-sex attraction and relationships in 13.2% of their teens (Holmes et al., 2020), with autistic females reporting lower levels of hetero-sexuality than autistic males or neurotypical females (Pecora et al., 2020). In adult-hood, 78% of respondents reported unwanted sexual contact beginning as young as age 14, which was at least partially mediated by low access to sex education (Brown-Lavoie et al., 2014). Autistic college students across genders reported higher rates of unwanted sexual contact on campus (8.2%) compared to neurotypical peers (4.6%) (Brown et al., 2017). An Australian twin study found a threefold increased risk of coercive sexual victimization prior to age 18 for autistic females (Gotby et al., 2018). Sexual activities can also be slightly different in autistic populations, with some reports of increased hypersexual and paraphilic fantasies or (for women) more solitary sexual behaviors (Schöttle et al., 2017).

Adults

Dewinter et al. (2017) reported more feelings of gender non-conformity in partici-pants assigned female at birth. Some individuals may also be incorrectly perceived as gender-diverse because they have difficulty filling expected gender roles. For example, some autistic women may not wear makeup due to sensory and/or execu-tive functioning difficulties, but may wish that they were able to do so. Others may be uninterested in adhering to gender norms but still feel at ease with their assigned gender. Gender identity does not predict sexuality, but is a factor in the amount of exposure to relevant sexual relationship models (Barnett & Maticka-Tyndale, 2015).

Bush et al. (2021) reported satisfaction and lower anxiety among a minority of autistic females who identify as asexual. Their sample also included a variety of sexual identities, including lesbian, gay, queer, and pansexual. Autistic women who were not heterosexual reported more negative or unwanted sexual experiences than their peers with and without autism, except for bisexual autistic women, who had fewer regrets related to sexual experiences (Pecora et al., 2020). In qualitative stud-ies, autistic women reported difficulty judging subtle social cues such as flirting, aggression, or coercion, also putting them at risk for sexual assault (Kanfiszer et al., 2017).

Partnering

First Person Narratives

> *Of course he broke up with me, no doubt smothered by my intense adoration and over-whelming need to be with him as often as possible. When he left me, I knew something in me had changed. I could feel my nerves start to unwind. I quit eating. Quit sleeping. Quit going to classes. Quit everything but breathing and sleeping, and frankly I didn't much care if I kept up with either of those chores either. Luckily, my counselor did care....I didn't have a conscious wish to give up. I just quit conscious living.* (Willey, 2012, p. 51)

> *I was diagnosed as being on the autism spectrum at age 54, after several very difficult years of self-discovery. I had always sensed that I was different. I just never understood how or why. I honestly thought that, once I had succeeded in learning the mechanics of socializing, I would be socializing. People would share information about themselves with me, yet I didn't know what I was supposed to do with it. People would call themselves my friends, but I couldn't figure out what I was supposed to do with a friend. Without this sharing of thoughts and feelings between myself and others, I had no clue just how much I thought or felt differently from others. It was quite a shock when I finally did discover how much of myself I had hidden even from myself all those years. - Susan Golubock* (Miller, 2015, p. 86)

> *But since we are emotionally naïve, very sense-oriented, have a lack of understanding of gender roles, and a fight-or-flight reaction to others, if we are romantically inclined, you might get a girl who chases boys with a dreamy idea of romance who can't actually stand to have a boyfriend.* (Simone, 2010, p. 79)

Couples

Roughly half of autism participants in one study were in a relationship, several with another individual with autism. While most desire relationships, many autistic women are single compared to neurotypical peers (DeWinter et al., 2017). A qualitative study of a handful of mixed-neurotype couples tells the story of how their partnerships were formed. They started with a honeymoon phase and then defined their relationship before establishing it. As the relationship deepened, conflicts and challenges with communication were encountered, as communication styles differed. Any camouflaging from earlier in the relationship would be harder to maintain as the relationship progressed (Smith et al., 2021). Partners used strength-based roles to facilitate partnership development as they encountered communication difficulties. Interpreting emotions was also difficult, as was understanding and accepting idiosyncratic characteristics of their partners.

Strunz et al. (2017) found 73% of autistic adults (60% female in the group) had intimate partnerships at one time, with 44% currently in a partnership. Only 7% of the sample had no desire for a romantic relationship. Partnerships in which both individuals were autistic were rated with higher satisfaction than if one partner was neurotypical.

Parenting

First Person Narratives

As an autistic woman, becoming a mum taught me an immense lesson in empathy, tolerance and care; a lesson in love. I learned that I can successfully ensure the survival and well-being of a creature who depends 100 percent on me. Now I know what it is like to love someone, I can apply that to other people, and I can measure, I can classify, I can understand the process of love and what is involved. Being a mum has made my emotional life much, much richer, and much clearer. And knowing that I am an Aspie mum, who can empathise with her autistic child like no other mum could, makes me feel empowered, and confident that I can raise a happy human. And that is no mean feat. Mother with autism (Hendrickx, 2015, p. 180)

Don't get me wrong. I love being her mother. She is a gorgeous human being in every way imaginable. But as an Aspergirl, I rail against assumptions of both gender and motherhood, and norms that I think are disrespectful and illogical, which, at their core, were created to keep good women down. (Simone, 2012, p. 80)

I was only 20 years old and happy to be having another baby... What I could not understand was why I was so extremely irritable and short tempered with everyone around me. I did not recognize that my son was having challenges in areas that might have been picked up by what we now call early intervention. I worked evening shifts so I would leave him with anyone I could find. I had no reason to enforce a bedtime, and didn't have any understanding why it was needed. There were no set rules and we ate when we wanted and what we felt like eating. Standards of nutrition were beyond my ability to comprehend. As long as there was food, I thought I was doing fine. - (Snyder, 2006, p. 129)

When I was carrying my baby, I didn't think of any of these. I didn't expect the baby to be this way or the other. All I wished for the baby was, to be healthy enough to grow and reach adulthood. Anticipating motherhood meant a strong feeling to protect and nurture. It came from the physical sensation of carrying my baby. The first feeling that I had for Ron was not really love, but an overwhelming sense of responsibility. - Sola Shelly (Miller, 2015, p. 242)

Overall, my sons appreciate my honesty, transparency, willingness to take responsibility for my actions, and ability to validate their own struggles and feelings. When they feel lonely or scared, they know I understand, and, more importantly, they know I believe them and validate their experience. They appreciate my consistency, my thorough explanations–the way I work to expose the unknowns. I have inspired in them the ideals of deep introspection and self-awareness. -Samantha Craft (Cook & Garnett, 2018, p. 116)

At this point, I hated my life. I was always angry at having to give up my wants and needs again and again. One day, I had a meltdown in my living room and heard myself say out loud that I hated my kids. Immediately, I knew I had gone too far. I loved my kids. I was just tired of my kids being the ones that were doing everything "wrong" and overwhelmed because I was the one expected to "fix" the situation. Couldn't anyone see that I was in over my head with my own issues much less able to handle theirs? It was as if I didn't even exist. - Kathryn Brewer (Kaim, 2017, p. 33)

Getting my own help was the only chance my children had for me to able to help them as well. I had to learn how to navigate me out of this mess if I was going to help them. They were beginning to cope and and navigate the world better than I was, and encounter problems that I could not assist them with, because I had not learned those skills myself. I was so fortunate to stumble on the Autism Women's Network (now the Autism Women & Nonbinary Network). - Jennifer St. Jude (Ballou et al., 2021, p. 60)

Positive and Also Challenging Experiences

See Chapter 9 for more on pregnancy and parenting experiences with newborns and very young children.

Parenting experiences for autistic people are just beginning to appear in the scientific literature. Some focus on autistic parents without specific reference to neurodiversity of the children, but others are specifically parent/child autistic dyads. This is described as both a help and a hindrance at times. Challenges include knowing how to model and teach positive behavior, how to understand their child's needs, controlling their own behaviors, and feeling connected to their children. There are also significant sensory demands in parents (Marriott et al., 2022). In qualitative interviews, these themes and additional information emerged about the mental health challenges of parenting, including trying to manage the complexities of the child's professional services. Positive aspects include the benefit of home being a place of acceptance of autistic traits for both parents and children (Marriott et al., 2022).

Winnard et al. (2022) interviewed autistic female adults who were and were not parents about parenting attitudes. Both positive and negative themes emerged. The first theme which was "fun and games," or the love that children give and the experiences of playing with children, was seen as positive. Giving and receiving support in a parent/child relationship was detailed as positive and an opportunity for growth for the parent. The need for routines was also mentioned as something that autistic parents do well and something that non-parents worried about (e.g., they worried their routines would be disrupted). Finally, the unique insight that an autistic parent may be able to offer an autistic child in parenting was listed as a benefit by parents and non-parents alike (Winnard et al., 2022).

Challenges identified by Winnard et al. (2022) included concerns about safety in typical childhood activities (mostly non-parents were concerned). Accessing services for their children was frequently mentioned as a challenge as well. Sensory sensitivities and overload were a universal challenge, viewed as unavoidable, but very difficult to manage with children. While many neurotypical parents may seek out other parents for support, the autistic parents in the study had significant difficulty interacting with other parents and communicating with teachers.

Dugdale et al. (2021) found many similar themes and added a call for service providers to receive training from autistic mothers on issues likely to need support during pregnancy and childrearing. In all studies, most participants found motherhood to be joyful and rewarding (85%; Pohl et al., 2020), but acknowledged the personal impact of parenting—benefitting from the intense connection, but needing to find a balance of meeting child and parent needs. The adjustment to parenting in the newborn and infant stages was noted as challenging in many ways. Sensory overload, loss of sleep, exhaustion, and disruption of routines were very difficult adjustments. When providers have more autism understanding, the mothers were seen as more "expert" about their child and received more support. There is often an expression of guilt or fear of judgment about having an autistic child or being an autistic parent and worry about parent ability to adequately support their child (not good enough) (Dugdale et al., 2021; Marriott et al., 2022; Pohl et al., 2020; Winnard et al., 2022). Participants almost universally acknowledged experiencing growth and change in parenting (Dugdale et al., 2021).

Autistic mothers report consistent difficulties with multitasking demands of parenting (Dugdale et al., 2021, Marriott et al., 2022; Pohl et al., 2020; Winnard et al., 2022), extending to domestic responsibilities and a lower sense of perceptions that they were organized. Pohl et al. (2020) reported more difficulties creating social opportunities for their children, but compared to neurotypical mothers, autistic mothers had similar opportunities to boost their child's self-confidence. Most autistic mothers (61%) felt like they should be offered extra support, but only 14% thought the supports they were receiving were adequate for their needs or their child's needs. This may be because more autistic mothers reported anxiety about inability to communicate effectively with professionals, leading to misunderstandings and conflict with professionals. The majority of autistic mothers did not disclose their own autism to their child's providers (Pohl et al., 2020). See Chap. 9 for more about pregnancy.

Living Authentically and Aging

God, what a relief being older is. I've become invisible. No-one expects anything of me anymore—I'm just old. Sad though that is in some ways, it's also a huge liberation: I can do whatever I like and nobody cares. Woman with autism (Hendrickx, 2015, p. 229)

What I have learned by the age of 55 is that one need not make a choice between learning to live in a social world one doesn't understand and living life in a way that makes sense and gives pleasure to the person that you are. - Susan Golubuck (Miller, 2015, p. 91))

Then, at age 74, I listened to my "savoir book" and learned about Asperger Syndrome. This knowledge has helped me to understand better the turmoils I experienced in the past and to understand that others think differently than I do; they don't process information the same way. I now try to modify my behavior towards others, and if a person is too difficult to socialize with, I don't continue to develop the relationship. I have a select circle of friends who understand me and take me for who I am without trying to change me. I am a person who enjoys being alone and enjoys my own company. I am quite comfortable in my skin. I tell most people about my Asperger's; I feel it is nothing to be ashamed of. There is nothing wrong with me; I just think differently than most. - Verne Kaminski (Kaim, 2017, p. 11)

Mid- and Late-Adult Development

Camouflaging has been discussed in Chaps. 5 and 11, detailing both advantages (acceptance) and costs (burnout). Even in adult relationships, camouflaging can be difficult to balance. With trusted family and friends, the "mask" can be dropped, and the authentic self can exist without threat of burnout in many cases. Sometimes, however, a partner may think the camouflaging is needed to maintain the relationship, or someone else in a social relationship may actually request that camouflaging continue (Mantzalas et al., 2022). Depending on the circumstance, (e.g. a workplace relationship), these demands may constitute discrimination.

Another approach to living authentically has been to consider living alone or to limit social contacts. Hwang et al. (2022) reported that although social contact and communication were welcome, there was a tendency among a sample of autistic adults (58% of whom were female) to prefer solitude (but not isolation). Interactions in which the social partner was respectful of the autistic adult's preferences and alignment of interests were more successful. The arenas in which most experiences were gained were in controlled environments (such as online) where the pace and method of communication were easier to navigate. Perceived stress has been found to show non-significant decreases as autistic people age, but the stress levels for autistic people assigned female at birth are significantly higher than for autistic people assigned male at birth and compared to the general population. Stress levels impact quality of life at all ages, so although it is still a significant factor compared to other populations, aging may show some promise with a small possible softening effect on previous stress levels (McQuaid et al., 2022). Aging can also bring an element of freedom from trying to conform or camouflage.

Even as children and young adults (<35 years), higher prevalence of chronic health conditions is documented in autistic populations (across genders). Statistics pulled from medical records showed more epilepsy, schizophrenia, inflammatory bowel disease, other bowel disorders, central nervous system disorders, diabetes mellitus type 1, sleep disorders, and muscular dystrophy (Kohane et al., 2012). In middle and later years, the most common medical conditions are more significantly present in the autistic sample, including some that are more rare (i.e., stroke and Parkinson's disease) (Croen et al., 2015). There are also significant genetic conditions such as Ehlers-Danlos syndrome that are associated with autism (Cederlöf et al., 2016). This is all to say that as autistic people age, healthcare concerns that have likely been present throughout adulthood will need particular attention and access to care to preserve quality of life.

Assessment Planning for Adult Autism and Social Connections

General assessment batteries for autism in adults can sometimes be misleading in our experience. A comprehensive assessment similar to the evaluation of an adolescent may result in conflicting and confusing results, as many of the measures have not been well-normed for females (particularly adult females). In our experience, additional time and interviews to gather more details about early life, social communication, and special interests can clarify the possibility of autism in an adult female. Partners, parents, and adult children can be excellent sources of information in addition to the individual. It is likely that adult female clients have done research on autism, which can cause some clinicians to question the genuineness of their reported history. In our clinical experience, it is overwhelmingly common for us to find adults who have "self-diagnosed" accurately, but professionals have not taken them seriously.

Although the ADOS-2, Module 4 (Lord et al., 2012), is designated for adults, there are some important caveats for its use in the cases of nuanced autism. There is an inherent bias in at least one of the interview questions regarding marriage that is asked in a way that assumes the person would not be married. In our clinical experience, women in particular have viewed some of the Module 4 tasks as infantilizing. Adjustments can be made by clinicians to reduce this effect, perhaps (e.g., introducing a children's book by commenting on the richness of the award-winning artwork). There is also an important issue that many clinicians outside of research settings are not yet aware. A revised algorithm for the Module 4 (Hus & Lord, 2014) has been published in the literature, jeopardizing the validity and reliability of resulting scores using the algorithms published on the Module 4 protocols. The original algorithm also does not include the standardized severity sores that are available across the other ADOS-2 modules, further complicating its use. Finally, in our experience, the one-hour duration of the ADOS-2 for adults is a short enough span of time that camouflaging can easily result in a low (i.e., insignificant) score. This became evident as the ADOS-2 concluded and soon afterward, changes in social communication and behaviors were evident, but not captured in the ADOS-2 scoring. It can absolutely be helpful in a comprehensive assessment, but *must be interpreted with caution.*

There is a newly released clinical interview for autism in adulthood (Wigham et al., 2020). Although large-scale trials are still ongoing, the tool is currently available without cost following an online training course (The Autism Clinical Interview for Adults; ACIA; Parr et al., 2021; Wigham et al., 2020). One of the ACIA authors, Ann Le Couteur, is the lead author on the ADI-R (Le Couteur et al., 2003), so this interview may also serve as a more accessible pathway to diagnosis for adults if their parents are not available for the extensive developmental interview required for the ADI-R. The ACIA approaches data collection by interviewing the individual and also someone who knows them well (not necessarily a parent). This feature allows for the diagnosis of adults who may not be able to respond to interview questions.

The ACIA features a pre-interview questionnaire (for subject and informant) to gather history, a clinical interview (for subject and informant), and a co-occurring interview (for subject and informant), acknowledging the complexity of social and emotional experiences and conditions in autistic adults that could also benefit from support. The ACIA was developed from the Family History Interview (Parr et al., 2021) and maps onto DSM-5-TR (APA, 2022) diagnostic criteria for autism. Time listed for the interview is 60–90 min (each) for the person and another informant. Scoring conventions are similar to ADOS-2 and ADI-R, with clinician ratings of 0 = no difficulties; 1 = difficulties; and 2 = frequent difficulties or impact on daily life. Scores are given for both Adulthood and Childhood for the person, patterned after the ADI-R Lifetime and Current algorithms. Specific cutoffs have not yet been established from a general population sample, but the information gathered through the interview is likely to inform both assessment and supports in ways that are more particularly suited to autistic adults (Parr et al., 2021).

Sexuality

Ask about sexual activity to ensure that the person has adequate healthcare information and access. Acknowledge the experiences of intersecting identities of autism and the LGBTQ+ community.

Partnering, Dating, and Victimization

Ask about experiences to assess the level of safety awareness and possible past trauma in current or past relationships. Ask specifically and explicitly about unwanted sexual contact, which may be more apparent in hindsight. Ask what the person's understanding of consent is.

Supports and Recommendations

Victimization and Vulnerability

In addition to sex education resources (below), there is a consistent thread in the research that more than education is needed. Some have strongly advocated for better education of caregivers and professionals (Cazalis et al., 2022). It is also possible that in addition to being autistic, just being female increases the risk of being a target of sexual violence, so supports targeted for all females would also be important. The Centers for Disease Control and Prevention Division of Violence Prevention (National Center for Injury Prevention and Control) has created a technical package of supports and guidance https://www.cdc.gov/violenceprevention/pdf/sv-prevention-technical-package.pdf (Basile et al., 2016). The World Health Organization (WHO) has a similar framework, titled RESPECT (WHO, 2021) https://www.who.int/publications/i/item/WHO-RHR-18.19. These resources provide action items and targets for improvement for women, educators, caregivers, and professionals.

Sexuality

Sources of information about sexuality can sometimes be limited for autistic adults. Although the internet is still a popular source of information for all, the availability of information from same-age friends and romantic partners about flirting, dating, and consent is much more limited than it is for neurotypical peers. This creates increased risk that requires better access to information about each of these topics, particularly consent (Crehan et al., 2022). Systematic access to sex education with consideration of autistic traits is the ideal solution, but until that happens, some resources have been developed by autistic self-advocates. The Organization for Autism Research (OAR, 2018) created a free audio-visual series called Sex Ed for Self-Advocates https://researchautism.org/self-advocates/sex-ed-for-self-advocates/, hosted by Amy Gravino and Peter Gerhardt, including a nine-episode podcast https://researchautism.org/self-advocates/sex-ed-for-self-advocates/sex-ed-for-self-advocates-podcast/.

Other resources include guidebooks such as *The Aspie Girl's Guide to Being Safe With Men: The Unwritten Safety Rules No-one is Telling You* by Debi Brown (2013) and *Safety Skills for Asperger Women: How to Save a Perfectly Good Female Life* by Liane Holliday Willey (2012).

Partnering and Dating

Clear communication is one of the most frequently mentioned keys to maintaining adult romantic relationships, allowing partners to not rely on theory of mind to guess what their partner needed or was thinking (Barnett & Maticka-Tyndale, 2015). In a study of neurotypical perceptions of autistic traits in dating relationships, NT women perceived autistic traits more negatively than men did. If both partners had some autistic traits, there were fewer problems (McMahon et al., 2021). Relationship communication problems may be another signal to at least consider autism communication differences as a possible reason for the difficulty.

Living Authentically and Aging

Waldron et al. (2021) gathered strategies to support older autistic populations, acknowledging the higher risk of physical and medical issues. Physical activity, nutrition, and spirituality and mindfulness were described by participants in the study (autistic adults age 50+) as supporting well-being and reducing health disparities as they got older. Unmet healthcare needs are a concern for autistic adults in general because of difficulties communicating, resulting in less access to preventive care, more emergency care, and less of a sense of self-efficacy about healthcare (Nicolaidis et al., 2013). Selected recommendations for healthcare providers are mentioned in Nicolaidis et al. (2014), giving details about the heterogeneity of communication strategies that could improve the quality of care. Some considerations are to use concrete and specific language and to slow down the speed of the interaction to allow for processing time. Avoid broad questions, or follow up with more closed-ended questions (e.g., examples of what you are asking about) to get more details. Don't require eye contact or overinterpret unusual body language. Attend to sensory sensitivities regarding light, sound, etc. and presentation of multiple stimuli at once. Accommodate needs for consistency and predictability, and allow for extension of communications to other modes if helpful (e.g., email or written lists). Make use of visual strategies to assist with executive function around healthcare. Autismandhealth. org is a resource developed in partnership with autistic adults, providing guidance for medical professionals and tools for autistic patients. See Table 12.1 for a summary of assessment strategies for adults.

Table 12.1 At-a-Glance Summary Adult Autism and Social Connections

Domain	Focus	Assessment planning and age ranges
Adult diagnosis	Age-appropriate diagnostic measure for adults and those who know them well	*Autism Clinical Interview for Adults* **ACIA** (Parr et al., 2021, 2015): ages 16+ Online Training through Newcastle Univ. materials provided free with training
Adult diagnosis	Social communication and behavioral observation	*Autism diagnostic observation schedule, Second Ed.* (**ADOS-2**) *module 4* **Interpret the ADOS-2 with caution**. It may result in a deceptively low score for multiple reasons (camouflaging, inherent bias, lack of awareness of the revised algorithm, etc.) (Lord et al., 2012; Hus & Lord, 2014, for revised algorithm)
Adult female diagnosis	No autism measure should be used in isolation, but this is one to consider adding to your assessment battery. This questionnaire was re-worded for adults	*Girls Questionnaire for Autism Spectrum Condition* (**GQ-ASC: Adult Women**) (Brown et al., 2020) https://tonyattwood.com.au/wp-content/uploads/2022/03/GQ-ASC-Adult-Women_.pdf
Data collection	Consider parents, partners, and adult children for interview	Extended interview data collection to follow up on individual interview
Victimization	Explore understanding of consent. The likelihood of non-consensual sexual contact may be high, but may not have been recognized at the time—There may be trauma as this is realized later in life	**Client interview**
Sexuality	There may not have been role models across the spectrum of sexuality	**Client interview**
Romantic partnering	Ask about navigating conflict and communication needs	**Client interview, partner interview**
Parenting	Parenting may be well-adapted to the family, but ask if there is stress about parenting that could be supported	**Interview**—Consider seeking training from autistic mothers to better understand needs and increase respect of mothers as experts
Healthcare for adults	Monitor carefully for a variety of health issues that will impact quality of life in adulthood	Academic Autism Spectrum Partnership in Research and Education **AASPIRE healthcare toolkit** https://autismandhealth.org/ Toolkits are available for providers and patients
Aging	Ask about health conditions and access to healthcare	**Interview**

References

American Psychiatric Association. (2022). *Diagnostic and Statistical Manual of Mental Disorders* Fifth Edition, Text Revision.

Ballou, E. P., da Vanport, S., & Onaiwu, M. G. (Eds.). (2021). *Sincerely, your autistic child.* Beacon Press.

Bargiela, S., Steward, R., & Mandy, W. (2016). The experiences of late-diagnosed women with autism spectrum conditions: An investigation of the female autism phenotype. *Journal of Autism and Developmental Disorders, 46*(10), 3281–3294. https://doi.org/10.1007/s10803-016-2872-8

Barnett, J. P., & Maticka-Tyndale, E. (2015). Qualitative exploration of sexual experiences among adults on the autism spectrum: Implications for sex education. *Perspectives on Sexual and Reproductive Health, 47*(4), 171–179. https://doi.org/10.1363/47e5715

Basile, K. C., DeGue, S., Jones, K., Freire, K., Dills, J., Smith, S. G., & Raiford, J. L. (2016). *STOP SV: A technical package to prevent sexual violence.* National Center for Injury Prevention and Control, Centers for Disease Control and Prevention. https://www.cdc.gov/violenceprevention/pdf/sv-prevention-technical-package.pdf

Brown, D. (2013). *The Aspie girl's guide to being safe with men: The unwritten safety rules no-one is telling you.* Jessica Kingsley.

Brown, K. R., Peña, E. V., & Rankin, S. (2017). Unwanted sexual contact: Students with autism and other disabilities at greater risk. *Journal of College Student Development, 58*, 771–776. https://doi.org/10.1353/csd.2017.0059

Brown, C. M., Attwood, T., Garnett, M., & Stokes, M. A. (2020). Am I autistic? Utility of the Girls Questionnaire for Autism Spectrum Condition as an autism assessment in adult women. *Autism in Adulthood: Challenges and Management, 2*(3), 216–226. https://doi.org/10.1089/aut.2019.0054

Brown-Lavoie, S. M., Viecili, M. A., & Weiss, J. A. (2014). Sexual knowledge and victimization in adults with autism spectrum disorders. *Journal of Autism and Developmental Disorders, 44*, 2185–2196. https://doi.org/10.1007/s10803-014-2093-y

Bush, H. H., Williams, L. W., & Mendes, E. (2021). Brief report: Asexuality and young women on the autism spectrum. *Journal of Autism and Developmental Disorders, 51*(2), 725–733. https://doi.org/10.1007/s10803-020-04565-6

Cazalis, F., Reyes, E., Leduc, S., & Gourion, D. (2022). Evidence that nine autistic women out of ten have been victims of sexual violence. *Frontiers in Behavioral Neuroscience, 16*. https://doi.org/10.3389/fnbeh.2022.852203

Cederlöf, M., Larsson, H., Lichtenstein, P., Almqvist, C., Serlachius, E., & Ludvigsson, J. F. (2016). Nationwide population-based cohort study of psychiatric disorders in individuals with Ehlers-Danlos syndrome or hypermobility syndrome and their siblings. *BMC Psychiatry, 16*, 207. https://doi.org/10.1186/s12888-016-0922-6

Cook, B., & Garnett, M. (Eds.). (2018). *Spectrum women: Walking to the beat of Autism.* Jessica Kingsley.

Crehan, E. T., Rocha, J., & Dufresne, S. (2022). Brief report: Sources of sexuality and relationship education for autistic and neurotypical adults in the U.S. and a call to action. *Journal of Autism and Developmental Disorders, 52*(2), 908–913. https://doi.org/10.1007/s10803-021-04992-z

Croen, L. A., Zerbo, O., Qian, Y., Massolo, M. L., Rich, S., Sidney, S., & Kripke, C. (2015). The health status of adults on the autism spectrum. *Autism, 19*(7), 814–823. https://doi.org/10.1177/1362361315577517

Dewinter, J., De Graaf, H., & Begeer, S. (2017). Sexual orientation, gender identity, and romantic relationships in adolescents and adults with autism spectrum disorder. *Journal of Autism and Developmental Disorders, 47*(9), 2927–2934. https://doi.org/10.1007/s10803-017-3199-9

Dugdale, A. S., Thompson, A. R., Leedham, A., Beail, N., & Freeth, M. (2021). Intense connection and love: The experiences of autistic mothers. *Autism: The International Journal of Research and Practice, 25*(7), 1973–1984. https://doi.org/10.1177/13623613211005987

Gotby, V. O., Lichtenstein, P., Långström, N., & Pettersson, E. (2018). Childhood neurodevelopmental disorders and risk of coercive sexual victimization in childhood and adolescence – a population-based prospective twin study. *Journal of Child Psychology & Psychiatry, 59*(9), 957–965. https://doi.org/10.1111/jcpp.12884

Hancock, G., Stokes, M. A., & Mesibov, G. (2020). Differences in romantic relationship experiences for individuals with an autism spectrum disorder. *Sexuality and Disability, 38*(2), 231–245. https://doi.org/10.1007/s11195-019-09573-8

Harris, K. M., & Udry, J. R. (2000). *National longitudinal study of adolescent to adult health (Add Health), 1994–2018* [Public Use]. Carolina Population Center, University of North Carolina-Chapel Hill [distributor], Inter-university Consortium for Political and Social Research [distributor], 2022-08-09. https://doi.org/10.3886/ICPSR21600.v25

Hendrickx, S. (2015). *Women and girls with autism spectrum disorder: Understanding life experiences from early childhood to old age.* Jessica Kingsley.

Holmes, L. G., Shattuck, P. T., Nilssen, A. R., Strassberg, D. S., & Himle, M. B. (2020). Sexual and reproductive health service utilization and sexuality for teens on the autism spectrum. *Journal of Developmental and Behavioral Pediatrics, 41*(9), 667–679. https://doi.org/10.1097/DBP.0000000000000838

Hus, V., & Lord, C. (2014). The Autism Diagnostic Observation Schedule, Module 4: Revised algorithm and standardized severity scores. *Journal of Autism and Developmental Disorders, 44*(8), 1996–2012. https://doi.org/10.1007/s10803-014-2080-3

Hwang, Y. I. J., Foley, K.-R., Elley, K., Brown, S., Joy-Leong, D., Li, X., Grove, R., Trollor, J., Pellicano, E., & Zheng, L. (2022). Experiences of performing daily activities in middle-aged and older autistic adults: A qualitative study. *Journal of Autism & Developmental Disorders,* 1–13. https://doi.org/10.1007/s10803-022-05473-7

Kaim, N. (Ed.) (2017). *In our own words: Women with Asperger/Autism profiles share their life stories.* Autism Asperger's Network. https://www.aane.org/wp-content/uploads/2017/03/20-Womens-Stories.pdf

Kanfiszer, L., Davies, F., & Collins, S. (2017). "I was just so different": The experiences of women diagnosed with an autism spectrum disorder in adulthood in relation to gender and social relationships. *Autism: The International Journal of Research and Practice, 21*(6), 661–669. https://doi.org/10.1177/1362361316687987

Kohane, I. S., McMurry, A., Weber, G., MacFadden, D., Rappaport, L., Kunkel, L., Bickel, J., Wattanasin, N., Spence, S., Murphy, S., & Churchill, S. (2012). The co-morbidity burden of children and young adults with autism spectrum disorders. *PLoS One, 7*(4), e33224. https://doi.org/10.1371/journal.pone.0033224

Le Couteur, A., Lord, C., & Rutter, M. (2003). *Autism Diagnostic Interview-Revised.* Western Psychological Services.

Lord, C., Rutter, M., DiLavore, P. C., Risi, S., Gotham, K., & Bishop, S. L. (2012). *Autism Diagnostic Observation Schedule* (2nd ed., pp. 1–4). Western Psychological Services.

Maddox, B. B., Crabbe, S., Beidas, R., Brookman-Frazee, L., Cannuscio, C. C., Miller, J. S., Nicolaidis, C., & Mandell, D. S. (2020). "I wouldn't know where to start": Perspectives from clinicians, agency leaders, and autistic adults on improving community mental health services for autistic adults. *Autism, 24*(4), 919–930. https://doi.org/10.1177/1362361319882227

Mantzalas, J., Richdale, A. L., Adikari, A., Lowe, J., & Dissanayake, C. (2022). What is autistic burnout? A thematic analysis of posts on two online platforms. *Autism in Adulthood, 4*(1), 52–65. https://doi.org/10.1089/aut.2021.0021

Marriott, E., Stacey, J., Hewitt, O. M., & Verkuijl, N. E. (2022). Parenting an autistic child: Experiences of parents with significant autistic traits. *Journal of Autism & Developmental Disorders, 52*(7), 3182–3193. https://doi.org/10.1007/s10803-021-05182-7

McMahon, C. M., Henry, S., Stoll, B., & Linthicum, M. (2021). Perceptions of dating behaviors among individuals in the general population with high and low autistic traits. *Sexuality & Disability, 39*(2), 309–325. https://doi.org/10.1007/s11195-020-09640-5

McQuaid, G. A., Weiss, C. H., Said, A. J., Pelphrey, K. A., Lee, N. R., & Wallace, G. L. (2022). Increased perceived stress is negatively associated with activities of daily living and subjective quality of life in younger, middle, and older autistic adults. *Autism Research: Official Journal of the International Society for Autism Research, 15*(8), 1535–1549. https://doi.org/10.1002/aur.2779

Miller, J.K. (Ed.). (2015). *Women from another planet? Our lives in the universe of autism.* AuthorHouse.

Nicolaidis, C., Raymaker, D., McDonald, K., Dern, S., Boisclair, W. C., Ashkenazy, E., & Baggs, A. (2013). Comparison of healthcare experiences in autistic and non-autistic adults: A cross-sectional online survey facilitated by an academic-community partnership. *Journal of General Internal Medicine, 28*(6), 761–769. https://doi.org/10.1007/s11606-012-2262-7

Nicolaidis, C., Kripke, C. C., & Raymaker, D. (2014). Primary care for adults on the autism spectrum. *The Medical Clinics of North America, 98*(5), 1169–1191. https://doi.org/10.1016/j.mcna.2014.06.011

Organization for Autism Research. (2018). *Sexuality on the spectrum.* https://researchautism.org/sexuality-on-the-spectrum/

Parr, J. R., De Jonge, M. V., Wallace, S., Pickles, A., Rutter, M. L., Le Couteur, A. S., van Engeland, H., Wittemeyer, K., McConachie, H., Roge, B., Mantoulan, C., Pedersen, L., Isager, T., Poustka, F., Bolte, S., Bolton, P., Weisblatt, E., Green, J., Papanikolaou, K., Baird, G., & Bailey, A. J. (2015). New interview and observation measures of the broader autism phenotype: Description of strategy and reliability findings for the interview measures. *Autism Research, 8*(5), 522–533. https://doi.org/10.1002/aur.1466

Parr, J., Wigham, S., Ingham, B., Berney, T., & LeCouteur, A. (2021). *The Autism Clinical Interview for Adults (ACIA) manual for administration. Newcastle University.* https://webstore.ncl.ac.uk/short-courses/faculty-of-medical-sciences/population-health-sciences-institute/autism-clinical-interview-for-adults-training-acia

Pearson, A., Rose, K., & Rees, J. (2023). 'I felt like I deserved it because I was autistic': Understanding the impact of interpersonal victimisation in the lives of autistic people. *Autism: The International Journal of Research and Practice, 27*(2), 500–511. https://doi.org/10.1177/13623613221104546

Pecora, L. A., Mesibov, G. B., & Stokes, M. A. (2016). Sexuality in high-functioning autism: A systematic review and meta-analysis. *Journal of Autism and Developmental Disorders, 46*(11), 3519–3556. https://doi.org/10.1007/s10803-016-2892-4

Pecora, L. A., Hancock, G. I., Hooley, M., MEsibov, G. G., & Stokes, M. A. (2020). Gender identity, sexual orientation and adverse sexual experiences in autistic females. *Molecular Autism, 11*, 57. https://doi.org/10.1186/s13229-020-00363-0

Pohl, A. L., Crockford, S. K., Blakemore, M., Allison, C., & Baron-Cohen, S. (2020). A comparative study of autistic and non-autistic women's experience of motherhood. *Molecular Autism, 11*(1), 3. https://doi.org/10.1186/s13229-019-0304-2

Rothman, E. F., Heller, S., & Graham Holmes, L. (2021). Sexual, physical, and emotional aggression, experienced by autistic vs non-autistic US college students. *Journal of American College Health,* 1–9. https://doi.org/10.1080/07448481.2021.1996373

Sagan, C., Druyan, A., Soter, S., & Malone, A. (2000). *Cosmos: a personal journey. Collector's ed.* Studio City, CA, Cosmos Studios.

Schöttle, D., Briken, P., Tüscher, O., & Turner, D. (2017). Sexuality in autism: Hypersexual and paraphilic behavior in women and men with high-functioning autism spectrum disorder. *Dialogues in Clinical Neuroscience, 19*(4), 381–393. https://doi.org/10.31887/dcns.2017.19.4

Simone, R. (2010). *Aspergirls: Empowering Females with Asperger Syndrome.* Jessica Kingsley.

Simone, R. (2012). *22 Things a woman with Asperger's Syndrome wants her partner to know.* Jessica Kingsley.

Smith, R., Netto, J., Gribble, N. C., & Falkmer, M. (2021). 'At the end of the day, it's love': An exploration of relationships in neurodiverse couples. *Journal of Autism and Developmental Disorders, 51*(9), 3311–3321. https://doi.org/10.1007/s10803-020-04790-z

Snyder, R. (2006). Maternal instincts in Asperger's Syndrome. In T. Attwood (Ed.), *Asperger's and Girls: World-renowned experts join those with Asperger's Syndrome to resolve issues that girls and women face every day!* (pp. 117–146). Future Horizons, Inc.

Strunz, S., Schermuck, C., Ballerstein, S., Ahlers, C. J., Dziobek, I., & Roepke, S. (2017). Romantic relationships and relationship satisfaction among adults with Asperger syndrome and high-functioning autism. *Journal of Clinical Psychology, 73*(1), 113–125. https://doi.org/10.1002/jclp.22319

Waldron, D. A., Coyle, C., & Kramer, J. (2021). Aging on the autism spectrum: Self-care practices and reported impact on well-being. *Journal of Autism and Developmental Disorders*, 1–11. https://doi.org/10.1007/s10803-021-05229-9

Wigham, S., Ingham, B., LeCouteur, A., Berney, T., Ensum, I., & Parr, J. (2020). Development and initial utility of the Autism Clinical Interview for Adults: A new adult autism diagnsotic measure. *Autism in Adulthood, 2*(1), 42–47. https://doi.org/10.1089/aut.2019.0052

Willey, L. H. (2012). *Safety skills for Asperger women: How to save a perfectly good female life.* Jessica Kingsley.

Willey, L.H. (2014) *Pretending to be normal: Living with Asperger's syndrome, Expanded edition.* Jessica Kingsley.

Winnard, R., Roy, M., & Butler-Coyne, H. (2022). Motherhood: Female perspectives and experiences of being a parent with ASC. *Journal of Autism and Developmental Disorders, 52*(5), 2314–2324. https://doi.org/10.1007/s10803-021-05122-5

World Health Organization (WHO). (2021, March 9). *RESPECT women: Preventing violence against women.* https://www.who.int/publications/i/item/WHO-RHR-18.19

Chapter 13
Advocacy for Neurodiversity

Introduction

The generation(s) of digital natives (those growing up with easy online internet access and tools) have an advantage over older women and others with nuanced autism who may never have encountered any information or role models for what this type of autism may look like. Finding someone who understands your experiences may be a rare event for some. For any generation, we have heard many women agree with the statement,

> *"Once women realize the truth, they can leap light-years ahead in their lives."* Nerenberg, 2021, p. 19).

As difficult as it may be to navigate the journey of identification or diagnosis, there is more work to be done. Learning how to advocate for themselves in light of their new self-knowledge can be empowering for autistic women and girls, and those with nuanced autism, but it also requires some extensive use of executive function to accomplish all of the goals a person seeks. Supports are still useful in self-advocacy.

> *Growing up, I wish my parents had known that teaching me to fight for my rights was more important than forcing me to fit in. I was conditioned early to know that my saying "no" was not an option, certain "atypical" behaviors needed to be eliminated, and being compliant made me "good." I spent a lot of time learning to deny my natural impulses and feelings in order to conform to what was expected of a "good girl." In doing so, I opened myself up to become a victim of both emotional and sexual abuse from adults and intense bullying from my peers. The way I experienced the world around me was supposedly wrong, and there was no argument. So, I remained silent. Always. Lei Wiley-Mydske* (Ballou et al., 2021, p. 31)

> *This tension between demanding official recognition and access to support on one hand and the seemingly opposite desire of wanting to be respected for neurological difference on the other hand is common across neurodivergences and in the conversations that make up the neurodiversity field. It's important to note that both desires are equally valid and can coexist.* (Nerenberg, 2021, p. 88)

© The Author(s), under exclusive license to Springer Nature Switzerland AG 2023
T. P. Gabrielsen et al., *Assessment of Autism in Females and Nuanced Presentations*, https://doi.org/10.1007/978-3-031-33969-1_13

Autism as Strength in Society and the Value of Role Models

A recent publication entitled, *Sincerely, Your Autistic Child: What People on the Autism Spectrum wish Their Parents Knew About Growing up, Acceptance, and Identity* (Ballou et al., 2021) embodies advocacy for the rising generation. The book's dedication reads,

> This book is dedicated to the autistic community of our past, present and future. Those we've known and those we haven't; those who have gone without recognition, support, or acceptance; those who are using their lives to be the change we all indeed; and for those to come who will build a better future.

With that in mind, many of the quotes listed here are framed as advice for advocacy for self and daughters. It is addressed to parents, but the messages apply to the professional community as well.

First Person Narratives

> By *cultivating the autistic mind on a brain-by-brain, strength-by-strength basis, we can reconceive autistic teens and adults in jobs and internships not as charity cases but as valuable, even essential, contributors to society.* (Grandin & Panek, 2013, p. 200)

> *I am discovering that my differences of being more open, more innocent, simpler, more honest, more gentle, less self-conscious and more childlike than most other adults can sometimes be real advantages in social interaction. These can be disarming and can get past other people's defences. After reading so much about Aspies being defined as having an impairment in social interaction, it is like an earthquake happening in my heart to realise the truth: that being an Aspie gives me some advantages in social interaction, too.* (Brown, 2013, p. 62)

> *"Being on the spectrum contributed to my success." She attributes much of that success to her not being bothered by the same superficial concerns as her peers when she was growing up. (speaking of Sara Seager)* (Nerenberg, 2021, p. 65)

> *Knowing an autistic adult who prioritized their happiness over typicality would have meant the world to me. Amethyst Schaber* (Ballou et al., 2021, p. 92)

> *I didn't meet any women my age who were Autistic and proud of it until my sophomore year of college. I think if I'd had more Autistic female role models, that would have helped me a lot. Heidi Wangelin* (Ballou et al., 2021, p. 46)

> *Make friends with autistic women. Your little girl needs to see adults she can be like. She needs to know adults who are profoundly joyful at minutia, who have executive functioning difficulties, who stim, who don't play the social games in the standard way. She needs to know adults like her exist. She needs us as a guide. And she needs to know her parents like the kind of person she will grow up to be. Thinking your family would avoid you if they weren't stuck with you? It aches. That "not the child my parents wanted" thing? It's easier to believe your mother when she tells you that you're exactly what she dreamed of when her friends get you and are on your wavelength. Kassianne Asasumasu* (Ballou et al., 2021, p. 23)

> *One of the best things about tapping into the resources that Autistic adults provide is that, unlike the experts, they don't insist that there is one way to learn and progress. They don't*

insist that rigid inflexible regimens be followed until a child is broken. Instead they seem to, almost universally, support the value of respecting individual needs. Beth Ryan (Ballou et al., 2021, p. 95)

Encourage your daughter to read autobiographies written by as many different Autistic women as you can. Maxfield Sparrow (Ballou et al., 2021, p. 147)

*My goal was not to raise my daughter to be like her peers, but to raise her to be herself--**an Autistic person with a love and understanding of who she is**--and autism is a big part of that. Anonymous* (Ballou et al., 2021, p. 152)

If I think of one thing I lack, one thing that could have made my life easier from the time I was a child up until recent days, it would be being a part of an autistic community. It is something that has been noticeably lacking from much of my life, and it is something I crave. - Jean Winegardner (Ballou et al., 2021)

Finding Community

Fortunately, there are many role models, mentors, and possible social relationships within the autism community and the broader neurodiversity movement. Online communities are listed here, but your local community may also have some small social groups. We have also seen book clubs, weekend workshops, conventions ("cons") and some long-term structured programs, included below as examples even if you are not in the geographic area.

Academic Autism Spectrum Partnership in Research and Education

https://aaspire.org/ Join participatory research, and benefit from past research, including health toolkits, inclusion tools, etc.

Autism Women's and Non-Binary Network (AWN) https://awnnetwork.org/

Webinars, newsletters, resource library, blogs, networking and social meet-ups, etc. on a variety of topics related to justice, including The Autistic People of Color Fund https://autismandrace.com/

Autism Asperger Network (AANE) https://www.aane.org/ Resources by group (e.g., adults, families, etc.) with an artist collaborative, women's stories, etc.

Autism Self-Advocacy Network (ASAN) https://autisticadvocacy.org/ Advocacy Action Center, Resource Library, Affiliate Groups by state and country. ASAN is a very active advocacy organization with policy briefs, commentary, and action items on current issues of the day as well as autism issues.

Felicity House in Manhattan, NY https://felicity-house.org/

Girls Night Out, University of Kansas, Lawrence, Kansas https://www.kumc.edu/school-of-medicine/academics/departments/pediatrics/outreach/girls-night-out-(gno).html

Advocating for Yourself and Your Rights

There is a sort of autism therapy, compliance therapy, that goes under many names, but the end goal is to ensure compliance with adult demands at the expense of the needs and emotional well-being of the patient. You will want to watch out for it because it is very dangerous to all Autistics and, in our culture, especially dangerous to female Autistics. Maxfield Sparrow (Ballou et al., 2021, p. 142)

Transitioning to high school was difficult, but it prepared me for the even more difficult transition to college. There are so many resources for autistic children, but people seem to forget that those kids grow into autistic adults, and we need support, too. I learned to advocate for myself, to ask for equal treatment and reasonable accommodations. I also learned to ask for help when I need it and to give help where I can. Most importantly, I learned to love myself. - Kennedy O. Onuoha (McCarthy, 2020)

My advice is, be vulnerable and courageous. Just as eye contact contains too much information, "life contact" seems to as well. (Simone, 2010, p. 216)

The climate at the time of this writing calls attention to the controversies of past and some existing intervention practices, focused primarily on applied behavior analysis or ABA practices (Leaf et al., 2022). In any care or therapy focused on autistic well-being, it is critical that the perspectives of autistic people be recognized, included, and prioritized. When some of these widely held practices are viewed from the lens of a vulnerable person, the risk of harm can seem considerable. Some first-person accounts describe traumatic experiences associated with aversive, coercive, and deprivation techniques used as treatment during childhood. Sometimes, the historical harm described in these accounts was not personally experienced, but the recognition of trauma to autistic children is described as feeling very immediate, personal, and threatening (Fahrenheit, 2020). There are many caring, compassionate autism providers providing ethical therapies and support, which may also include some evidence-based ABA providers who are client-focused and value individual dignity and independence. The fit between provider and the individual and an individual goal-centered approach for any type of support or therapy are important targets for advocacy regardless of the type of supports. Families and autistic people have the right to choose the approaches that work best for themselves.

We have received questions from many adults and their loved ones related to adult success in the world. These questions revolve around keeping a job, getting into a graduate program, developing relationships, or a new housing situation. There is a common worry behind these conversations—how do we help the people in a new environment to understand and support us? There is one technique that we became acquainted with at some point in our careers and have not been able to find citations for, unfortunately. It builds upon the concept of Social Stories™ by Carol Gray (2015), but there is a twist. To advocate for yourself in a new environment or relationship, think about a way to tell *your* story in a way that helps others to not misunderstand you. We have used the term "personal" or "reverse" social story about how you "work." The basics to include would be explaining things like "These are the conditions I work best in" and "This is the kind of feedback or communication style that I respond best to" and possibly something like "These are the strengths that I can bring to this work/relationship/apartment." You can consider expanding to "I can work longer if I can take short breaks here and there," or "If I am not talking much, I may need time to process something," or "I am sensitive to loud sounds, so you will often see me with ear buds or ear plugs so I can concentrate in a noisy environment." These are just examples, and do not require disclosures of diagnoses, but may ease transitions and help you to advocate for what you need to thrive. There is no need to "create" the type of visuals often used in Carol Gray's Social Stories™; these can be short conversations that you choose to have all at once or as needed to advocate for yourself.

Educating Professional Communities

There are three resources recently published in the scientific literature that address the lack of awareness of what nuanced autism looks like, each taking a different tactic to educate the gatekeepers of identification, those in professional communities. While there are some who maintain that official diagnosis is not necessary for someone to proceed with their life with the self-knowledge of autism (Price, 2022), in our experiences, people describe the freedom of self-understanding when they were identified with autism. We are also aware of people in our practices who have strong self-understanding, but still await an official diagnosis. They tell us they are seeking the official or final identification, not because they question the outcome, but so that they can move forward. Barriers have been financial (young adults without the means to pay for evaluations not covered by insurance) and time-related (wait lists that are typically much longer for adults).

The first of these resources is Duvall et al. (2021). See Table 13.1 for an excerpt from their road map for identifying autism spectrum disorder, which describes red or "pink" flags to guide accurate differential diagnosis.

The second paper (Lai et al., 2022) took this idea further and mapped examples of nuanced presentations onto DSM-5 (2013) diagnostic criteria (this article also includes the same information for ADHD). Using extensive data from research, the table gives examples of behaviors that meet the DSM-5-TR (2022) diagnostic criteria that may not yet be in the community clinician's exemplar sets for autism (Table 13.2).

The third resource (Suckle, 2021) organized a call for action based on evidence, with suggested policy and practice changes (amendments) with desired outcomes. The impetus for these calls is to alleviate suffering. The author points out that persistent anxiety and/or severe mental crises such as suicidal thoughts and behaviors can "open a door, but why should girls and young women need to spiral downwards before help is given?" (Horlock, 2019, p. 50 as quoted in Suckle, 2021) (Fig. 13.1).

Table 13.1 Symptoms of autism spectrum disorder: real-life examples of red flags and pink flags from expert clinicians (Duvall et al. 2022).

Symptom type	Red flag	Pink flag
Restricted, repetitive patterns of behavior, interests, or activities		
Restricted interests and play	*Exhaustive and obsessive interest in highly specific, atypical topics. For example, dishwasher models, electric blanket controls, state license plates, WWII war planes, recites the Latin names of dinosaurs to strangers at the grocery store, carries doorstopper with them at all times or memorizes bus routes as a hobby.*	*Really likes to learn about and talk about certain niche topics. For example, Minecraft, Dinosaurs, Thomas the Train, Five Nights at Freddy's, US History, Aviation , My Little Pony or Psychology.*
Repetitive movements	Stereotyped pacing that wears a route into the carpet due to frequency, whole body spinning and/or rocking in conjunction with head banging when content or bored or to wind down or pink flag movements combined with associated visual regard.	Non-specific pacing, toe-walking, head banging when upset or frustrated, shaking legs up and down, wringing hands, hand flapping (not uncommon in young children), subtle finger posturing while talking or completing tasks.
Sensory seeking behaviors	Licking sandpaper, cannot go for walks on rainy days because child lies face down in puddles to feel water on lips, repeated smelling of items with no odor (e.g., puzzle pieces). Lining up items and looking along the line (gets down on the floor to look at objects at eye level), peering out of corner of eyes (visual regard). Backing one's body into another to request frequent and intense squeezing.	Likes rolling down hills, rollercoasters, always wants to spin in tire swings or office chairs, loves water play, seeks out spicy or crunchy foods, seeks out mirrors or bright lights, prefers tight clothes, likes tight hugs/squeezes, heavy blankets or weighted vests, likes walking barefoot, likes to stroke or rub hair.
Sensory under sensitivity, over sensitivity (sensory avoidant behaviors)	Underresponsive: Major injury occurred without display of pain or sharing with adult (burned hand on stove, broken toe, needed stitches when closed hand in car door). Oversensitive: Avoids favorite places because cannot stand the hum of neon lights, extreme distress with daily noises so these cannot occur in their presence (e.g., vacuum), repulsed by the smell of people who are eating mints or have recently bathed and smell of soap, since infancy has avoided or resisted all physical contact (touch).	Underresponsive: High pain tolerance for minor injuries (skinned knee, bruises). Oversensitive: Picky eater; dislikes soft texture or mixed texture food; refuses hot or cold food (insists on room temperature); dislikes tags in clothes; hates having hair washed or cut; refuses to wear jeans, shoes, or jackets; resists change of clothes with change of seasons. Dislikes or is distressed by loud noises (fire alarm, sirens), covers ears with blender. Likes to be squeezed or tapped but not touched softly or stroked. Will initiate touch with others but dislikes others to initiate touch.

Difficulty with transitions and change, rigidity, or inflexibility	Severe distress with trivial changes (e.g., home décor is moved, need to take alternate route due to roadwork), even switching from non-preferred activities is hard (e.g., Let's skip teeth brushing tonight and read an extra book instead). Refuses to eat from bowls, always walks on the left side of sidewalk.	Adjusting to new teachers (or substitutes or returning to school after a holiday) is stressful, switching from preferred to non-preferred activities is hard (e.g., time to turn off TV and get ready for bed), has to complete activities (TV program, game, worksheet). Needs special lovey to fall asleep, preference for a certain seat in the car or favorite plate.
Play, whole and part relationships	Little functional use of toys as they are intended to be used (e.g., exclusively spins wheels on cars but never "drive them"). Interest in objects to the exclusion of people or the social world.	Poor-quality pretend play (pretend play by him-/herself but not with others, pretends the same scenario over and over), wants others/caregiver to participate in play but only in certain ways (e.g., may be very directive).

Social communication and social interaction

Social relationships	Seeks out relationships for primarily rational reasons (e.g., cites tax benefits of marriage). Talks incessantly about preferred topics regardless of partner's interest. Not easily comforted by caregiver, and distress may have no obvious cause.	Trouble understanding and expressing feelings or emotions (e.g., alexithymia), trouble reading the tone of a room, gravitates to adults or much younger children. May be difficult to comfort but caregivers usually know what the trigger for distress is. A history of difficulties maintaining friendships (often without understanding why they end).
Verbal social communication	Asks perseverative questions he/she already knows the answer to (not reassurance seeking), pronoun reversal (e.g., says "she wants water," instead of "I want water"). Immediate and delayed echolalia of content and tone (e.g., parroting repetitively without context, responds to "How are you?" with "Whenever you're in trouble, just yelp for help!"). Pervasive atypical prosody with combinations of ASD-specific patterns (mid-word dysfluencies/breathy breaks, poor inflection, mis-assigned stress) present since early childhood or marked language regression (loss of skill).	Scripted questions of others (asks new people same set of questions: What do you like to do? Did you have a nice weekend?), pedantic, overly formal speech (e.g., like a little professor). Immediate echolalia of content (e.g., responds to other's comment of "I like cows," with "cows," can be common in language delays). Subtle vocal quality differences or atypical prosody (e.g., tends to be flat, often exaggerated or frequent sarcastic tone). Speaks too loud or too soft for the social context, language delay with plateau of skills.

(continued)

Table 13.1 (continued)

Symptom type	Red flag	Pink flag
Nonverbal social communication	Using another person's hand as a tool (e.g., manipulates another's hand to operate a toy without eye contact), does not point to items just to show and share (e.g., points and looks to airplane, then looks to parent with smile, then looks to airplane), regularly avoids eye contact and does not smile with eye contact to share enjoyment, even with preferred adults.	Leads others by the hand to what they want. Limited gestures, variable or poorly modulated eye contact. Does not respect the usual personal space boundaries. Has flat or inappropriate facial expressions.
Social responsiveness, social initiation, and social maintenance	Poor reciprocity (does not roll ball back and forth or respond to name when younger), never responds to comments made by others only direct questions, does not even notice if others are in obvious distress. Initiates with others solely to get needs met (e.g., requests). May tolerate (or enjoy) if caregiver or others join in child's play but child does not readily seek out the caregiver to share pleasurable activities or seek to maintain interaction if caregiver stops attending.	*Trouble keeping a conversation going, only understands others' emotions if obviously displayed. Passive, abrasive, aggressive or disruptive when approaching another for social interaction. Described as being ignored by peers (due to passive presentation). Difficulty with reading nuances of peer relationships (e.g., is bullied OR reports being bullied even when that is not the intent; misunderstandings related to misinterpreting others' cues).*

Duvall et al. (2021, p. 1175–1176), used with permission

Table 13.2 Nuanced autism phenotypes that tend to be modulated by sex and gender (e.g., more likely to present in under-recognized individuals such as girls/women) (Lai et al., 2022. p. 93–94)

DSM-5 criteria	Diagnostic considerations for nuanced presentation
A1: Social-emotional reciprocity	Attention and interest to social stimuli can be present to some extent and modulated by gendered contexts and upbringing
	Conversation may be superficially back and forth (sometimes with scripted politeness, well-rehearsed in asking questions, or seemingly four-way but mostly offering own experiences/views), but reciprocity difficulty arises with topic shifting, unfamiliar contexts, or increasing complexity (e.g., more than two people conversing)
	Conversation reciprocity improves and becomes more natural when talking about interests
	Can have intact affective empathy and show sympathy (including toward animals)
A2: Nonverbal communication	Nonverbal expressions (e.g., eye contact, facial expression orientation, and conventional, descriptive, and emphatic gestures) can be superficially present, though can be exaggerated, inflexible, or with insufficient integration across modalities and with verbalization
	Understanding neurotypical nonverbal communications may be the main challenge
	Subjectively reporting learned and forced alternative ways of making eye contact (e.g., looking at other's forehead or nose) and facial expression orientation throughout childhood/teenage—this effort can disrupt verbal exchange, objectively shown as reduced integration of verbal and nonverbal communication
A3: Developing, maintaining, and understanding relationships	Interests to social relationships and peer interaction can be present, with developmentally appropriate desire for friendships, yet finding them difficult to navigate and manage
	Social awareness can be present to certain levels
	Tend to be naive in relationships
	May prefer to be alone in neurotypical social situations, but can have close friends especially when there are shared characteristics or interests
	Can figure out neurotypical others' thoughts and feelings with deliberate efforts and sufficient processing time, but intuitive understanding is still challenging
	Can invest large amounts of energy preparing for social interactions and feeling exhausted and drained afterward
B1: Stereotypy or repetitiveness	Repetitiveness may not be apparent motor mannerisms
	Stereotypy can manifest as idiosyncratic language expression, including unusually formal, pedantic, detailed, or precise language

(continued)

Table 13.2 (continued)

DSM-5 criteria	Diagnostic considerations for nuanced presentation
B2: Insistence on sameness	Can be perceived as perfectionism or preoccupation with details Can manifest as strictly following rules, "black and white" thinking, or insisting on believed truth (especially when co-existing with A3 features)
B3: Fixated interests	Content of circumscribed interest can be typical to neurotypical and gendered contexts Despite ego-syntonic, engagement with circumscribed interest can be exhaustive Circumscribed interests can be used as social currency
B4: Idiosyncratic sensory responses	Both hyper- and hypo-responsivity can be present within the same or across different sensory modalities Can also present as enhanced perception Can also present as difficulties in interoception Can manifest as eating problems Can be associated with choices of clothing and appearance not fitting stereotypical gender expectations
C: Evident characteristics in early developmental period but may not fully manifest until demands exceed capacity or masked by learned strategies	Impression management of the individual following sociocultural (including gendered) expectations may lead to learned modification of own behaviors across development, resulting in attenuated autistic behavioral presentations (a process termed "autistic camouflaging," "masking," "passing as non-autistic," etc. [16■,65■■]) that render some, but not all, cardinal features of autism less apparent However, impression management is not autism-specific nor diagnostic for autism. Positive subjective reports of developmental experiences of intention and efforts to "camouflage/mask/pass" and the cognitively taxing nature due to autistic cognition and executive function challenges, alongside collateral information of evident autistic features in early years (i.e., childhood), are key to autism diagnostics in this scenario [17■] Autistic "camouflaging/masking/passing" should be recognizable. First, there should be autistic features early in life to be masked or compensated for, when camouflaging efforts started. Further, there should be repeated camouflaging practices/rehearsals that the individual exercised over time, so it was less successful initially but over time they were better at it. Finally, even when an autistic person masters camouflaging, there should still be observable signs of this effort, including (i) the exhaustion and withdrawal afterward (e.g., signs of "autistic burnout" [43■]), (ii) inflexibility across contexts (e.g., much more difficult in the "cocktail party" scenario), and (iii) subtle de-synchronization during interpersonal interactions, "out-of-sync" episodes, and efforts to keep up with synchronization—hence, social-behavioral differences may manifest and become more observable over time during long interactions and especially in novel or unpredictable settings

D: Clinically significant impairment in current functioning	Despite superficially intact functioning, can easily feel exhausted due to impression management efforts [43*]
	Subjective distress should also be considered for making a clinical diagnosis
	Context dependence of functioning is not uncommon: e.g., keeping oneself together in public (e.g., at school, workplace) but experiencing/expressing substantial emotion regulation challenges (e.g., burnout, meltdown) in private settings (e.g., at home)
	Frequently requiring time alone to recover and restore energy
	Overall, the clinical diagnosis is based on the Gestalt of behavioral cognitive patterns and their developmental profiles and that functional and well-being impacts are directly associated with this Gestalt in neurotypical contexts
Associated features that commonly co-exist	Can have co-existing difficulties in understanding own emotions (i.e., alexithymia) and other's emotions, accompanied by long processing time or difficulty differentiating emotions
	Childhood imaginative/pretend play (e.g., doll play) can be present, but is often predominated by setting up toys and scenes, scripted (even interactive), and with limited reciprocity (even with the presence of agency using dolls/figures)
	Good structural language ability, especially in expression (including hyperlexia)
	Executive function difficulties, motor difficulties, and emotion regulation challenges may be common and can substantially cloud the clinical picture
	Body-focused repetitive behaviors may be common
	Do not reach the level of adaptation or achievement expected given the intelligence level
	Increased variance and fluidity in gender expression and identity, as well as sexual orientation and sexual identity

Lai et al. (2022), *Towards equitable diagnosis for autism and attention-deficit/hyperactivity disorder across sexes and genders. Current Opinion in Psychiatry, 35*(2), 90–100. https://doi.org/10.1097/YCO.0000000000000770. Used with permission

The third resource organized a call for action based on evidence, with suggested policy and practice changes (amendments) with desired outcomes. The impetus for these calls is to alleviate suffering. The author points out that persistent anxiety, and/or severe mental crises such as suicidal thoughts and behaviors can "open a door, but why should girls and young women need to spiral downwards before help is given?" (Horlock, 2019, p. 50 as quoted in Suckle, 2021).

Evidence-base	Policy amendments	Practice amendments	Intended result
		NECESSARY ACTION	
The nature of the neuro-cognitive architecture of autism results in a wide range of behavioural evidence in both males and females	Stronger emphasis on the underlying cognitive similarities within autism over assumed behavioural similarities (between autistics)	Standardised consistent program of training on female autism presentations to be delivered to educational and clinical gatekeepers as part of regular compliance training	Autistic females being identified as autistic despite not meeting prototypical behavioural patterns.
Complex and multifaceted use of masking can feature heavily in emerging understanding of female autism	Acknowledgment of the many types and functions of masking, including masking throughout the diagnostic pathway	Greater validity to self-reporting alongside observed behavioural evidence.	A reflective diagnostic pathway, adapted to account for the multifaceted nature of masking, which gives greater weight to self-reported evidence
Diagnostic overshadowing is a prevailing and significant factor that can impede the identification of female autistics	Charting of key secondary symptoms associated with female autism (for example, eating disorders, self-harm and obsessive compulsive disorder)	Sensitive and timely preliminary screening for autism in the key conditions where significant diagnostic overshadowing occurs with immediate clinical referral if needed	Autistic females will receive earlier identification and appropriate autism-centred treatment for co-morbid secondary symptoms
Certain life-stages and events may present as particularly challenging for autistic females (for example, adolescence, pregnancy or illness) and this may increase autistic symptoms and concurrent needs	Recognition that whilst autism is pervasive, capacities to cope and compensatory strategies might obscure difficulties (both to the self and the local environment) and therefore delay or preclude diagnosis	Practitioners need training that highlights the fluid and fluctuating needs of autistic females. Furthermore, self-reported evidence should be accepted where compensatory strategies have concealed lifelong difficulties	Better understanding of apparent 'peaks' in the life-stages of autistic females, where female autistics that display a greater need for diagnosis at particular junctures are given full evaluation
Socio-environmental factors have a considerable impact on how female autistics present, as difficulties and challenges might only be apparent in 'safe' environments	Acknowledgment that the 'multiple context' stipulation may slow down identification, in particular if local gatekeepers lack training in the complexities of diagnosing female autism	Consistent training on how autism might present differently in different contexts. Validity to self-reporting across contexts	Autistic females being identified as autistic despite their capacity to mask or present differently in different socio-environmental contexts

Fig. 13.1 Summary of evidence-driven amendments to female autism identification (Suckle, 2021, used with permission).

The Future

We anticipate rapid change among the autistic and professional communities in the next few years. As we have presented the research and our clinical experiences to varied professional audiences over the last few years, we have been encouraged to hear the professional community coming on board with many of the recommendations put forth by the autistic community. There is a palpable hunger for more information to better guide the experiences in assessment for the autistic and professional communities. Disagreements about how to accomplish everyone's goals will likely continue to exist, but our hope is that the quality of lives for autistic women and those with nuanced autism will be better in meaningful ways moving forward.

References

American Psychiatric Association. (2013). *Diagnostic and statistical manual of mental disorders* (5th ed.). Author.

American Psychiatric Association. (2022). *Diagnostic and statistical manual of mental disorders* (5th, Text Rev ed.). Author.

Ballou, E. P., daVanport, S., & Onaiwu, M. G. (Eds.). (2021). *Sincerely, your autistic child.* Beacon Press.

Brown, D. (2013). *The Aspie girl's guide to being safe with men: The unwritten safety rules no-one is telling you.* Jessica Kingsley Publishers.

Duvall, S., Armstrong, K., Shahabuddin, A., Grantz, C., Fein, D., & Lord, C. (2021). A road map for identifying autism spectrum disorder: Recognizing and evaluating characteristics that should raise red or "pink" flags to guide accurate differential diagnosis. *The Clinical Neuropsychologist, 36*(5), 1172–1207. https://doi.org/10.1080/13854046.2021.1921276

Fahrenheit, F. (2020, January 11). *An open letter to the NYT: Acknowledge the controversy surrounding ABA, neuroclastic: The autism spectrum according to autistic people.* https://neuroclastic.com/an-open-letter-to-the-nyt-acknowledge-the-controversy-surrounding-aba/

Grandin, T., & Panek, R. (2013). *The autistic brain: Helping different kinds of minds succeed.* Mariner Books.

Gray, C. (2015). *The new social story book, revised and expanded 15th anniversary edition: Over 150 social stories that teach everyday social skills to children and adults with autism and their peers.* Future Horizons.

Horlock, S. (2019). Girls group respecting the female identity of girls with autism in a school setting. In B. Carpenter, F. Happé, & J. Egerton (Eds.), *Girls and autism educational, family and personal perspectives* (pp. 48–55). Routledge.

Lai, M. C., Lin, H. Y., & Ameis, S. H. (2022). Towards equitable diagnoses for autism and attention-deficit/hyperactivity disorder across sexes and genders. *Current Opinion in Psychiatry, 35*(2), 90–100. https://doi.org/10.1097/YCO.0000000000000770

Leaf, J. B., Cihon, J. H., Leaf, R., McEachin, J., Liu, N., Russell, N., Unumb, L., Shapiro, S., & Khosrowshahi, D. (2022). Concerns about ABA-based intervention: An evaluation and recommendations. *Journal of Autism and Developmental Disorders, 52*(6), 2838–2853. https://doi.org/10.1007/s10803-021-05137-y

McCarthy, T. (2020). Autism after 21 Stories / Kennedy O. Onuoha | Grateful for my 'sticky brain'. Madison House Autism Foundation. https://madisonhouseautism.org/autism-after-21-stories/kennedy-onuoha/

Nerenberg, J. (2021). *Divergent mind: Thriving in a world that wasn't designed for you*. HarperOne.

Price, D. (2022). *Unmasking autism: Discovering the new faces of neurodiversity*. Harmony.

Simone, R. (2010). *Aspergirls: Empowering females with Asperger syndrome*. Jessica Kingsley Publishers.

Suckle, E. K. (2021). DSM-5 and challenges to female autism identification. *Journal of Autism and Developmental Disorders, 51*, 754–759. https://doi.org/10.1007/s10803-020-04574-5

Index

The manufacturer's authorised representative in the EU is Springer
Nature Customer Service Centre GmbH, Europaplatz 3, 69115 Heidelberg,
Germany. If you have any concerns regarding our products, please
contact ProductSafety@springernature.com

Printed and bound by CPI Group (UK) Ltd, Croydon, CR0 4YY

24/04/2026

02096348-0006